Physician Productivity and the Demand for Health Manpower

Physician Productivity and the Demand for Health Manpower

An Economic Analysis

Uwe E. Reinhardt
Department of Economics and
Woodrow Wilson School of
Public and International Affairs
Princeton University

Ballinger Publishing Company ● Cambridge, Mass.
A Subsidiary of J.B. Lippincott Company

This book is printed on recycled paper.

International Standard Book Number: 0-88410-103-7

Library of Congress Catalog Card Number: 74-7465

Printed in the United States of America

Library of Congress Cataloging in Publication Data

Reinhardt, Uwe E
  Physician productivity and the demand for health manpower.

  Bibliography: p.
  1. Physicians—United States. 2. Medical personnel—United States.
3. Medical economics—United States. I. Title. [DNLM: 1. Physicians—
Supply and distribution—United States. W76 R369p 1974]
RA410.7.R47   331.1'26   74-7465
ISBN 0-88410-103-7

In fond memory
of my father,
Wilhelm Reinhardt, 1900–1973

Contents

vii

List of Figures

List of Tables

Preface

Economists generally write for one of three audiences: their professional peers, their students, and policymakers—notably those in the public sector. This book is addressed to the latter two audiences. It is an attempt to bring certain insights gained from economic theory and applied economic research to the task of formulating the nation's health manpower policy during the next several decades.

The book has three major parts. Part I is essentially a review of health manpower policy during the past few decades and a survey of alternative proposals to increase the productivity of American physicians. Part II presents an empirical analysis of health-care production in private medical practices. Part III summarizes the salient conclusions from that analysis and evaluates their implications for federal health manpower policy.

Parts I and III form the main body of the book. Together these two parts present a self-contained discussion oriented towards readers unfamiliar with economic theory or uncomfortable with the use of calculus and matrix notation as expository devices. Among these readers will be public-policy makers in the health field and students of public policy, for example, students of the type the author has regularly taught at Princeton's Woodrow Wilson School of Public and International Affairs. Beneath virtually every proposition advanced in Parts I and III there lurks formal economic theory or applied econometric research, yet a serious effort has been made to develop these propositions in language accessible to readers not formally trained in economics. Where formal theory or economic jargon are used, they are explained as part of the narrative. Where cumbersome mathematical notation is unavoidable, the discussion has been relegated to a technical appendix.

The discussion in Part II, however, does presuppose some familiarity with economic theory and econometrics. These chapters are intended for readers who would like to see a more formal exposition of the assumptions and methodology underlying other parts of the book, such as senior undergraduates or graduate students in economics interested in applying their skills to problems in the production of health services. One may go lightly on Part II, or skip it altogether, without losing the main thread of the analysis developed in Parts I and III.

No pretense is made that the book offers a perfectly balanced view of health manpower policy. The discussion throughout reflects an economist's view of the world and focuses solely on economic variables as potential targets for public policy. The author is aware that analyses of this sort abstract from the myriad of noneconomic factors that influence the decisions of the providers and consumers of health care, factors that may frequently overshadow any purely economic considerations. The author is also aware that the economist's perspective on health policy is occasionally seen as amusing or even offensive, particularly among medical practitioners. Some bemusement, for example, may be triggered by the image of a critically injured patient consuming his or her last energy in the complex hedonistic calculus that culminates in what economists call the "price-elasticity of the demand for medical care." Some irritation, on the other hand, may be expressed by physicians who, like other professionals, pride themselves of a relentless dedication to the substance of their profession—the alleviation or prevention of human suffering—and who deem their professional conduct to be impervious to the pecuniary incentives thought to motivate the classical *homo economicus.*

In offering his analysis, an economist never pretends that economic factors are all that matter in shaping human behavior. All he assumes is that, among many variables, economic factors are also important, and that the marginal impact economic incentives have on human behavior tends to be sufficiently pronounced to be of interest to public policymakers—even in the context of medical practice. To abandon that precept would, of course, rob economic analysis of the main contribution it can make to the evaluation of public policies in the health area. Besides, there is ample empirical evidence that the economist's instincts in this respect are basically sound.

The policy prescriptions offered by economists frequently strike other social thinkers as unduly hardnosed. Perhaps this is why economics is sometimes referred to as "the dismal science." Economists are trained to remind their audiences of the cost of ostensibly benign social policies, costs that are often so subtle as to be hidden from view and hence conveniently overlooked. Thus, economists will invariably think of any public subsidy to some members of society as an implicit redistribution of wealth coming at the expense of someone else. They are acutely aware of the financial incentives inevitably embodied in any flow of funds between the public and private sectors, and do not hesitate to recommend exploitation of these incentives for the purpose of reaching stated social objectives. They base their analysis on the assumption that public policymakers should use the funds entrusted to them wisely, that is, efficiently. And, finally, they are not enamored with the notion that social problems can be solved simply by injecting generous doses of unrestricted public funds into perceived problem areas, as so many social commentators still seem to be.

Many of the policy prescriptions offered in this book reflect this philosophical bent. These recommendations should not be mistaken for political conservatism. Far from it, they are intended to reflect concern for efficiency in the management of society's resources. They are occasionally also intended to correct mistaken beliefs about the equity of current public policies, especially those dealing with financing the education of health professionals.

Acknowledgments

The basic research material underlying this book was accumulated over a number of years. In the course of that research, I have benefitted greatly from an ongoing dialog with fellow economists working in the health manpower area, notably Stuart Altman, Martin Feldstein, Paul Feldstein, John O'Rourke, Mark Pauly, Frank Sloan, Kenneth Smith and Stanley Wallack. At Princeton I have, over the years, had many stimulating conversations on health policy with my colleague Herman Somers, whose office happens to contain the finest health economics library on our campus and whose intimate knowledge of all aspects of the health-care sector never ceases to amaze me.

Dennis Epple, formerly a graduate student in our department, read the entire manuscript and offered many helpful suggestions concerning both style and substance. Michael Schiffres, my research assistant during the summer of 1973, traced down much of the basic source material used in Chapter Two and prepared a number of tables included in that chapter. The manuscript was typed, with great care, by Elizabeth Miller of the Woodrow Wilson School. It is said that the completing of almost any manuscript sooner or later becomes a pain in the anatomy. This one, at any rate, did. The pain was greatly eased by Ms. Miller's expertise in the preparation of manuscripts, by her attention to detail, and by her always cheerful cooperation in the enterprise.

All of these direct and indirect inputs into my research effort are acknowledged with gratitude.

Financing for the writing of this book has come from a variety of sources. Many of the chapters were written while I was on a leave of absence from Princeton University. The leave was made possible by a Bicentennial Preceptorship endowed by Princeton's Class of 1931. This is a good opportunity to thank these faithful alumni for their generosity. Additional research support was provided by the Department of Health, Education and Welfare under contract HSM-110-73-354. The statistical estimates presented in Chapter Six are taken from my doctoral dissertation at Yale University. These estimates were developed at the Human Resources Research Center of the University of Southern California, with data and financial support from Medical Economics, Inc., and with some additional support from the Community Profile Data Center of the Department of Health, Education and Welfare. The research support provided by HEW and by Medical Economics, Inc. is greatly appreciated. In as controversial an area as health manpower policy, however, it bears stressing that the interpretation of any statistical results presented in this book and the policy prescriptions based thereon reflect strictly my own views and not necessarily those of these sponsors.

A large measure of gratitude is due my wife, Tsung-mei. I thank her not so much for the good companionship and the compassion many authors acknowledge in their wives. She gives all that, but hardly expects to be thanked for it in print. Rather, I thank her for her valuable direct contributions to earlier parts of my research and for her assistance in completing the manuscript. I am very much in her debt and hope that she will write a book one day so I can return the favor.

Finally, I expressly wish not to thank my son, Hsiao Nio, for his peculiar contribution to my research efforts. As little sons go, Hsiao Nio has been nothing short of a prince ever since he was born some eighteen months ago. As an input into the book-production process, however, his marginal productivity appears to be strictly < 0 for every waking hour he contributes. He shares with me responsibility for any errors or shortcomings that remain in the manuscript.

Princeton, New Jersey
July 1974

Part One

Physician Productivity and Health Manpower Projections

Chapter One

Issues in Health Manpower Policy

Ever since the end of World War II, and especially since the introduction of the publicly financed Medicare and Medicaid programs, Americans have been concerned over a doctor shortage. Deficits in physician manpower have been forecast, for successive decades, by a number of government commissions, government agencies, and public health specialists. The rapid postwar rise in physician fees, the often crowded appointment calendars and waiting rooms of primary care physicians, the paucity of health personnel in rural areas or urban slums, and a substantial and sustained influx of foreign-trained physicians into the United States are all widely taken as evidence that the shortage is real and acute. In the face of these symptoms, only a few heretics—for example, Ginzberg [1966] and Schwartz [1972]—have had the temerity to suggest otherwise.

These heretics ought not be dismissed too lightly. The fact is that the United States enjoys one of the highest physician-population ratios in the industrialized world (see Table 2-2). Nations whose health-care systems are regularly cited as models worth emulating (e.g., Sweden, Great Britain, or the Netherlands) somehow seem to make do with far fewer physicians per capita than does the United States. Although Sweden, for one, has for many years tried to catch up with the United States ratio [Anderson, 1972, pp. 123-4], there is no evidence that the relatively lower physician-population ratios in these European nations have come at the price of lower health standards.

The already favorable relative standing of the United States is likely to be enhanced further by the massive federal support to medical education legislated during the late 1960s and early 1970s. Figure 1-1 shows the impact of this support on the capacity of American medical schools. Between 1965 and 1973 the size of the entering class in American schools of medicine and osteopathy increased by over 60 percent, and further increases are expected under health manpower legislation already enacted.

3

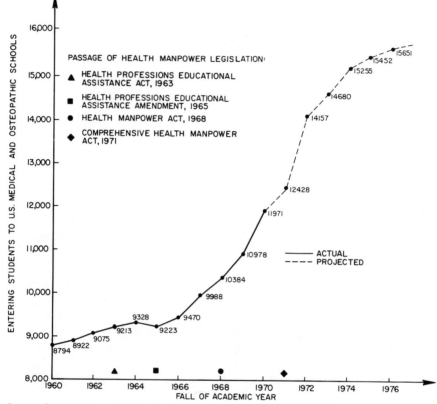

Source: Private Communication from the U.S. Department of Health, Education and Welfare, Division of Manpower Intelligence.

Figure 1-1.   Federal Health Manpower Legislation and Its Impact on Medical School Capacity.

An expansion program of this sort has long-run implications that are sometimes overlooked. During the next two decades, for example, there will occur a drastic change in the age distribution of the nation's physicians. Each year many more physicians will enter the profession than will retire. As a result, the aggregate supply of physicians and physician-population ratio in this country will increase for decades to come even if after 1975 the capacity of American medical schools were to be frozen at the currently projected level of about 15,500 entering students.

The contribution of American medical schools to the future supply of active physicians in this country is shown in Figure 1-2. It is assumed that for the remainder of this century the capacity of American schools is held

constant at its 1975 level. In order to highlight the contribution solely of
American medical schools to the physician supply, the diagram reflects only
those foreign medical graduates already practicing in the United States by the
end of 1970. From 1971 on, gross additions to the supply of physicians exclude
any inflow of foreign-trained physicians. Consequently the supply trends shown
in the diagram understate the supply that can actually be expected, for in the
two-year period 1971–72 alone, the United States admitted about 13,000 foreign
medical graduates on permanent resident visas. The forecasting equation underlying Figure 1–2, the derivation of age-specific attrition rates for physicians
and a number of tables containing the raw data for this forecast are presented in
Appendix A.

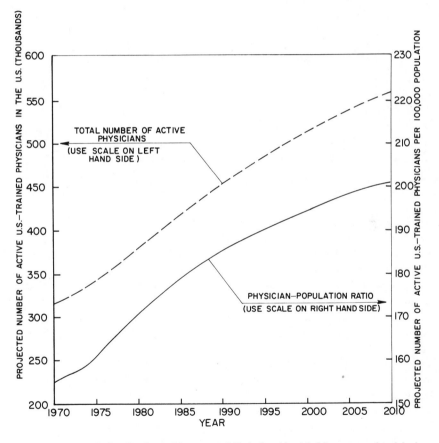

Figure 1–2. Projected Impact of Existing Health Manpower Legislation
on the Supply of Active U.S.-Trained Physicians, United States, 1970–
2010

A medical education is enormously expensive, perhaps in excess of $50,000 per physician.[1] Higher still are the human resource costs of an ever-increasing supply of physicians, for medical students are drawn from a pool of highly talented manpower that could serve society well, and conceivably better, in other professions. The mere cost of training and maintaining large numbers of physicians is, of course, not in itself an argument against such a program. This author, at any rate, is not prepared to argue that the expansion program reflected in Figure 1-1 was either wholly or partly unnecessary. The problem is that even the current, already much expanded capacity of American medical schools is viewed by many as inadequate. Authoritative voices call for yet another round of medical school expansion, some for as much as a doubling of existing capacity.[2] Before the nation commits itself to such a program, now may be the time to ask: How much is enough? Now may even be the time to ask: Is there already too much?

Many observers of the United States health system find such questions irritatingly irrelevant. These observers point out, first of all, that all the symptoms of a doctor shortage are still very much in evidence: physician fees are still rising, appointment calendars and waiting rooms are still crowded, some areas are still without physician manpower altogether, and the influx of foreign-trained physicians continues unabated. It is argued that only a massive increase in American-trained physicians can ultimately eliminate these symptoms, and that such an increase may very well require a doubling of medical school enrollments.

Aside from the alleged shortage of physicians' services, a sustained expansion of medical schools is also widely urged on the ground that the demand for medical training far exceeds its supply. Traditionally only about half the applicants to American medical schools have been accepted, a proportion that has decreased markedly during recent years. In 1972, for example, there were 36,135 applicants for 13,757 available places in the entering class,[3] and in 1973, 40,500 applicants competed for 14,124 first-year places.[4] In a recent editorial on this issue, the American Medical Association estimated that, in addition to the 113 medical schools already in existence, another 100 schools of the present average size would be needed to accommodate the current number of *qualified* yet rejected applicants [Egan, 1973, p. 991]. Medical educators in particular view this trend with alarm. It is argued that to deny qualified Americans the opportunity to pursue the career of their choice is a "national shame" [5] and "inimical to our democratic institutions" [Gerber, 1973a, p. 15]. One's sense of shame is heightened, according to this view, because the United States has for years raided the physician supply of less developed nations that have invested vast amounts of their own scarce resources in the development of this human capital. Some medical educators have called for the drastic step of prohibiting the inflow of foreign-trained physicians altogether,[6] presumably for the benefit of both the United States and the donor countries.

Finally, there is the notion that even if too many American-trained physicians were produced at some point in the future, that development could hardly be viewed as a social problem. First, the United States would be able to compete more effectively for the hearts and minds of foreign people by exporting physicians to needy nations, a competition the Soviet Union is said to have won hands down so far [Gerber, 1973, p. 13]. But even in the absence of any outflow of physicians, it is argued, the social and economic consequences of a doctor surplus can hardly be as serious as those of a physician shortage. To sound the alarm before any doctor surplus actually becomes manifest, in this view, is therefore not only foolhardy but downright irresponsible. It is playing with the health of the American people.

These arguments spring from good intentions and, given their objective, are apt to strike a responsive chord among concerned citizens and policymakers. Unfortunately, the case for continued expansion of medical schools seems to rest on a quite unrealistic picture of the market for physician services, a lack of realism that oddly enough lends the argument its intuitive appeal. Furthermore, parts of the case rest on normative premises that can at least be questioned.

THE MARKET FOR PHYSICIAN SERVICES

Those who would seek to contain the rising cost of physician services and to solve the problem of maldistribution through massive increases in the aggregate supply of physicians seem to structure their case on a rather idealistic picture of the medical-care marketplace, a picture with which true-blooded economists should feel comfortable, but one with which, after some empirical research, they have become disenchanted. Crucial to the "expansionists'" argument is the theory that increases in the aggregate physician-population ratio will engender fierce competition among medical practitioners, which in turn will generate all the traditional side effects, in textbook fashion. Thus it is thought that through price-competition the level of physician fees (and hence the cost of health maintenance) will be forced down and that competitive pressure will force reluctant practitioners into the nation's cultural hinterland or into medical specialties endowed with relatively moderate degrees of social prestige. The widely held theory that for many years in the past the American Medical Association has maintained the physician's favorable income position through artificial constraints on the capacity of medical schools lends credence to this hypothesis.[7] It is a theory in need of a review.

If the market for physician services conformed to the textbook model of perfect competition, the previous scenario would be believable. Among the essential characteristics of a competitive market are (1) that individual sellers or buyers have no discretionary power over the price of the commodity being traded; and (2) that changes in supply do not influence the quantity consumers demand at any given market price—that is, that demand and supply are independently determined. Many markets for commodities, labor services or even some professional services (e.g., aerospace engineers or college teachers) satisfy these conditions. An increase in the supply of these types of manpower tends to generate downward pressure on hourly remuneration or, if hourly remuneration is downwardly inflexible, some of these professionals simply go unemployed. Whatever the actual outcome may be, however, the economic consequences of any excess supply fall primarily on the professionals themselves. Although the spectacle of unemployed engineers or taxi drivers with Ph.D.'s may be viewed as a social problem of sorts,[a] policymakers concerned with the supply of these professionals can quite legitimately claim that those who suffer the economic hardships of excess supply must ultimately bear responsibility for their own occupational choice. Besides, the majority of such professionals typically succeed in finding alternative employment, often at no pecuniary sacrifice.

One's prior knowledge about medical practice in this country suggests that the market for physician services differs fundamentally from the competitive norm, as do the economic consequences of excess supply. The first distinct feature of the market for physician services is that demand is not independent of supply. The second is that physicians probably have considerable discretion in the pricing of their own services; there is evidence that within fairly wide limits physicians can set their fees so as to attain a chosen target income [Feldstein, 1970]. Given these market characteristics, an excess supply of physicians is likely to generate *upward* rather than downward pressure on the cost of health maintenance and at most some disguised underemployment among physicians. But where fees can be raised to generate a target income, physicians obviously can protect themselves from any major loss of income even in case of overt or disguised underemployment. Physicians themselves are thus unlikely to suffer seriously from the economic consequences of a physician surplus. Instead, the economic costs of excess supply are likely to fall primarily on individual consumers of health care or, through insurance premiums and taxes, on society at large.

This rather bold and disturbing prognosis requires added explanation. Strictly speaking, the consumer of physician services is fully autonomous only in the decision whether or not to seek contact with the medical-care system. Once that contact is made, the physician becomes the patient's "management consultant" and assumes responsibility for specifying the set of services going into the treatment of the patient's medical condition. Although the patient may participate in this decision process, the physician naturally dominates by virtue

[a]One economic consequence that might be viewed as a loss to society as a whole is the service these professionals might have rendered society had they chosen a different occupation. In most instances, however, an alternative employment will in fact be chosen *ex post*.

of his technical competence in medical matters. He is, in effect, the patient's agent. Under the American practice pattern, however, the physician usually acts also as a profit-oriented entrepreneur who produces and sells at least part of the medical services he recommends. This dual role of the physician, combined with the fact that most physician services in this country are rendered on a fee-for-service basis, inevitably subjects him to a potential conflict of interest and destroys the postulated independence between supply and demand (if only in principle). In other words, the market for physician services is one in which suppliers can to a considerable extent create the demand for their own services and any objectively determinable, real surplus of physicians can usually be made to disappear through physician-induced increases in demand. As Fuchs and Kramer put it in their study of the determinants of expenditures for physician services in the United States:

> The most striking finding of this study is that supply factors (technology and *number of physicians*) appear to be of decisive importance in determining the utilization of and expenditures for physician services. . . . Because physicians can and do determine the demand for their own services to a considerable extent, we should be wary of plans which assume that the cost of medical care would be reduced by increasing the supply of physicians. [1972, p. 2; emphasis added.]

Physicians may take offense at the thrust of this argument. The conduct of medical practice, they may argue, is subject to a far stricter code of ethics than almost any other agency relationship in the economy, a code that expressly forbids the compromising of medical science for the sake of pecuniary gain. Besides, they may add, given the typically heavy patient load of physicians and the satisfactory income that can be earned without resort to unethical conduct, economic conflicts of interest are surely more imagined than real. Under these circumstances, it may be held, it is patently absurd to depict medical practice as the economic analog of, say, an automobile or television repair shop.

Although some authors have sought to demonstrate empirically that not all physicians invariably stand above the economic conflict of interest alluded to above,[8] there is actually no need to press that theme any further here. In postulating the likelihood of physician-induced increases in the demand for their services, one need not really appeal to baser economic motives: the application of medical science to human illness is a sufficiently imprecise enterprise to permit great leeway in practice patterns even on purely medical grounds. After all, a good part of medical practice involves decisionmaking on the basis of empirical information concerning the patient's health status, and it can rightly be held that the more information the better. Since both patients and physicians are conditioned to view the resource intensity of medical treatment as an important index of its quality, it is only reasonable to assume that, where physicians are in ample supply, even marginally beneficial diagnostic or therapeutic procedures will be performed, and that the normal physician-patient encounter will be lengthened to absorb the available physician time. This development is even more probable when patients are covered by health insurance and do not directly or indirectly bear the full cost of their treatment. In short, there is no reason to suppose that medical practice is immune from Parkinson's Law.

It may be argued that any physician-induced increase in the "demand" for physician services is apt also to increase the quality of the treatment being dispensed, even if the extra services are not absolutely necessary. If one excepts from this assertion elective surgery, this may be a valid point and one an economist is not equipped to dispute. An economist can point out, however, that the added quality comes at a price, and that it is pertinent always to ask whether the quality so added is worth that price.

The ability of patients to absorb added physician services must have a limit. Once that limit is reached, it may be argued, *price competition* among physicians will surely set in; it is then that the benefits from an expanded physician supply will become more visible. Unfortunately, neither economic theory nor the available evidence on this point are at all reassuring. Over the country's various regions or states, for example, one observes a strong *positive* correlation between the average level of physician fees and the physician-population ratio [9] (see Tables 2-5 and 2-6). Even within states or regions, fees tend to be high in metropolitan areas (where physician-population ratios are high) and low in rural areas (where physician density is low). Unfortunately, these data are consistent with two rival theories on the behavior of physician prices, one that may be referred to as the competitive model and the other as the price-setter model. These two theories lead to completely different predictions concerning the response of physician fees to increases in the physician-population ratio; the first theory suggests that fees will decline, the second that fees will rise. Since the behavior of physician fees is highly relevant to health manpower policy, it is worth dwelling a bit on these theories.

The competitive model is based on the hypothesis that the individual physician is essentially a price-taker; that is, that he charges customary local fees and cannot unilaterally deviate from them.[10] Implicit in the model is the assumption that local fees are set by the interaction of local supply and demand conditions so as to equate the quantity of care demanded with the quantity supplied. It is assumed that the community's demand for an *individual* physician's services is highly price-sensitive (price-elastic) even if the community's demand for physician services in general is price-insensitive (price-inelastic). This assumption, in turn, is based on the notion that consumers in the market for physician services possess a considerable degree of sovereignty. At the very least, it must be assumed that consumers shop around for low-priced physicians when making initial contact with the medical system, and that they are prepared to leave their customary physician when the latter's fees are perceived to rise above those charged by similar physicians elsewhere in the community. In assessing the realism of the competitive and the price-setter models, one should keep these assumptions in mind.

According to the competitive model, the observed positive correlation between fees and physician density simply reflects the fact that physicians respond to market-determined local fees in their location decision. Higher fees in some locations are thought to reflect higher effective demand (need backed up by ability and willingness to pay) in these areas, and not discretionary pricing power on the part of physicians. The fact that fees are not the same in all areas merely indicates that factors other than the level of fees loom large in the physician's location decision. If this theory were a correct model of reality, then an increase in the physician-population ratio in a given region would be expected ultimately to drive down the customary level of fees in that region, the observed positive correlation between fees and physician density across regions notwithstanding.

The alternative hypothesis is that the individual physician usually does have a fair degree of discretion over the level of his fees and that he can alter these fees to change his income.[11] A number of institutional factors lend plausibility to this theory. First, physicians themselves are not permitted to advertise openly and may, in fact, not adhere to a standard price per procedure. Second, few consumers take the time or muster the courage to shop around for low-priced physicians. Physicians themselves are not accustomed to quoting prices on the telephone, and consumers may even feel that low fees betray low quality. For these reasons it is fair to assume that a community's effective demand for physician services can at best set very vague upper limits to the range of fees that can be charged in a given locality. Since consumers are assumed to be ill-informed about relative physician fees in their locality, the theory posits a price-insensitive demand curve even for the individual physician. Practically this means that even the individual physician can raise his fees without triggering significant reductions in his patient load.

Precisely how the individual physician sets his fees under the price-setter theory is an open question. One possible hypothesis might be that the physician sets his fees as would a profit-maximizing monopolist,[b] or perhaps even a price-discriminating monopolist [Kessel, 1958]. An alternative hypothesis, and one that seems to have gained wide currency in recent years, is that physicians do not generally try to charge all the traffic can bear, but instead set their fees so as to attain a desired *target income*, to maintain sufficient excess demand for their services to allow them to be selective about patients and to enjoy the prestige that comes with being slightly overbooked. From an analytic viewpoint, this is clearly a rather loose and unsatisfying theory, for it leaves unspecified how the target income is set. The most plausible assumption is that

[b]Technically speaking, this hypothesis is inconsistent with the assumptions that the demand for the individual physician's services is price-inelastic at his observed fees [Arrow, 1963, p. 957].

the target is set with reference to the local income distribution or to the modal physician income in the region. If so, physicians within a given locality probably do adhere to a rather narrow range of fees in spite of the discretionary pricing power they may possess. This outcome, incidentally, would be strikingly similar to the price behavior one would observe in competitive markets, although the determination of the narrow range of fees would clearly be quite different and so would be the response of fees to changes in supply.

The "price-setter" model also is consistent with the observed positive correlation between fees and physician density. If that theory is an accurate description of the real world, then an increase in the physician-population ratio can be expected to exert *upward* pressure on medical costs. The physicians' initial reaction to increased physician density is likely to be an increase in the services rendered per patient, either by meeting excess demand or by inducing demand. These added services may initially be rendered at given fee levels, but if the patient-load per physician drops off sufficiently, physicians may seek to augment their income by raising fees, either individually or perhaps even through a collective agreement. Such price inflation would obviously exacerbate the cost-push from any physician-induced increase in the per capita demand for physician services. It is a prospect that should give policymakers pause.

How are policymakers to choose among rival theories all of which appear to be compatible with a given body of empirical information? One approach would be to identify the assumptions on which these theories rest, to examine these assumptions in the light of one's knowledge of the real world, and to proceed on the theory embodying the most realistic assumptions. This approach has intuitive appeal and is often followed in practice, even by economists. However, a good many economists—notably those associated with the so-called Chicago School—frown upon that procedure because (a) one's assessment of relative degrees of realism tends to be subjective; (b) each of the theories may embody both realistic and unrealistic assumptions, so that one must weigh the importance of each assumption before arriving at a clear-cut choice; and (c) the true test of a theory is how well it predicts.

The scientifically soundest method of testing a theory is to explore its predictions within a carefully structured experimental design. Few social scientists are afforded this luxury, not only because experimental designs tend to be expensive, but especially because the subjects to be analyzed—in this case physicians—refuse to hold still for such experiments. A second-best solution is to pretend that the empirical information routinely generated by the health-care sector can be treated as results from an experimental design. Economists do this by constructing mathematical models of rival theories and by estimating these models statistically from the available nonexperimental data. Once the models are estimated, their compatibility with the real world can be evaluated in two ways. First, there are statistical tests indicating how well the estimated model itself fits the underlying data base. Second, one may use the model to predict interesting target variables for a time period (or a cross-section sample of physicians) different from that underlying the estimated model itself. The relative validity of alternative models can then be assessed by comparing these predictions with the values actually observed in the time period (or cross-section sample).

In the area of physician price behavior, econometric research of the sort just described has begun only recently. In this research, physician fees are related not only to physician-population ratios, but also to a variety of other variables which, according to one's model, may have a direct or indirect influence on fees. By including these variables in one's analysis one can, in principle, control for their influence and examine the relationship between fees and the physician-population ratio on the assumption that all other factors remain constant. Unfortunately, the data so far available to economists have been rather crude, so that the statistical results derived therefrom are anything but robust.[12] By and large, these results appear to lend relatively more support to the price-setter model and, specifically, to the hypothesis that physicians set their prices so as to maintain a certain income position over time. It bears repeating, however, that these results are less than conclusive and that further research in this area would be highly desirable.

One particular difficulty with econometric research on physician fees is that the economic context in which fees are determined may vary from region to region and certainly from one time period to another. (For a more extensive discussion of this problem, see Appendix B.) Economic models estimated from data from one economic context may not give a reliable clue to the behavior of fees under another context. Prior to the 1960s, for example, individual patients paid a large portion of the physician's bill; since then the proportion covered by private insurance carriers and the public sector has been steadily increasing. In the foreseeable future, the nation is likely to adopt a comprehensive national health insurance program that may once more drastically alter the market for physician services. A change in insurance coverage does not merely alter the net price consumers pay for physician care. Such a change is likely to alter the physicians' basic philosophy of fee-setting, as well as the market and even political constraints on his pricing decision. Since national health insurance appears to be virtually upon us, that context may well be the most relevant one for current health manpower policy.

How physician fees would behave under a national health insurance scheme with fee-for-service reimbursement of physicians is an interesting question. Much would depend on the bargaining posture adopted by the third-party payers—insurance companies or public agencies. It must be remembered that a medical education is arduous and imposes upon the individual trainee enormous personal costs, especially in foregone earnings. One suspects that much would be made of this point in any negotiations over fee schedules. Given the usually beneficial and highly personal role physicians play in their patients' lives, one may suppose that both the public and the third-party payers can be persuaded that once individuals have put twelve or more years of their lives into medical training, society more or less owes them a decent living. And if one may judge by other countries operating under similar regimes—Canada or West Germany, for example [13]—it may be supposed that a "decent living" will always refer to a position somewhere in the top 5 or 10 percent of the nation's income distribution. If fee schedules under a national health insurance plan were negotiated on the notion that society owes the medical graduate a secure economic position—and one must suspect that they would be negotiated on this basis in America—then any increase in the number of medical schools automatically represents a tacit commitment to furnish an equal number of additional "decent" annual incomes that would have to be transferred from society as a whole to physicians as a group, regardless of supply conditions. Those who would seek to encourage, through continued federal assistance, a sustained expansion of American medical schools almost invariably seem to overlook this economic aspect of the proposed manpower policy.[c]

THE PROBLEM OF MALDISTRIBUTION

The behavioral models considered above also bear directly on the problem of the alleged maldistribution of medical manpower. Virtually all research on the locational decisions of physicians has indicated that physicians do not generally locate where the need for their services is most acute, but instead gravitate toward geographically and culturally attractive areas (mostly urban or suburban) where per capita income is high and the effective demand for their services (perceived need backed up by purchasing power) is correspondingly strong.[14] Figure 1–3 and Table 1–1 illustrate this pattern.

The locational preferences exhibited by physicians are neither surprising nor reprehensible; they are those of highly educated professionals in general. As already noted, however, unlike most other professionals, physicians individually and collectively tend to enjoy substantial control over the demand for their services and over the level of their fees. If the current situation in general surgery (a specialty widely thought to be in oversupply in many regions) is any guide at all, one suspects that physicians will generally be able to earn satisfactory incomes even in relatively overdoctored areas. One should therefore not expect increases in the aggregate supply of medical manpower to spill over into the now underserved areas unless the contemplated increases were truly staggering. Such increases would, of course, lead to widespread oversupply in the relatively attractive regions, saddling consumers there (or taxpayers paying

[c]Much could be learned in this respect from Canada, where a physician surplus seems to be in the offing. Nearly all Canadians are now covered by comprehensive health insurance. Under the provincially administered insurance plans, physicians are paid on a fee-for-service basis according to fee schedules periodically negotiated with the provincial insurance commissions. The physician-population ratio in Canada has increased rapidly in recent years and continues to do so. It would be illuminating to monitor the response of negotiated fee schedules to these increases in the physician supply.

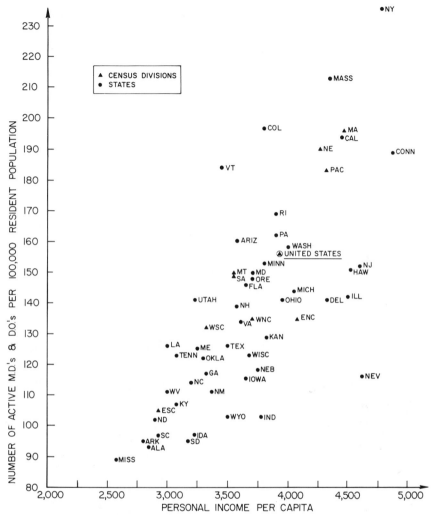

Source: Data on Physicians—U.S. National Center for Health Statistics 1972, Table 83, p. 149. Data on Population from U.S. Bureau of the Census 1972a. Data on per Capita Income from U.S. Bureau of the Census, *United States Statistical Abstract 1971,* Table 519, p. 319.

Figure 1-3. Physician Density and Personal Income per Capita by Census Division and by States (United States, 1970).

on these consumers' behalf) with the cost inflation likely to be triggered by a physician surplus.

For these reasons, a policy that seeks to achieve a more desirable geographic distribution of medical manpower simply by adding to the existing

Table 1-1.   Distribution of Nonfederal Physicians in Patient-Care Activities by Demographic County Classification, United States, 1970

Demographic County Classification[a]	Nonfederal Physicians in Patient-Care per 100,000 Residents	Income per Capita
Nonmetropolitan:		
Less than 10,000	40	$2,419
10,000–24,999	51	2,394
25,000–49,000	64	2,621
50,000 or more	87	2,821
Potential Metropolitan	124	3,086
Metropolitan:		
50,000–499,000	107	3,114
500,000–999,999	141	3,404
1,000,000–4,999,999	150	3,714
5,000,000–or more	192	4,165

[a]Numbers refer to size of resident population.
Source: American Medical Association [1972], Table 55.

capacity of medical schools is unlikely to be cost-effective. Indeed, one is entitled to wonder whether that policy would ever be effective at all, even if one did not insist on strict cost-effectiveness. This conclusion leads one to consider health manpower policies more narrowly targeted on (1) the medical school; (2) the medical student; and (3) the practicing physician. Unfortunately, a penetrating exploration of these policies would soon lead beyond the intended focus of this book. The following discussion is therefore confined to some general (and necessarily rather superficial) remarks on the issue. Furthermore, the focus of the discussion is primarily on the problem of the alleged *geographic maldistribution* of physicians. It will be apparent, however, that any policy prescriptions in that area can, generally, also be applied—with obvious alterations —to the problem perceived in connection with the *specialty distribution* of physicians. Broadly speaking, the latter problem is thought to be a relative over-emphasis on specialty training and a shortage of primary-care physicians.

Public policies addressed to the maldistribution problem may seek to modify the behavior of medical schools, of medical students, and of practicing physicians either *directly* through public regulation—for example, through the allocation of residencies among regions and among institutions according to some preconceived allocation scheme, through a draft of physicians for service in shortage areas, through allocation of medical practitioners among counties on the basis of certificates of need, and so on—or more *indirectly* through the provision of financial incentives designed to elicit the desired behavior.

A case can be made for treating direct public regulation in this area as an instrument of last resort. It is difficult to find instances in other areas of economic activity where public regulation has ever come close to reaching its ostensible objectives. By contrast, it is fairly easy to compile a list of glaring failures headed, no doubt, by public regulation of the transportation industry. These failures do not warrant the conclusion that public regulators are inherently incompetent or wicked. The problem lies in the nature of the regulatory process itself.

First, the potential force and the directness of public regulation presupposes that the regulator be given a clear mandate, one capable of staying attuned to changes in technology and economic circumstances. The definition of this mandate is no easy task. One remarkable feature of the ongoing debate over the geographic (and specialty) distribution of physicians, for example, is that no one has so far been able to suggest a hypothetical distribution that might be considered ideal or even adequate. In the absence of such a standard it will be virtually impossible to develop a universally acceptable regulatory response to the maldistribution problem. All that can really be done at this time is to move gingerly in what one deems to be the right *direction*—for example, in the direction of increasing the number of physicians available to rural popula- tions or in the direction of increasing the proportion of physicians in family practice. For a regulatory approach to be successful, the regulator must clearly be given more precise marching orders than these.

Second, the implementation of public regulation typically requires the skills of the very people one seeks to regulate. This requirement leaves the regulatory process open to capture by the targets of regulation—in the present case, the medical profession and its various specialty associations. Even if a deliberate takeover of the regulatory process does not take place, it is almost inevitable that the predilections of the regulated predominate in that process. As a result, the edicts issued under direct public regulation may turn out to be essentially a political compromise on the part of particular interest groups among those to be regulated, a compromise that abstracts unduly from the consumers' needs and preferences. Public regulation of the transportation industry is rife with such instances. It is not difficult to imagine them in the health-care sector as well. (For a careful and lucid exploration of this issue, see Havighurst [1973] and Noll [1974].)

Finally, where public regulation actually does threaten to constrain the regulated in ways they find uncomfortable, it typically elicits ingenious stratagems for working around the constraints. Although in some instances such defeats of public regulation may be judged a public good, they do in almost all instances come at a stiff price: the fees paid to that army of professionals— mainly lawyers, but occasionally also accountants and economists—who make a profitable lifetime career by protecting individual clients from the impact of public regulation. From the viewpoint of individual clients the private benefits so reaped may well justify these professionals' fees. From the viewpoint of society, however, the effort of professionals on both sides of the regulatory process often amounts to a waste of talent as glaring as the waste of advertising in the soap industry. The consumer who ultimately foots the bill is not amiss in judging the hardworking professionals who nourish themselves on the regulatory process as effectively parasitic. Public policy ought not to encourage that kind of waste.

Failures of direct regulation elsewhere is admittedly no conclusive argument against public regulation of the health-care sector if such regulation is found to be the only practical approach to the maldistribution problem. These failures should, however, serve as a general warning that public regulation of any private economic activity is never to be undertaken lightly, and that its introduction in each instance warrants a strong and explicit defense. Such caution seems all the more advisable because this type of policy seems ill-suited to the American temperament, especially to professionals in the health-care sector.

Policies working more indirectly through changes in financial incentives have the advantage of being less forceful and less pointed than direct regulation of economic behavior. This lack of precision and of forcefulness may be judged a disadvantage by some. It appears more advantageous when it is recalled that those who issue regulatory edicts can and often do make mistakes, and that public policymakers often know merely the direction in which they wish the targets of their policies to move rather than the ultimate destination to be reached. Unfortunately financial incentives have potency only where those expected to react to them are under strong economic pressure. In the context of the health-care sector, this circumstance may require considerable political courage on the part of policymakers.

A good number of proposals are currently being discussed to tie federal support of medical schools to some index of desired conduct, the latter being thought of as the recruitment and training of a student body whose ultimate choice of specialty and practice-location conforms to the direction public policy seeks to encourage. There seems little doubt that enormous financial pressure could be brought to bear on medical schools, especially if state governments were prepared to coordinate their budget policies in this respect with federal health manpower policy. But even if it were politically feasible to make the threat of fiscal sanction credible—an assumption not to be taken for granted—there remain a number of problems with this approach. First, it would be extremely difficult to develop a sensible formula linking financial support to medical school performance. Since it is presumably actual rather than predicted outcome that is to be rewarded, and the geographic-specialty distribution of a graduating class can be satisfactorily ascertained only years after completion of formal medical training, a medical school may find itself fiscally penalized in one year for sins committed years earlier.

Aside from the administrative problem of devising an equitable formula for public support, there is the question of how much control medical schools actually have over the locational and specialty choices of their students. Spokesmen for medical schools deny that this control is strong enough to make any significant difference.[15] Such protestations, however, are apt to be self-serving and are therefore to be taken with a grain of salt.

It can perhaps be held that a medical school does not really have any control over the ultimate locational choices of their graduates. Although it is sometimes suggested that a medical school could identify candidates likely to practice in the now underserved areas—if only medical educators were willing to deviate somewhat from traditional measures of academic excellence in selecting their students—one does have little assurance that original intentions or imputed preferences will actually survive medical training. Medical educators could therefore argue that performance with respect to the ultimate geographic distribution of their graduates is essentially a matter of luck, and that one ought not to accompany the incidence of luck with fiscal sanctions or rewards.

It is not clear that medical schools are equally powerless in determining their students' specialty choice. Granted, it could be argued that the *demand* for specialty training ultimately reflects the students' own preferences. But that argument hardly absolves medical schools from responsibility for the mix of specialists they train. First, one suspects that medical educators actually do have at least some influence—and perhaps a quite strong influence—over their students' preferences concerning specialty choice. More important, medical educators are instrumental in determining the *supply* of residencies in the various medical specialties, and in the long run the number and mix of residencies supplied ultimately determines the specialty mix of the overall physician population. If one accepts the assertion that the latter deviates substantially from the mix that would be optimal from society's viewpoint, one implicitly judges the supply of residencies to be unresponsive to society's need. Precisely what causes this lack of responsiveness is, of course, an interesting question.

In a properly functioning market environment, society's demand for productive factors (e.g., a particular type of manpower) is signalled to the producers of these factors (e.g., a training institution) through signals that travel from consumers to the producers of consumable commodities via the commodity markets, from these producers to the owners of productive factors (e.g., workers who in a sense own their own human capital) via the so-called factor markets, and, in the case of manpower, from the latter to the educational sector via the markets for vocational training. It is generally agreed that in the United States this information flow works reasonably well in many areas of economic activity, and that it tends to evoke the appropriate response from those who are touched by it. As noted above, in the health-care sector these signals do not seem to travel smoothly. Alternatively, if the signals are somehow transmitted through public statements, the producers of health services or the producers of health manpower seem to find themselves in an economic position that shields them from the discipline of the marketplace. As a result, they can ignore signals conveying information about society's needs without suffering the traditional economic consequences of such behavior.

In the previous section a number of serious flaws in the market for physician services were suggested, flaws that permit a disturbing deviation between consumers' needs and the medical profession's response to them. Medical educators might argue that this is the source of the maldistribution problem. More specifically, they might define their own social obligation as responding primarily to the revealed preferences of their students, leaving it to the latter to respond appropriately to the health-care needs of patients. On that theory, medical educators may think of themselves as quite responsive to social needs *as they perceive them*, and they may argue—as some educators do [16]—that the medical student rather than the medical school is the proper target of public policy in this respect.

As already noted, however, in their capacity as department chiefs in teaching hospitals medical educators do determine the number of residencies supplied by their departments, albeit in negotiation with hospital administrators. One suspects that in these negotiations the educators' views carry a heavy weight, especially if the fiscal situation of the hospital permits the administrator to be generous. Before declaring medical educators as completely innocent and helpless bystanders in their students' specialty choice—and before therefore declaring a policy of fiscal sanction against medical schools as futile—this author would certainly wish to gain a better understanding of the motives and incentives underlying this negotiation process. It is sometimes said that a staff physician's professional satisfaction derives to some extent from the sophistication of the equipment in his hospital. It might similarly be hypothesized that, in his role as department chief, the medical educator derives satisfaction from controlling a relatively large number of residencies. If so, one can posit the alternative hypothesis that the mix of specialists produced by a teaching hospital reflects not really the adaptive response of medical educators to their students' intrinsic professional interests, but instead the students' adaptation to their professors' professional predilections—predilections that may be quite impervious to the interests of both students and society at large. If that hypothesis is valid, the medical school would quite clearly be an inviting target for a policy that seeks to alter the specialty mix of the physician supply.

It is not yet clear which of the two preceding hypotheses is more nearly correct. Unfortunately, few insights on this issue can be gained from the published literature; they await much needed future research. But it is clear that one ought not to dismiss too readily the notion that medical schools are a proper target for health manpower policies related to the maldistribution problem. For the moment one had best preserve an open mind on the issue.

If medical schools either cannot or simply will not respond appropriately to threats of fiscal sanction—or if public policymakers should be too timid to make such threats—one might try to direct such policies at the medical student instead. As will be argued shortly, a case can be made on ethical and economic grounds to force a substantial increase in the tuition charged medical students, perhaps even to 100 percent of the long-run average cost of a medical education. Such a change from current practice would be a desirable first step in developing any policy aimed at influencing the behavior of medical students through financial incentives. Given the heightened economic pressure so generated, one might then grant generous loans or scholarships to those students likely to select the now understaffed specialties or to locate in now under-served regions. Once again, however, this approach is contingent on one's ability to identify such students. As noted above, one has no assurance that original preferences concerning location or specialty will remain stable over time. Furthermore, such a policy might force medical schools to accept candidates from the now rejected strata of MCAT scores, a compromise medical educators might be loath to make.

An alternative to unconditional loans or scholarships would be to grant financial assistance only in response to an overt promise by recipients to practice in now understaffed areas or specialties. Unfortunately, this policy leads to problems at both the ethical and practical levels. At the ethical level, one suspects that, even if the policy were effective, it would tend to condemn students from the lower income strata to relatively unattractive practices, leaving the choice selections to the offspring of more opulent parents. Members of minority groups, in particular, might reject the very idea of tied assistance. At the practical level, there is the problem of enforcing such promises. Under the nation's laws, the government could at most recover tuition plus interest if the promise is broken. In most cases, the financial lever that could be so employed would therefore not exceed $50,000 or so. At customary and prospective levels of physician remuneration, however, a sum of $50,000 is not likely to strike medical graduates as a terribly imposing portion of their expected lifetime income, especially if such costs can be passed through to consumers via professional fees. The probability that medical graduates will simply buy out of an earlier promise is therefore high. This hypothesis finds some support in the mixed results achieved with existing programs of tied assistance to medical students, although the maximum financial lever under these programs has not been as high as $50,000.

If neither the medical school nor the medical student furnish responsive targets for a policy working through financial incentives, one is left to attack the maldistribution problem either through direct public regulation—including perhaps outright franchising of medical practices—or through the manipulation of financial incentives faced by practicing physicians. (For a more extended discussion of such policies, see Reinhardt [1974].) The obvious policy lever in this case would be the price (fees) of physician services. An alternative might be the income tax rates imposed on physicians.

In connection with physician fees it may be observed that, quite aside from the professional and cultural attractions of, say, New York City, the fact that physician fees there are often several times those paid in, say, the rural South for the same precedure can certainly not be said to enhance the relative attractiveness of medical practice in the rural South. While a reversal of these relative fee levels might not trigger a mass migration of physicians toward the South, one certainly cannot escape the feeling that such a change—or even merely greater equality of absolute fee-levels across the nation—would enhance the relative attraction of the now shunned locations to physicians at the margin. It would hence be a policy move in the right direction.

A similar observation can be offered in connection with specialty choice. The fact that remuneration per hour effectively worked in surgery tends to be many times that per hour worked on preventive care in family practice can certainly not serve as an inducement to leave the relatively overpopulated specialty of surgery in favor of family practice. Here appropriate differentials in hourly pay would certainly trigger the desired marginal shift in specialty choice, even if not every medical graduate were responsive to such financial signals.

Proposals to seek a redistribution of medical manpower across regions (or across specialties) through changes in the relative level of fees paid in various regions (or in various specialties) are frequently met with skepticism. Quite aside from the administrative or political feasibility of the proposal, it is argued, the typical physician is motivated by a good many factors other than income, and only an economist would ever dream that income by itself could serve as a sufficiently strong and reliable policy lever. To bolster this argument, it is pointed out that a failure of economic incentives to work in this area has been amply demonstrated by the failure of existing tied-loan programs to elicit the desired behavior from medical students.

Two comments may be offered in response to these observations. First, policies using medical school tuition (even at 100 percent of cost) as a policy lever involve only a relatively modest amount of money and have an impact of only short duration on the physician's economic position. By contrast, policies working through the reimbursement mechanism can be made to involve substantial changes in annual physician income, and furthermore will affect the physician's income throughout his or her working life. Second, the power of interregional fee differentials to alter the locational choices of medical practitioners—or of interspecialty fee differentials to alter their specialty choices—is clearly a function not only of the absolute size of these differentials, but also of the average income that can be earned in relatively overstaffed areas (or specialties). In this connection it is useful to think of the "other factors" often said to dominate the physician's choices as "luxuries" of which more is consumed as income rises, and which pale in significance as income falls. It can readily be conceded that a doubling of medical fees in, say, the rural South, would fail to draw a substantial number of physicians to that region if fee levels in New England or California were kept at levels sufficiently high to afford physicians there the luxury of an income in the top 5 percent of the local income distribution, even in the face of overt or disguised under-employment. Similarly, it is not reasonable to expect physicians to leave general surgery for the less prestigious family practice if, regardless of fees in family practice, fees for surgery remain sufficiently high to afford even a severely underemployed surgeon a position near the top of the national income scale. It is no paradox that persons with high incomes are relatively insensitive to economic incentives at the margin. Economic theory predicts precisely such behavior. That theory, however, also suggests that the sensitivity to economic incentives is heightened when these incentives become large relative to income, and herein lie some possibilities.

A serious effort to use the reimbursement mechanism as a vehicle for altering the distribution of medical manpower across regions, or across specialties, would hardly proceed on a basis that affords even the most ineffi-cient or underemployed practitioner a comfortable income. Such a policy would have to establish fees at which overt or disguised underemployment would imply mediocre incomes and hence strong economic pressure for medical students to choose relatively understaffed specialties, and for physicians to locate in relatively underserved areas. In other words, the policy would attempt to stimulate precisely the kind of economic pressures automatically generated in competitive labor markets in which remuneration tends to rise in the face of excess demand, and to fall in the face of excess supply. If these pressures were strong enough, they should work in the health-care sector just as they do in other sectors of the economy.

The author is well aware that the policy of "economic pressure" sketched out above would not be administratively feasible at this time, because even the publicly financed Medicare/Medicaid programs cover only a part of the otherwise private market for physician services. The Medicare/Medicaid pro-grams can obviously not move completely in abstraction from general market conditions. And in the U.S., where legislators tend to be highly responsive to small but vocal interest groups, such a policy may not be politically acceptable even under a publicly financed system of comprehensive and universal health insurance, although then the policy would be at least administratively feasible. It would therefore not be unjust to judge this policy proposal as politically naive. These reservations notwithstanding, there may nevertheless be some merit in letting one's mind wander now and then outside the bounds of contemporary political parameters and to explore rather bold policy moves that may become feasible in the future. After all, who is to say that one day's heresy may not become another day's forklore, and thus a third day's statute? It has happened before and it may happen again.

Finally, in thinking about the maldistribution problem one should never lose sight of the fact that the problem manifests itself for the most part as a shortage of *primary* health services in *some* locations. Once contact with a primary-care facility has been made, it is usually not too difficult to transport the patient to a specialist's location, should intervention by the latter be found necessary. In fact, there may be sound medical and economic reasons for permitting specialists to concentrate in certain locations where sophisticated support facilities can be shared. Nations that plan their health sectors under a central authority have long recognized this *desideratum*. The ideal geographic distribution of physicians is thus not likely to be one assuring all counties (or even states) a single standard mix of specialists and a single standard physician-population ratio.

There can be little doubt that the alleged maldistribution of primary care in this country has been able to persist on the strength of the nation's medical licensure laws, which have traditionally accorded to physicians the exclusive right of acting as the sole legitimate entry into the medical system. It can be argued that the very existence of the maldistribution problem points to a failure on the part of the medical profession to live up to the responsibility implicit in its exclusive franchise on health-care delivery. The profession could be said to have forfeited that privilege and could be forced to share the responsibility for primary health care with paramedical professionals—for example, nurse practitioners or the various types of health workers commonly lumped together under the label "physician extenders." Since the power to license health workers rests with the public sector, that sector also has the power to remove the bottlenecks generated by current licensure laws and to encourage deployment of physician substitutes where physicians refuse to serve.

It is now widely recognized that the training of physician substitutes is desirable, a recognition that has reflected itself in generous federal support for experimental training programs. Controversies remain, however, concerning the legal status of these new types of manpower. These controversies originate partly in concern about the quality of medical care. As might be expected, they also spring from certain economic conflicts between the medical and paramedical professions.

In principle there is no reason why a pediatric nurse practitioner, a midwife, or any other formally trained physician extender should not deliver primary health care as an *independent* practitioner, even on a fee-for-service basis (although preferably not so). Under appropriate statutory safeguards—expressed perhaps through mandatory or permissive licensure—such practitioners could introduce a healthy element of competition into the otherwise flawed market for health services. They could provide consumers who have seemingly minor medical problems with an alternative to higher-priced physician care. Should certain problems not be minor after all, the paramedics could then refer patients to full-fledged medical practitioners. One suspects that an ample supply of independently practicing paramedics might in this way be used to eliminate much of the maldistribution problem now perceived, unless, of course, the paramedics are also drawn from social classes that can thrive only in well-to-do urban areas.

The danger inherent in this approach is, of course, that a paramedic may fail to recognize a serious medical condition if confronted with one, thus prolonging the waiting time to proper medical care. Indeed, if paramedics render services on a fee-for-service basis, they may, under conditions of excess supply, have an economic incentive to delay referral to a physician. That possibility, however, exists also at other levels in the medical hierarchy. A general practitioner, for example, also may fail to recognize the need for a specialist's intervention when that intervention would be most appropriate, and a general practitioner also may face economic incentives to delay referral. Society has long learned to live with these dangers inherent in the current delivery system. It would probably become accustomed also to those inherent in a regime of independent paramedic practices.

The alternative to independent paramedical practice is obviously to place the paramedic under the medical and economic control of a fully licensed physician. Not surprisingly this is the approach favored by the medical profession and in current legislation concerning paramedics. The strategy presumably provides better guarantees against low-quality primary care. (It also, of course, serves to protect the medical profession from unwelcome competition.) The strategy, however, does create some problems that may ultimately defeat the original intent of training physician extenders.

First, if physician extenders must remain under visual supervision of a physician, their spatial and specialty distribution will necessarily parallel those of physicians and thus permit continued existence of gaps in access to primary care. If, on the other hand, the paramedic administers care in spatial separation from the employing physician, the probability of erroneous diagnoses may approximate that experienced under independent paramedic practice unless the paramedic is linked to the physician by two-way audio-visual communication. Experiments with such systems are underway in several places in the United States (see, for example, Geomet, Inc. [1972, Chapter 4]).

Second, there arises the question of how much consumers (or third-party payers) should pay the physician for services performed solely by a physician extender in the physician's employ. Current thinking in Congress appears to gravitate to the notion that a physician ought not to reap the economic fruits of the paramedic's labors. At the ethical level this sentiment has a certain appeal. Its translation into a reimbursement strategy, however, is apt to eliminate much of the economic incentive physicians have in hiring physician extenders in the first place. As is so often the case, what is ethically appealing in this case appears to clash with what is economically sound. This issue is clearly an important problem in the formulation of health manpower policy; we therefore return to it for a fuller discussion toward the end of the book (see Chapter Seven).

FOREIGN-TRAINED PHYSICIANS AND THE
PHYSICIAN SHORTAGE

By the end of 1970, about 63,000 of the 348,000 active and inactive physicians in the United States had graduated from a foreign medical school. About 39 percent of these physicians received their medical education in Europe; 33 percent in Asia—mainly the Philippines (12 percent), India (6 percent) and South Korea (3 percent); 16 percent in Latin America; about 10 percent in Canada; and 2 percent in Africa and Oceania. Over 80 percent of these physicians were engaged in patient care as their primary activity, a disproportionate number in hospital-based practice. For example, although foreign-trained physicians in 1970 represented only about 18 percent of all physicians in the United States, they represented about 32 per cent of all hospital-based physicians and only 11 percent of all office-based physicians. It is also noteworthy that they amounted to about 27 percent of all physicians engaged in medical research.[17]

Many foreign-trained physicians initially come to this country on student exchange visas for graduate medical education in internships and residencies. Having been trained in the sophisticated and capital-intensive pattern of American medical practice, they find no outlet for their skills in their home countries and prefer to remain in the United States where adequate support facilities are more readily available. In making that decision, they are undoubtedly lured also by the relatively high income and prestige associated with medical practice in this country. The same lure has undoubtedly also attracted those foreign-trained physicians who have entered the United States directly on immigrant visas. With the lifting of the national quota system in 1968, a large number of Asian physicians have come to the United States via this route. Finally, about 10 percent of all foreign-trained physicians are actually American-born citizens who have studied medicine abroad (mostly in Europe), presumably after being rejected by American medical schools.

Although there has always been some immigration of foreign-trained physicians into the United States, the trend appears to have accelerated during the 1960s. Between 1962 and 1971, about 47,000 foreign-trained physicians entered the country on exchange visas. During the same period, about 29,000 entered on permanent-resident visas including, however, exchange visitors who subsequently switched to that status [Stevens and Vermeulen, 1972, p. 96, Table A2]. This development seems to reflect the liberalization of U.S. immigration laws for physicians during the late 1960s, for between 1968 and 1971 alone 33,000 foreign medical graduates came to this country.

It must be assumed that the liberalization of the immigration laws was a deliberate attempt by the United States to cope with the physician shortage perceived in the late 1960s. Hospitals in particular offered many more residencies and internships than could be filled with American medical school graduates, and there was a perceived shortage also of housestaff physicians. The fact that a disproportionate number of foreign-trained physicians are in hospital-based practice suggests that they have, in fact, served to fill some of the voids left by the uneven distribution of American-trained physicians over regions and provider facilities. But if the open-door policy was thought to solve the wider problem of maldistribution, its success has not been spectacular. As a study by Butter and Schaffner (1971) has indicated, the distributional impact of foreign-trained physicians has generally been to *increase* rather than decrease the inequality among states and between rural and urban areas. Disproportionate numbers of these physicians have located in the already well-endowed northeastern United States, in California, and in Hawaii. The relatively under-doctored southern states have received disproportionately few.

As already noted, many commentators on the United States health system find its heavy reliance on foreign-trained physicians disgraceful. It is argued that the country's open-door immigration and educational exchange policies for physicians robs less developed nations of badly needed medical manpower and in effect constitutes foreign aid in reverse. It has been estimated, for example, that the migration of Philippine physicians to the United States contributes roughly $1.5 million annually to the U.S. economy, and that the long-run human resource costs to India of 1,000 physician emigrants per year may be as much as $35 million if one considers the economic potential of such manpower.[18] There obviously is something to the charge that the United States posture in this respect must appear callous in the eyes of the Third World. Whether restrictions to this migration would actually help the donor countries, however, is not quite so obvious, for it is unclear just who in the donor countries is actually being deprived by the outflow of their physicians.

It was shown in the preceding section that physicians in the United States have a penchant for locations in which money can readily be earned and in which it can be well spent. This locational preference among physicians seems to be universal. As Eli Ginzberg has noted on this point, "Israel has more doctors per head of population than any other country in the world; there is more than one physician for every 500 persons. Nevertheless, rural coverage in Israel is inadequate; physicians do not want to live in the country" [1969, p. 113]. Ginzberg adds that the problem exists even in the socialist countries of Eastern Europe, and that almost all of the three hundred physicians serving Ethiopia's 25 million people live in the country's two major cities [p. 114]. Elsewhere it has been estimated that roughly 95 percent of the physicians in Iran serve no more than 24 percent of the population, leaving the other 5 percent to care for the remaining 76 percent of the population; and that in general roughly 90 to 95 percent of the physicians in the less developed donor countries practice in urban areas where the physician-population ratio is often higher than in many United States cities.[19] Finally, in their study of foreign-trained physicians in the United States, Stevens and Vermeulen come to the disturbing conclusion that

> medical schools in Third World countries, while offering a valuable base for the training of medical specialists, scientists, and teachers, are too often not producing physicians who are appropriate for, or motivated toward, the major health care needs of their own nation.
>
> In this sense, it is not always appropriate to speak of a "drain" of high-level manpower from a developing country to the United States. There may in fact be insufficient posts in the developing country for physicians who are in essence qualified in urban medicine [1972, p. 76].

These findings throw a different light on the thesis that United States reliance on foreign-trained physicians deprives the donor countries of badly needed medical manpower. It is true that the implications of physician migration on the health systems of the donor countries have not been explored as fully as they should be,[20] and that circumspection must be used in the interpretation of the data cited in the preceding paragraph. Even so, available data suggest at least tentatively that the migration of foreign-trained physicians into the United States effectively constitutes a transfer of medical manpower from reasonably well-to-do urbanites in the donor countries to well-to-do and sometimes not so well-to-do urbanites in the United States. That flow has admittedly served to fill certain gaps in the distribution of American physicians and has hence been welcomed by the formulators of health manpower policy in this country; but the flow also seems to represent the product of a push away from relatively over-doctored centers in countries that cannot fully absorb their own physicians to the latters' satisfaction, and of the pull towards the economic rewards and professional prestige associated with medical practice in the United States.

In the final analysis, it may be asked why the less-developed countries themselves have done so little in the past to discourage the emigration of their physicians, as they undoubtedly could, or to alleviate the glaring maldistribution of medical manpower in their own society. The proposition that the United States solve these problems for them by prohibiting the immigration of foreign-trained physicians does not strike one as morally compelling, at least not until these countries themselves make greater efforts to gear their medical training programs and health manpower policies to the health needs of their own people.

While the case for United States restrictions on the immigration of foreign-trained physicians *in the interest of potential donor countries* seems rather less than compelling, it may one day be in the interest of the United States itself to restrict that flow. Such a policy may be adopted either as part of a more general policy to limit the supply of physicians in this country, or in response to the common complaint that the training of foreign medical graduates often falls short of American standards. In the meantime, it seems neither irrational nor ironical to follow an open-door policy vis à vis foreign medical graduates, or to send American citizens to European medical schools, while at the same time restricting the capacity of American medical schools to its currently planned level. As indicated in Figure 1-2, the ratio of American-trained physicians per 100,000 U.S. residents can be expected to increase throughout the next four decades without further expansion of American medical schools above the level projected for 1975. Even if one accepted the assertion that there is now an acute shortage of physicians at the aggregate level—an assertion this author does not accept—one would surely have to admit that sooner or later the shortage will be overcome with currently planned indigenous medical school capacity. From this perspective, the importation of foreign medical education or of foreign-trained physicians can be viewed simply as the most economic way of meeting the perceived physician shortage in the short run. Indeed, in comparison with continued construction of American schools, such a policy would be a more economic solution to a short-run physician shortage even if the United States reimbursed the donor countries for the education of the imported manpower. Although payment for a nation's investment in individual emigrants—either on the part of the emigrant or by the recipient nation—is not customary, it can certainly be argued on moral grounds that the United States repay at least the less-developed donor countries for the human capital it imports from them.

THE SUPPLY OF AND DEMAND FOR MEDICAL EDUCATIONS

There remains the proposition that to deny qualified Americans the career of their choice is a national shame and inimical to our democratic institutions. This is a peculiar argument. There are probably many Americans qualified and willing to become airline pilots who are denied the opportunity to do so. There are many qualified Americans desirous of becoming college professors, but are also denied that opportunity. There are many qualified people who want to become high school teachers, lawyers, bricklayers, bus drivers, astronauts, aerospace engineers or movie stars—and many of them are denied the opportunity to pursue the career of their first choice. This is neither a national shame nor undemocratic: there simply is a limit to the demand for these candidates' potential contribution.

Those who decry the high rejection rates of American medical schools fail to perceive, first of all, that the decision to pursue a particular career reflects at once the desire to practice in the chosen occupation, a yearning for the prestige (if any) associated with that career, and the hope for the income stream it is expected to generate. Which of these desires dominates in particular instances is not always clear, particularly not from a routine application form.

It has been estimated that the annual rate of return to a college graduate on his or her own investment (including foregone earnings) in four years of medical school and one year of internship is approximately 25 percent [Sloan, 1970]. This is an attractive yield by almost any standard. In view of these high returns one suspects that at least some applicants to medical school— and perhaps many—seek access not so much to a medical career but to a sound investment to which the career is more or less incidental. This motivation, once again, is not reprehensible. The search for good investments is as American as the proverbial apple pie. The point is that failure on the part of many Americans to gain access to such investments is not necessarily a source of national disgrace, so long as all qualified applicants are given a fair chance to compete for them. This argument is all the more compelling when one considers the enormous public subsidies to investments in medical training.

As a first step in thinking about this issue, it is useful to view a medical education as a "commodity" being traded in a competitive market. In the absence of outside support, the supply of medical educations (that is, the number of places offered by medical schools at given levels of tuition) would depend primarily on the cost of producing medical educations. The demand for medical educations, on the other hand (that is, the annual number of applicants at given levels of tuition) is a function of the applicants' intrinsic interest in medical science, of the nontuition costs (especially foregone earnings) of that education, and, of course, of the monetary rewards expected from a medical career. If the number of qualified applicants were relatively large, there would presumably emerge an equilibrium tuition at which the number of qualified applicants just matches the places being offered. If the argument is that neither the government, nor organized medicine, nor any other interest group ought to constrain acceptances below the freely determined equilibrium, one cannot but agree. It is hard to think of an ethical foundation on which such restrictions could rest.

In the real world, however, there is extensive outside intervention in the market for medical educations. Medical schools are highly subsidized, largely with public funds. As a result, the regular tuition charged by medical schools covers only a fraction of their instructional budgets, and even some portion of that tuition is sometimes subsidized through scholarships. Oddly enough, physicians themselves seem rarely aware of how much of the returns on their investment comes courtesy of the public purse, even though physicians have long been among the staunchest supporters of the free-enterprise system. Strictly speaking, the subsidies they receive ought not to be taken for granted: on their face they constitute a transfer of wealth from some members of society to others and as such require explicit justification.

One can think of a number of reasons for public subsidies to a professional education. Such subsidies may be a redistributive device aimed at making professional careers accessible to lower income classes or particular ethnic groups, especially in cases where loans for investments in human capital are not readily made available. Such subsidies could also be justified if the training of the individual ultimately bestows benefits on society that will not be reflected in the income society pays the professional for his or her services. In the case of medical education, for example, these services may consist of a draft into military service in an otherwise all-volunteer armed force.

As a first principle, however, it would seem fairer to require that the professional amortize out of his or her own income the great bulk (if not all) of the costs that can be identified with his or her training. If general or selective subsidies were felt desirable, they could then be examined on their own merit and granted where deemed appropriate. Although this proposition may seem radical to some, it is surely not as far-fetched as the notion that the nation is morally obligated to grant every otherwise qualified American access to highly subsidized physician-income streams. If subsidize one must, one should at most permit all qualified applicants to compete freely for the number of medical educations that can reasonably be justified. And that justification cannot rest on emotional appeals to the nation's sense of shame; it must be based instead on society's objective need for physician services.

SUMMARY AND OVERVIEW

The rising cost of physician services, the unavailability of physician services in some areas of the country, the influx of foreign-trained physicians into the United States, or the desire of American college graduates to become physicians do not necessarily make the case for continued expansion of American medical schools. Such an expansion may do little to eliminate acute shortages where they exist; it may simply generate an excess supply of physicians in already well-endowed locations. A surplus of physicians, however, is apt to be a mixed blessing. Both economic theory and available empirical evidence suggest that such a surplus may translate into unnecessarily high per-capita consumption of medical care and into inflated professional fees.

It is difficult to accept that a nation already enjoying one of the highest physician-population ratios in the world suffers from an acute shortage of medical manpower *at the aggregate level.* Particular areas in the United States are undoubtedly understaffed, and certain segments of the population lack adequate medical care, even in regions whose overall physician-population ratio is high. Certainly there are physician shortages in particular medical specialties (such as family practice) or provider facilities (such as municipal hospitals). These shortages, however, reflect primarily a *maldistribution* of the existing supply of medical manpower and should not be confused with an aggregate physician shortage.

Any perceived shortage of medical manpower is, of course, nothing but a perceived shortage of the type of medical services that have *traditionally* been furnished by medical practices in a manner to which both the physician and his patients have become habituated. Nothing in the nature of medical practice in this country persuades one that the habitual in this context is in fact optimal. On the contrary, there is persuasive evidence (to be presented later) that in the conduct of his practice the typical American physician is rather wasteful of his own (expensive) time, and that many so-called "physician services" actually need not be produced by physicians at all. Thus even if one accepted the assertion that, quite aside from the problem of maldistribution, the United States suffers also from an *overall* shortage of "physician services," it is far from obvious that the appropriate solution to this problem would be an increase in the supply of physicians. Such a policy would undoubtedly be expedient; its implementation would require little more than a generous dole of public funds to medical educators and students. Unfortunately, the policy would also rob the health-care sector of one of the more powerful incentives to rationalize its use of health manpower. It would perpetuate an environment that has long been hospitable to a wasteful use of physician time and, as the behavioral models considered earlier suggest, it might encourage even greater waste in the future. As Eli Ginzberg has correctly observed on this point, "It may well be that the effective use of physician manpower depends in the first instance on a taut supply of physicians" [1969, p. 10].

A more rational health manpower policy—one advocated in a number of recent publications [21] —would clearly be one aimed at moving the health-care sector toward greater efficiency in its use of physician manpower. Such a mandate is obviously far more complex than the task of merely generating ample numbers of physicians. It requires, first of all, that technically feasible ways of increasing the average productivity of American physicians be discovered. Next it is necessary to assess the economic merits of technically feasible avenues. (One tends to be instinctively in favor of increases in manpower productivity, and thus often forgets that such gains are usually achieved only through greater use of other resources, either capital equipment or, in the case of medical practice, paramedical and clerical manpower. Some technically feasible gains in physician productivity may actually not be worth their cost.) Finally, one must gain a firm understanding of the incentives to which physicians respond in the organization and conduct of their practice. The aim of the exercise is, of course, to discover policy levers through which physicians can be induced to exploit productivity gains that are technically feasible and that make economic sense.

In the remainder of this book, the potential for future gains in physician productivity, its implication for future physician requirements, and its implication for health manpower policy are examined in greater depth. The focus throughout the analysis is on *aggregate* manpower requirements. Local shortages resulting from the maldistribution of medical manpower, either geographically or across specialties, are viewed as a problem more or less distinct from the problem of overall supply and will be touched upon only tangentially.

The analysis begins in Chapter Two with a brief review of health-manpower forecasting during the last several decades. This review is offered in order to highlight certain methodological features the various forecasts have had in common. These features, it appears, have strongly colored the definition of the "doctor shortage" as that term is used in public statements and have inevitably influenced also the policy responses to those statements. In particular, they seem to have diverted attention from the organization of medical practice in this country and thus from the relationship between physician productivity and physician requirements. As is shown at the end of Chapter Two, the projected future need of physicians is enormously sensitive to one's assumptions about the productivity of physicians.

The very mention of the term "physician productivity" confronts one with the difficult problem of defining the output from the physician's professional activities. As is well known, or can at least be well imagined, this problem leads to a number of conceptual issues that have never been and are not likely ever to be resolved to everyone's satisfaction. Even so, it behooves anyone who proposes to discourse upon physician productivity to lay bare the premises on which his use of that term is based. This is done at the beginning of Chapter Three. The remainder of that chapter is given to a brief analysis of the magnitude and sources of growth in physician productivity during the past several decades, primarily in order to establish a basis from which to speculate about the potential for future productivity growth.

It seems widely agreed that the average productivity of American physicians has grown significantly during the postwar years, sufficiently rapid, in fact, to permit a more or less constant number of physicians per capita during most of these years to cope with an ever-increasing per capita demand for physician services. Opinions differ sharply, however, on the likelihood of future productivity gains. One school of thought deems it virtually impossible to increase the patient load of the average American physician further without seriously impairing the quality of his services, and regards any policy predicated on the realization of future productivity gains a dangerous pipedream. The preponderant view—certainly among health economists—is that physicians have not even begun to exploit the productivity potential actually within their reach. Among the more commonly mentioned measures of reaping this potential are (1) the consolidation of traditional solo practices into large-scale multispecialty group practices; (2) greater reliance on capital equipment in the delivery of medical care; (3) the substitution of paramedical and clerical for medical manpower; and (4) a shift from fee-for-service reimbursement toward prepayment for comprehensive health care.

There has long been some controversy about the relative effectiveness of these proposed changes. They are therefore examined in broad overview in Chapter Four. On the basis of the available empirical evidence it is concluded that, contrary to widely held opinion, neither the formation of group medical practices per se nor greater use of capital equipment in medical practice is likely to yield substantial economies in the medical manpower required to serve given population groups. There *is* persuasive evidence—drawn largely from existing prepaid group practice plans—that the prepayment feature as such tends to yield economies in the use of medical manpower—primarily, however, through induced reduction in the per capita utilization of in-patient physician services and, oddly enough, not through greater efficiency in the production of physician services. One's main hope for economies of the latter sort, it is concluded in Chapter Four, rests in the potential of health manpower substitution.

In Chapters Five, Six and Seven, the effect of health manpower substitution on physician productivity is examined within a formal production-function framework. Chapter Five presents that framework at the conceptual level. Empirical estimates of production functions for physician services are presented in Chapter Six. In Chapter Seven the economic properties of these estimates are explored in some detail. The policy implications emerging from this research are examined in the concluding chapter. That chapter ends with some thoughts on the relationship—real or imagined—between *efficiency* and *quality* in the context of health-care production.

As indicated earlier, the idea to meet the nation's future need for medical services through more effective use of medical manpower rather than mere increases in the supply of physicians is not new. It can be discerned in the report of the National Advisory Commission on Health Manpower (1967), in the so-called Gorham Report (1967), in the writings of Weiss (1966), Monsma (1969), and notably in Rashi Fein's *The Doctor Shortage* (1967). When these publications were written, however, the empirical evidence bearing on the issue was scanty indeed, and their authors had to proceed as much on the basis of intuition as on solid facts. Perhaps as a result, their views have sometimes been set aside as either invalid or impractical [Gerber 1967]. In the meantime much new evidence has been gathered. At the same time, the supply of medical manpower in this country has been increasing at a pace that exceeds earlier expectations, while the rate of population growth has slowed. A fresh and critical look at the "doctor shortage" is therefore in order.

NOTES

1. Medical schools produce medical training, medical research, and various forms of patient care. The allocation of total costs to each of these production activities is inevitably somewhat arbitrary. Consequently, it is not easy to identify the short-run and long-run average cost of a medical education as such. A figure of $100,000 has been cited by Gerber [1973, p. 13] and is consistent with cost data made public by the Association of American Medical Colleges [1973]. According to the Association, the institutional cost of an undergraduate medical education are between $16,000 and $26,000 per student per year, depending on the individual school being considered.

In a subsequent report published by the Institute of Medicine of the National Academy of Sciences [1974], the average annual cost of an undergraduate medical education is estimated to be only about $12,600 per student. The Institute's definition of cost is based on a narrower definition of the teaching activity of medical school faculty, and hence allocates a smaller proportion of faculty salaries to medical education as such.

2. See, for example Alex Gerber [1973]. The long-run implications of such proposals are examined in Chapter 2.

3. Data presented in "Medical Education in the United States 1972–73," *Journal of the American Medical Association* (November 19, 1973), p. 909.

4. Verbal communication from Dr. P. Rosenthal, Association of American Medical Colleges, Washington, D.C., June 26, 1974.

5. Dr. Robert A. Chase of Stanford University, as quoted by the *New York Times*, October 17, 1973.

6. Dr. Richard Warren of Harvard University, as quoted in *ibid.*

7. This thesis is most clearly set forth in Friedman [1962], pp. 137–60. In this connection see also Friedman and Kuznets [1945], Hyde et al. [1954], and Rayack [1965].

8. One of the boldest papers of this genre is Monsma's "Marginal Revenue and the Demand for Physicians' Services" [1970].

9. In this connection a careful distinction must be drawn between the fees for particular medical services and physician earnings per hour or per week. In his analysis of physician supply behavior, for example, Sloan [1973] finds a strong and significant negative correlation between the physician-population ratio in an area and weekly earnings per physician. A mildly negative though statistically insignificant correlation is also found between hourly physician earnings and the physician-population ratio in the area. To the extent that Sloan's findings are reliable they suggest that a physician hour in areas with high physician density may be somewhat "cheaper" than an hour of physician time in relatively under-doctored areas. From society's viewpoint, however, this is hardly relevant. The important point from society's perspective is how the physician hour is used— and how it is used reflects itself in the price of the services produced with physician time. An inefficient producer may quite possibly earn relatively little per hour of his time and yet charge an unnecessarily high price per unit of output.

10. The most explicit statement of this model is found in the *Report of the Commission on the Cost of Medical Care* by the American Medical Association [1964], Chapter 2. Other authors who seem to posit that model, at least implicitly, are Frech and Ginsburg [1972], Fuchs and Kramer [1972], and Ruffin and Leigh [1969].

11. That school of thought is represented in Feldstein [1970]; Jones, Struve and Stefani [1967]; Kessel [1958]; Newhouse [1970]; and Newhouse and Sloan [1972].

12. In his "The Rising Cost of Physician Services," Martin Feldstein [1970] concludes that a competitive-market model is simply incompatible with observed behavior of physician fees. He notes that the physician's pricing decision is best understood within a target-income model. Newhouse [1970] and Newhouse and Sloan [1972] reach a similar conclusion in their analyses of physician fees. They point out that the target-income model is implicit also in statements on fee-setting offered by physicians.

   More recent work by Sloan throws some doubt on the *universal* validity of the target-income hypothesis. In Steinwald and Sloan [1973] and Sloan [1974], the fees charged by individual physicians in a nationwide cross-section sample of physicians are statistically related to the number of physicians in the physician's "market area" (presumably the state in which he practices, or his county—it is not clear from the paper) and to some fifteen other variables that may conceivably influence the physician's fees. The physician density in the physician's market area is represented by two variables: (1) the number of physicians in the physician's own specialty; and (2) the number of physicians in other specialities not necessarily competing with the physician. The statistical results from this research are mixed. After controlling for all other factors likely to affect fees, a positive partial correlation between fees and the number of potentially competing plysicians in the market area is found for internists, obstetricians-gynecologists, and pediatricians. These results are fully consistent with the target-income hypothesis. For general surgeons and general practitioners, on the other hand, fees for some procedures exhibit a positive partial correlation with the number of potential competitors in the area (thus supporting the target-income hypothesis), while fees for other procedures exhibit a negative partial correlation with physician density, a result more consistent with a competitive-market model. It is these results that compel one to declare the empirical research on the matter as less than conclusive, although on balance the estimates presented in Steinwald and Sloan [1973], Table II, are more supportive of the target-income than of the competitive-market model.

   The target-income hypothesis finds further support in a study on physician pricing by Kehrer and Knowles [1973]. The authors' statistical approach is quite similar to that adopted in Steinwald and Sloan. In characterizing physician density in the individual physician's market area (his county), Kehrer and Knowles also distinguish between physicians who are potential substitutes for or competitors of one another, and physicians in other specialties. Using once again a nationwide cross-section sample of physicians, they estimate statistical relationships between fees or markup (average revenue divided by average cost), on the one hand, and physician density and a host of other variables on the other. After controlling for the potential influence of all these other variables on physician fees (or on his markup), the authors' estimates appear to lend support to the target-income hypothesis "since in some specialties (general practice, internal medicine, pediatrics, opthalmology, general practice-general surgery groups, and diversified group practices), prices (fees) are positively and statistically significantly related to ratios of competitive-specialty physicians to population" in the physician's county [p. 6–3]. The authors caution, however, that the observed higher fees in areas with high physician density may reflect services of a correspondingly higher resource intensity. The authors arrive at this conclusion after noting that the physicians' markup does not appear to vary significantly with physician density.

Kehrer and Knowles, incidentally, equate increased resource intensity of physician services with higher quality. As is noted in the text, higher resource intensity need not imply higher quality; it may reflect waste. And even higher quality must be able to justify its higher costs. This is a point made quite forcefully also by Evans et al. [1973], whose analysis of medical practices in the Canadian province of British Columbia indicates a substantial positive correlation between interregional physician density and the number of physician services consumed per capita under the province's comprehensive health insurance plan. Evans interprets this phenomenon as physician-induced increases in demand [pp. 389–393]. In an earlier analysis of the behavior of physician fees prior to the introduction of universal health insurance in Canada, Evans also comes down on the side of the target-income hypothesis (see Evans [1972]).

In short, then, while results from research to date leave enough open questions on the behavior of physician fees to point up the need for further research, the available evidence tends to support the notion that increases in the physician population ratio are likely to exert upward rather than downward pressure on fees.

13. About 98 percent of the West German population is covered by comprehensive health insurance. The insurance system is operated by a network of 900 separate insurance companies and "sickness funds" (*Krankenkassen*) closely supervised by the West German government. Primary-care physicians are paid by these funds on a fee-for-service basis according to fee schedules negotiated between regional medical associations and regional associations of the insurance carriers, and ratified by the government. The fee schedules have not worked any hardship on German physicians—their average income in 1971 is reported to have been in excess of $65,000, and their average net taxable income about $54,000, figures that are high by U.S. standards and even higher by West German standards. Between 1953 and 1973, medical fees in West Germany rose by about 700 percent; during the same period, the cost of living rose 48 percent. It would seem, then, that organized medicine in West Germany has been

very persuasive in making the case for "adequate" physician remuneration. In 1972, incidentally, West Germany is reported to have
had 191 physicians per 100,000 population, a sharp increase from
the ratio of 166 per 100,000 reported in 1966. Data taken from
Gonzales [1973], pp. 40–1.

14. For examples of this type of research, see Benham, Maurizi and Reder
[1968]; Fuchs and Kramer [1972]; and Rimlinger and Steele
[1963].

15. Verbal communication from John A. D. Cooper, M.D., President, Association of American Medical Colleges, during a presentation to the
George Washington University Health Staff Seminar, February 20,
1974.

16. Ibid.

17. Data developed in Stevens and Vermeulen [1972], Appendixes A to D.

18. Quoted in ibid., p. 81.

19. Estimates quoted in the *Journal of the American Medical Association*
(October 22, 1973), p. 463.

20. This, at any rate, is one of the conclusions reached by Stevens and Vermeulen [1972] in their study of foreign-trained physicians in the
United States.

21. See Fein [1967]; Monsma [1969]; Jones, Struve and Stefani [1967]; and
Weiss [1966].

Chapter Two

The Dynamics of Health
Manpower Forecasting

I. AN HISTORICAL SYNOPSIS

Studies pointing to an existing or impending shortage of physicians in this country have been published with remarkable regularity. As early as 1933, for example, Drs. Roger Lee and Lewis Jones had argued that as of that year the nation had 13,000 fewer physicians than could be considered adequate on strictly medical grounds. The Lee-Jones study was followed, after the war, by the Ewing Report in 1948, the Mountin-Pennell-Berger study in 1949, and the report of the President's Commission on the Health Needs of the Nation in 1953. These reports offered alternative projections for a variety of normative physician-population ratios, although one gathers that among these, the physician-population ratio actually enjoyed by the most richly endowed region during the year the forecast was made tended to be the preferred standard. On that basis, the three postwar reports projected a 1960 deficit of between 42,000 and 59,000 M.D.'s, and called for direct federal support of *medical education* in addition to the government's long-standing support of *medical research.* Congress did not respond positively to these recommendations, in spite of several administration attempts to introduce appropriate legislation. Even so, the actual supply of physicians in 1960 did turn out to exceed by about 30,000 the supply projected a decade earlier. During the same period, however, physician requirements also appear to have risen beyond earlier expectations—partly because of unanticipated population growth and no doubt also because of upward revisions in the definition of "need." By the end of the 1950s, at any rate, there was renewed concern over the "doctor shortage," and new studies of the health manpower situation were launched.

In 1958, the Department of Health, Education and Welfare issued the so-called Bayne-Jones Report in which it was argued that a decline in the

M.D.-population ratio below its 1955 level[a] would be against the national interest, and that maintenance of that ratio would require an increase in annual graduations from medical schools from about 6,800 in 1955 to 8,700 in 1970.[b] This report was followed one year later by the report of the Surgeon General's Consultant Group on Medical Education [1959], widely known as the Bane Committee Report. The Bane Committee held that maintenance of the 1950 ratio of 148 physicians per 100,000 population—with physicians defined to include doctors of osteopathy (D.O.'s)—was a minimum essential to protect the health of the American people. On that basis, a minimum requirement of 299,000 physicians was forecast for 1970 and 330,000 for 1975. The corresponding supply figures, however, were estimated to be at most 296,000 and 318,000, respectively. The actual statistics for 1970 and current projection for 1975 provide an interesting contrast to these projections. As is seen in Table 2-1, the Bane Committee's targets have been or will be exceeded by comfortable margins.

Table 2-1. Physician Supply and Physician-Population Ratio, United States, 1970 and 1975

	1970	*1975*
All Physicians, Active and Inactive	348,000	N/A
per 100,000 Population	166	—
Professionally Active Physicians	323,000	367,000
per 100,000 Population	155	170

Physician and population data are for the United States, Puerto Rico and U.S. outlying areas. The population in 1975 is assumed to be 216 million.

Sources: Data for 1970—U.S. National Center for Health Statistics [1972], Table 81. Projected physician supply for 1975—U.S. Congress, House [1971], p. 943. Projected population for 1975—U.S. Department of Commerce, Bureau of the Census [1972], Series E, Table 1.

To cover the manpower deficits suggested by its forecasting model, the Bane Committee had called, once again, for direct federal intervention in the financing of medical education. Federal support, it was argued, should be aimed at increasing graduations from medical and osteopathic schools from about 7,400 in 1959 to 11,000 in 1975. Legislative response to this recommendation was slow in coming, but when it did come it was vigorous. In 1963, Congress passed the Health Professions Educational Assistance Act authorizing, for the first time, direct federal support for the *teaching* activities of medical schools. The act provided for a three-year program of matching grants for the construction, expansion or renovation of teaching facilities for medical doctors,

[a]In 1955, the number of active M.D.'s per 100,000 population in the United States and possessions was about 134. This figure excludes doctors of osteopathy.
[b]Actual graduations in 1970 were close to 8,500.

osteopaths, dentists, nurses, and other types of health personnel. In addition
to these institutional grants, the act also authorized the federal government
to grant loans and scholarships to students in medicine, osteopathy, and dentist-
ry. The program was modified and extended to fiscal years 1967–69 by the
Health Professions Educational Assistance Amendment of 1965, to fiscal
years 1970–71 by the Health Manpower Act of 1968, and to fiscal years 1972–74
by the Comprehensive Health Manpower Act of 1971. Together these acts triggered a substantial influx of federal funds into medical education.[c] As was shown
in Figure 1-1, this influx of funds had a commensurate impact on first-year
medical school enrollments. Although some growth in medical school capacity
was evident even prior to direct federal support, the presumption is justified
that growth since 1965 is directly attributable to federal intervention and
would probably not have been nearly as remarkable in the absence of that
support.[1]

Passage of the 1968 and 1971 legislation was undoubtedly much
encouraged by yet another series of health manpower studies published during
the late 1960s. Shortly after passage of the Medicare/Medicaid legislation in
1966, President Johnson established the National Advisory Commission on
Health Manpower to develop appropriate policy recommendations for improving the availability and utilization of health manpower. In its report [1967],
the commission concluded that the expected growth of the future physician
supply, combined with continued productivity increases of about 4 percent
per year, could certainly be expected to keep up with future population growth;
in fact, from the report it may be inferred that the commission implicitly forecast a *surplus* of 14,000 physicians by 1975.[2] Even so, to permit more substantial increases in per capita utilization of health services than were implicit
in that forecast, the commission recommended "a substantial expansion in the
capacity of existing medical schools" and "continued development of new
schools" [Vol. I, p. 19]. At about the same time the Bureau of Labor Statistics
(BLS) offered similar advice. According to the BLS forecast, total needs for
M.D.'s and D.O.'s in 1975 was expected to be 390,000; that is, 60,000 more
than had earlier been estimated by the Bane Committee. To meet this requirement solely with graduates from American medical schools, the BLS argued,
would require average annual graduations during 1966–75 to be 80 percent
higher than the 8,000 physicians actually graduated in 1966 [1967, p. 2].

In recent years, public statements on the physician shortage have
commonly made reference to a deficit of 50,000 physicians, a figure whose
origin and factual basis appears to have remained something of a mystery.[d]
Actually that figure is an estimate prepared by the U.S. Public Health Service

[c]It has been estimated that nearly $3 billion have been provided under the
program [Stewart and Siddayao, 1973, p. 65].

[d]See, for example, Blumberg [1971, p. 12] and Schwartz [1972, p. 60]. Both
writers profess puzzlement over the origin of the figure and suggest that it has no reference
date.

(PHS). As early as 1966, and only months after the publication of the BLS forecast, the PHS had predicted a requirement of between 400,000 and 425,000 physicians by 1975 [1967, p. 10]. Underlying the higher of these figures was the norm that, by 1975, the nation attain the highest physician-population ratio actually attained, in 1966, by the four major regions in the United States. The lower estimate was obtained by extrapolating the staffing pattern of comprehensive prepaid group practices—suggesting roughly 100 physicians per 100,000 population at risk—to the United States population as a whole [p. 9]. Using the latter of these norms, and taking account of estimated manpower shortages in psychiatry (15,000), in rural areas and urban ghettos (8,000), in hospital residencies and internships (10,000), and in teaching, research and administration (5,000) the PHS identified an overall shortage of 50,000 physicians as of 1969,[3] and that appears to be the origin of the widely cited and mysterious figure of 50,000. This estimate subsequently found its way into the *1970 Manpower Report of the President* [p. 175] and, by the way of an interview with Dr. Roger Egeberg, then Assistant Secretary of Health, into the well-known Carnegie Commission report on medical education [1970, p. 18]. The Carnegie Commission, in turn, seems to have used that estimate as a basis for its recommendation that "the number of medical school entrants or their equivalent should be increased from the 10,800 estimated for 1970–71 to about 15,300 by 1976 and to about 16,400 by 1978 [pp. 2 and 43]. In Figure 1–1 it can be seen that the first of these targets will virtually have been met by 1976.

During the congressional hearings on the Health Professions Educational Assistance Amendments of 1971—legislation subsequently passed as the Comprehensive Health Manpower Act of 1971—the Department of Health, Education and Welfare submitted a medical manpower forecast, reproduced in Figure 2–1. The supply forecast "based on students in the pipeline and current [1970] supply" reflects construction grants and institutional support already provided in legislation prior to 1971. The "additional physicians under the proposed administration program" are increments implied by the new funding under the legislation proposed in 1971. In Figure 2–1, it is further assumed that nonfederal support of medical education will be continued, but that there will be no increases in enrollment that do not reflect federal support. Finally, it is assumed that foreign medical schools will supply a total of 3,000 physicians a year to the United States pool.[e] The implications of this forecast are interesting. As can be seen in Figure 2–1, even in the absence of the Comprehensive Health Manpower Act of 1971, the estimated deficit of 50,000 physicians would have been eliminated by 1980. Since the act was actually passed in 1971, the shortage will be eliminated even sooner. Passage of the act, according

[e]The latter two assumptions are clearly conservative. First, under sufficient demand pressure it should be entirely feasible to increase medical school enrollments somewhat even in the absence of federal support; such increases were, after all, achieved even prior to federal intervention. Second, it was shown in Chapter One that the annual influx of foreign-trained physicians has exceeded 3,000 by a considerable margin in recent years.

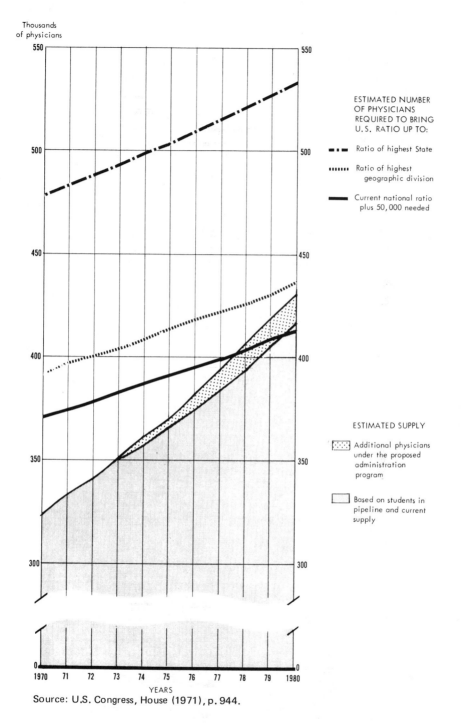

Thousands
of physicians

ESTIMATED NUMBER
OF PHYSICIANS
REQUIRED TO BRING
U.S. RATIO UP TO:

— ·— Ratio of highest State

▪▪▪▪▪▪ Ratio of highest
geographic division

▬▬ Current national ratio
plus 50,000 needed

ESTIMATED SUPPLY

Additional physicians
under the proposed
administration
program

Based on students in
pipeline and current
supply

YEARS

Source: U.S. Congress, House (1971), p. 944.

Figure 2-1. Projected Supply and Requirements of Physicians,
United States, 1970–80.

43

to the estimate, will eliminate even the projected shortage based on the highest physician-population ratio among the nine census regions (the Middle-Atlantic Region including New York, New Jersey and Pennsylvania). This rather sanguine conclusion, incidentally, is reiterated also in the *1972 Manpower Report of the President* [pp. 130-1].

The supply of 430,000 active physicians forecast under the Comprehensive Health Manpower Act for 1980 implies a ratio of about 190 physicians per 100,000 population.[4] As is apparent from Tables 2-2 and 2-3 below, this is a high ratio, not only by historical standards for the United States alone, but also on an international basis. Even excluding from the supply forecast any net additions of foreign-trained physicians during 1973-80, and allowing for the contingency that not all funds authorized under the 1971 legislation will actually be appropriated or spent, a ratio of at least 170 active physicians per 100,000 population can reasonably be projected for 1980. That ratio also is high by any standard.

Table 2-2. Number of Physicians Per 100,000 Population, United States, 1950-70[a]

Year	Active and Inactive	Active Only
1950	149	141
1955	150	141
1960	148	140
1965	153	145
1967	158	150
1970	166	155[b]

[a]Includes federal and nonfederal M.D.'s and D.O.'s in the U.S., Puerto Rico and all other U.S. outlying areas. The population figure includes all civilian and military personnel in the U.S., Puerto Rico and U.S. outlying areas.

[b]Estimated as the sum of 311,203 active M.D.'s and 0.85 X 14,300 active and inactive D.O.'s, and based on a population of 209.5 million.

Source: U.S. National Center for Health Statistics [1970, 1972], Table 81.

And yet it is a safe bet that, toward the end of this decade, there will come still another round of statements alerting the American public to an existing or impending "doctor shortage," each buttressed by one or the other manpower projection, and each issued along with urgent pleas for an expansion of medical school capacity. Indeed, there is no need to wait until the end of the decade. A suitable forecast of manpower "needs" is already built into the Public Health Service projections of 1971; in Figure 2-1 this forecast is represented by the line labeled "Ratio of Highest State" (New York), implying a normative ratio of about 237 physicians per 100,000 population by 1980 under most recent population projections. Nor need one wait for statements alerting us to the implied physician shortage. In an article published in August 1973 entitled "Yes, There is a Doctor Shortage," Professor Alex Gerber of the University of Southern California Medical School asserts:

Table 2-3. International Comparison of Reported Physician-Population Ratios, 1969 (number of physicians per 100,000 population)

North America		Eastern Europe	
Canada	141	Bulgaria	183*
United States[a]	155	Czechoslovakia	145
		Hungary	191*
Western Europe		Poland	146
Austria	182*	Romania	129
Belgium	155	Yugoslavia	95
Denmark	145		
Finland	95	Other	
France	130	Australia	118
Fed. Rep. of Germany	170*	Israel[b]	245*
Netherlands	122	Japan	111
Norway	141	New Zealand	115
Sweden	130	U.S.S.R.	231*
Switzerland	138		
United Kingdom:			
England & Wales	121		
Northern Ireland	131		
Scotland	133		

[a]This ratio includes only professionally active physicians. It is not clear whether figures for the other nations have been similarly adjusted.

[b]Includes physicians who are registered in Israel but do not reside or practice there.

*Denotes nations reporting a higher physician-population ratio than was reported by the United States.

Source: World Health Organization [1972], Table 2.1.

> the preponderance of evidence suggests to me that this country suffers from both a maldistribution and a[n aggregate] shortage of physicians. . . . I believe that in the long run this shortage can only be remedied by a federal commitment to fund a huge medical school expansion program. . . . *Such a policy calls for a doubling of our present medical school facilities.* [1973a, pp. 13 and 60; emphasis added.]

It is not altogether clear from the statement what Professor Gerber means by a "doubling of our present medical school facilities." One interpretation might be that he proposes to double the size of the entering class. In 1973, that figure stood at about 14,400 if one includes in it first-year enrollments in osteopathic schools. A more conservative interpretation would be that he proposes a doubling of total enrollments, or, equivalently, of the average class size in 1973. Including once again enrollments in osteopathic schools, that figure was about 13,460.[5] If one assumes that this entire enrollment figure is subject to an attrition rate of about 5 percent, then Gerber's *desideratum* would appear to be a long-run annual graduating class of about 25,600 physicians.

The approximate long-run implications of Professor Gerber's proposal on the physician-population ratio in this country are suggested by

Figure 2-2. In that diagram the lower of the two curves represents the probable physician-population ratio generated by currently projected graduations from American medical and osteopathic schools. This projection includes foreign-trained physicians already practicing in the United States by the end of 1970. However, it excludes the inflow of foreign medical graduates from 1971 onward, primarily because it is anybody's guess what the future inflow of these physicians into the United States will be. The base line time series on graduations from American medical and osteopathic schools was developed by the Department of Health, Education and Welfare and appears to be the best and most plausible projection currently available.[6] The projection calls for a gradual increase of annual graduations from about 10,400 in 1973 to 16,800 by 1990.

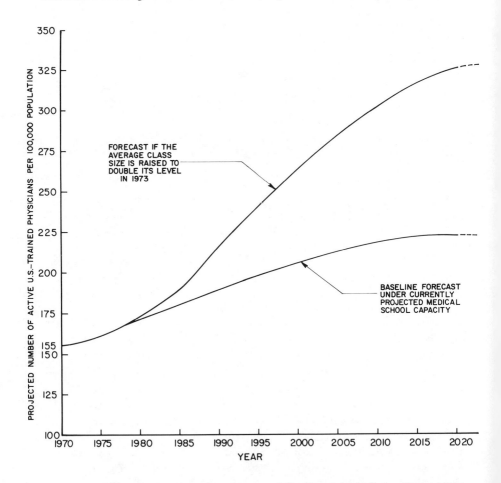

Figure 2-2.   Long-Run Impact of Medical School Expansion on the Supply of Active U.S.–Trained Physicians, United States, 1970-2020

The higher of the two curves is based on the assumption that the target level of graduations proposed by Professor Gerber is reached by 1988. It is assumed that there will be a combination of massive new construction and of expansion in the class size of already established medical schools. In his supply projections for physicians in the United States, Blumberg [1971, p. 27] has suggested that annual rates of increase in entering-class size can vary from 400 to 1,300. Between 1971–72, the entering-class size of American medical schools actually increased by 1,365 [*Journal of the American Medical Association*, November 19, 1973, p. 985]. In postulating the time path for annual graduations under the Gerber proposal, we have assumed that some of the momentum of recent medical school expansion will be maintained, and that annual increases in the size of the entering class vary between 500 and 1,300 places. Specifically, the following additions to the annual graduating classes have been postulated: 1978–82—each year 500 more graduations than in the previous year; 1983–84— each year 1,000 more graduations than in the previous year; 1985–87—each year 1,250 more graduations than in the previous year; and 1988—924 more graduations than in the previous year. This brings the total number of graduations to 25,600 by 1988. It is assumed that thereafter annual graduations will remain at that level. This series of graduations, incidentally, also excludes the inflow of foreign-trained medical graduates from 1971 onward. The upper curve in Figure 2–2 therefore also underestimates the supply that could be expected under the proposed regime.

The supply projections in Figure 2–2 are based, once again, on the forecasting framework developed in Appendix A. Further particulars underlying the forecast are presented in Table A–7. The projections necessarily involve a number of assumptions that may or may not be borne out by future events; they are therefore to be viewed as rough indicators only. Since the projections are, if anything, underestimates of likely future supply conditions, however, they do point up sharply the normative proposition Professor Gerber seems to be offering. If Professor Gerber is serious, and if we have interpreted him correctly, he appears to be advocating a ratio in excess of 215 active U.S.-trained physicians per 100,000 population by 1990, and in excess of 262 by the year 2000. At currently projected population growth, the peak ratio one should ultimately expect to follow from this scheme would be in excess of 325 U.S.-trained physicians per 100,000 population, for the physician-population ratio continues to rise after the year 2000. (A ratio of 300 would be reached by the year 2010.)

These numbers, it bears repeating, are conservative. They exclude the annual inflow of foreign-trained physicians from 1971 onwards, an inflow that actually amounted to about 13,000 physicians in 1971–72 alone. Although it may be doubted that the immigration of foreign medical graduates can continue at this high a rate in the future, it can also be doubted that this flow will become trivial in the foreseeable future (unless, of course, Congress decides to restrict that flow through changes in the immigration laws). That Professor Gerber *is* serious, incidentally, and that we have indeed interpreted him correctly (perhaps conservatively), seems confirmed by his plaintive question: "If Russia can graduate 30,000 doctors annually, why can't we?"[f] [Gerber 1973b, p. 7].

Cynics may associate Professor Gerber with the "medical education complex" and attribute to his proposal roughly the same ethical content as is commonly attributed to concern by aerospace engineers over an alleged "national security gap" and to the attendant calls for higher defense budgets. Careful reading of Gerber's writings, however, persuades one that he ought not to be so dismissed; his proposal does not strike one as self-serving.[7] Attainment of a physician-population ratio of 250 or even 300 physicians per 100,000 population would certainly make medical services more readily available to some segments of the population—perhaps, though not necessarily, even to those now under served. This is the apparent objective of Gerber's proposal. What Gerber and others arguing in this vein seem to overlook is that implementation of such a proposal would also obligate society to furnish between 250 to 300 *physician incomes* per 100,000 population. And, given the characteristics of the medical care market, the average level of these incomes would undoubtedly remain somewhere near the top of the national income scale.[g] Suppose, for example, that the average professionally active physician will continue to require a *net* income (after professional expenses) of at least $45,000 in equivalent 1973 dollars, a figure that is not unrealistic in the light of recent statistics on physician incomes. On this assumption the annual cost simply of maintaining 250 to 300 physicians per 100,000 population at their customary station in life would amount to $113 to $135 for every man, woman and child in that population, or to $450 to $540 for the average family of four.[h] These figures do not even cover the physician's professional expenses (including his automobile), which tend

[f]In answer to Professor Gerber's question, Russian physicians are salaried and their salaries tend to be relatively modest. To sustain 231 physicians per 100,000 population (the physician-population ratio in the Soviet Union) therefore requires a much smaller transfer of goods and services from society at large to physicians as a group than would be the case under the United States health system. Quite aside from this transfer, however, it is not obvious why the manpower allocation chosen by Russian planners (or, for that matter, any other decision made by them) should be taken as an appropriate standard for the United States. The use of talented manpower in any particular activity has opportunity costs and one has no assurance that Russian planners have taken these costs properly into account— that is, that they invariably plan *efficiently*.

[g]According to statistics published by the American Medical Association [1973, p. 66] the average net income of medical practitioners was $39,727 in 1969 and $41,789 in 1970. It may be argued that a vastly increased pool of physician manpower will automatically exert downward pressure on physician fees and incomes. As was noted in Chapter One, however, the market for physician services is not a truly competitive one and physicians are likely to maintain their favorable income position even under conditions of excess supply.

[h]The argument advanced above should not be construed as an implicit criticism of the income level enjoyed by the average American physician. American physicians work hard and may justly feel entitled to the incomes they receive. The argument does, however,

to average about 60 percent of net income [American Medical Association 1973, pp. 71–2] , and at least some of which would not have to be incurred at all if the physician ceased to practice.[i]

These figures raise two important questions: First, even if one assumed that the health services delivered by these 250 to 300 physicians per 100,000 population were absolutely necessary, it can be asked whether they could not be produced more cheaply under a less physician-intensive delivery mode. In addition, it may also be asked whether all the services that would be delivered under the regime proposed by Professor Gerber would indeed be absolutely necessary. At any rate, a nation already devoting over 7 percent of its gross national product to health services and viewing the ever-rising cost of health maintenance as one of its many crises surely ought to think twice before rushing headlong into the expansion program Gerber proposes.

The preceding illustration may be criticized for overlooking the fact that not all professionally active physicians render patient care. Somers and Somers, for example, have pointed out that during the postwar years "a declining proportion of doctors has been engaged in patient care" and that "these trends . . . are likely to continue in the years ahead" [1961, p. 121] . To illustrate this point, the authors draw attention to the fact that between 1931 and 1957 the percentage of (active and inactive) physicians engaged in private practice dropped from 85.9 to 68.8, and that the percentage active in teaching, research, public health and in the federal government increased from 4.1 to 10.5. In their analysis of expenditures on physician services during the postwar period, Fuchs and Kramer make the same point. According to their data, the percentage of professionally *active* physicians actually engaged in patient care dropped from 91.5 in 1949 to 85.5 in 1967 [1972, p. 16] . On the strength of these data, it may be suggested that the physician-population ratios in Figure 2–2 overstate the true availability of physician services in future years. This is an important caveat, but not one to blunt the thrust of the argument developed here.

First, it is not clear that the trends perceived during the 1950s and 1960s will actually persist in future years. According to recent statistics furnished by the American Medical Association, the number of active M.D.'s involved in direct patient care as their *primary activity* actually increased slightly during the period 1968–72, as may be seen from Table 2–4. Whether that trend should

---

raise the question whether under the regime proposed by Professor Gerber—a regime under which physician time would quite probably be used inefficiently—consumers of physician services would receive their money's worth.

[i]It is recognized that not all of a physician's professional expenses would be eliminated were he to withdraw from medical practice. Some of his aides, for example, might have to be transferred to lend greater support to the remaining pool of medical manpower. Also, a portion of the gross transfer to physicians is indirectly returned to the general fund through taxes, although consumers are not likely to appreciate this fact.

Table 2-4.   Percentage Distribution of Professionally Active Federal and Nonfederal M.D.'s, by Activity, 1969-1972

Activity	1969	1970	1971	1972
Patient Care[a]				
Office-Based	62.1	61.9	62.0	62.7
Hospital-Based	27.3	27.7	28.1	28.3
	89.4	89.6	90.1	91.1
Non-Patient Care				
Medical Teaching	1.7	1.8	1.8	1.8
Administration	4.0	3.9	3.8	3.4
Research	4.1	3.8	3.4	2.9
Other	0.8	0.9	0.9	0.8
	10.6	10.4	9.9	8.9
Total Active M.D.'s				
(in thousands)	(303.0)	(310.8)	(318.7)	(320.9)
	100%	100%	100%	100%

[a]Physicians reporting the direct delivery of patient care as their *primary activity*.

Sources: Calculated from data in the following publications by the American Medical Association: Haug and Roback [1970], Vol. I, table A; American Medical Association [1971], p. 1; [1972], p. 1; [1973], p. 1.

be extrapolated into the future is, of course, not clear either. It may be suggested, for example, that physicians in future years might virtually be driven into administrative or research positions, should the available supply of physicians exceed the absorptive capacity of the medical care market in culturally attractive locations. If the public sector is accommodating in this respect—that is, if it offers physicians for administrative or research services a remuneration competitive with the income that could be earned by practicing medicine in relatively less attractive locations—then an increasing penchant for nonpatient-care activities could well be kindled in physicians. But in that case the average annual per capita cost of maintaining, say, 250 to 300 "professionally active" physicians per 100,000 population at their customary station in life would still remain somewhere in the neighborhood of the figures suggested earlier. The only difference would be that society would not receive in return a commensurate flow of patient-care; it would purchase administrative and research services instead.

This turn of events, however, should lead one to wonder whether the administrative and research services so acquired have, in fact, been obtained as cheaply as they could have been had from nonmedical personnel (for example, from personnel trained in health administration or natural scientists, either of whom tend to work at lower salaries). After all, the extent to which the public sector competes with the private market for physician manpower is a policy decision surely as much as is public support of medical schools. It is really part and parcel of a comprehensive health manpower policy and ought to be consistent with the latter.

From the congressional hearings prior to passage of the Comprehensive Health Manpower Act of 1971 one notes that the potential for overshoot made graphic in Figure 2-2 is actually not unappreciated by health manpower policymakers, although an open voicing of that concern is clearly viewed as risky. The following exchange between Congressman Paul G. Rogers (then Chairman of the House Subcommittee on Health and Environment) and Dr. Kenneth M. Endicott (then Director of the Bureau of Health Manpower Education in the Department of Health, Education and Welfare) is illuminating.[8]

> *Dr. Endicott.* Well, sir, the experience over the past several decades would suggest that no matter how hard you run you lose ground. The number of physicians per capita has increased substantially and, yet, at this time we recognize generally, I think, a greater shortage than we had before. The thing which has, I think, concerned us in attempting to plan for the future is a question not of reaching adequacy, but perhaps overshooting in view of the very costly business of building and operating medical schools.
>
> *Mr. Rogers.* Now, let me understand. You say you are afraid of overshooting rather than reaching adequacy?
>
> *Dr. Endicott.* Well, this has been a concern which has been expressed to me on a number of occasions by economists and so on. But—
>
> *Mr. Rogers.* Well now, this concerns me.
>
> *Dr. Endicott.* It is concerning me too.
>
> *Mr. Rogers.* If that is the philosophy that is prevailing in the department—
>
> *Dr. Endicott.* No, sir.

Dr. Endicott, it appears, was expressing an entirely legitimate concern.

II. HEALTH MANPOWER FORECASTING AND THE ESCALATION OF PHYSICIAN "REQUIREMENTS"

The objective of the preceding survey has been to indicate a certain pattern underlying the dynamics of health manpower planning. If the time path of the actual physician supply in past years is compared with requirements projected earlier for those years, it will be noted that actual supply typically has come close to or even exceeded projected requirements. Oddly enough, this fortunate turn of events has never been a source of satisfaction, for in the meantime the definition of requirements has been changed and new manpower forecasts have been issued, each pointing either to an existing or impending physician shortage. The pattern seems to conform to the motto *plus ça change, plus c'est la même chose.* The problem of the "doctor shortage" appears to be one incapable of solution.

A part of the historical pattern can, of course, be explained by the introduction in the late 1960s of the Medicare and Medicaid programs, a development that could probably not have been foreseen in the political climate of the 1950s (when the Bane Committee Report was issued). In response to increases in health care utilization under these programs, some upward revision in estimated manpower requirements was clearly in order. There is no reason to assume, however, that taking account of this legislation, or even of future legislation in this area, will in itself eliminate further escalation in estimated physician requirements. Such escalation appears to be guaranteed by the methodology typically employed in health manpower forecasting.

Although there has been some variation in the models underlying the forecasts cited above, it is probably fair to say that most of these models have been patterned closely on the general forecasting equation

$$M_t = R_t P_t \tag{2-1}$$

where P_t denotes the size of the population to be served at time t, M_t is the required number of physicians at time t, and R_t is some normative physician-population ratio, usually held constant over time. As noted in the previous section, the *minimum* acceptable value of R has usually been the physician-population ratio actually observed during the year of forecast; the *desirable* norm has typically been the highest ratio observed among the states or the major geographic regions. This definition of future physician requirements is somewhat unfortunate, for it tends to obscure the fact that the requirement of physicians is merely a derivative of a requirement of "physician services," more precisely defined as "the kind of medical services normally provided by physicians' practices, including services rendered by physicians to inpatients."[j]

To make the relationship between "physician services" and "physician manpower" required more explicit, it is useful to express the physician-population ratio in equation (2-1) as

$$R_t = \left(\frac{D_t}{Q_t}\right) \tag{2-2}$$

where D_t denotes the projected per-capita utilization of physician services at time t, and Q_t the average annual number of physician services produced per physician in year t.[k] Variable Q_t may be referred to as *average annual physician*

---

[j]This definition should be thought to include any medical service produced on the premises or under the auspices of the physician's practice, whether or not the physician himself produced these services.

[k]Of the manpower forecasts cited earlier, only those produced by Rashi Fein (1967), by Jones, Struve and Stefani (1967), and Monsma (1969) are based on separate

productivity and is obviously a function of both the average *hourly physician productivity* and of the number of hours physicians work per year. The tendency of conventional health manpower forecasts toward escalation in manpower requirements appears to originate in both the definition and measurement of D_t and in the assumptions and policy recommendations made concerning the productivity variable, Q_t.

The Definition of Need

In Chapter One a distinction was made between "need" and "effective demand," the latter being defined as "need as perceived by the consumer and backed up by an ability and willingness to pay." This distinction is not always made clear in the literature and perhaps not fully appreciated, for the two concepts are frequently and quite illegitimately used as synonyms.

Economic analyses of the physician shortage are typically based on the concept of effective demand.[9] Use of this concept has several advantages. First, the effective demand for any good or service is an objectively determined function of some set of socioeconomic and demographic variables, a function that can be estimated empirically, at least in principle. Second, if this demand function is known, it may be viewed as an indication of the value society collectively places on the consumption of the good or service in question. This index of value, however, reflects the prevailing distribution of purchasing power as much as or more than the consumers' perception of need. While the ethical precepts underlying this valuation principle are generally accepted for most ordinary commodities, the modern view holds them to be inapplicable to health services, whose consumption has come to be viewed as a basic human right rather than a privilege. For this reason most public health specialists have based their manpower forecasts on the concept of need. This is probably as it should be, at least as long as the distribution of purchasing power in this country remains as uneven as it is today.

Unfortunately the concept of medical need is highly subjective, an attribute that is necessarily transferred to any health manpower forecast based on that concept. First, it is not clear whether the need for medical care should reflect the very subjective perception of consumers or the more objective perception of medical practitioners, who presumably know better what the consumer's medical needs may be. Most manpower forecasts, one gathers, have opted for the latter conception of need. But that definition also remains rather subjective, for one would expect even medical experts to develop their notions of medical need partly with reference to the socioeconomic and cultural context in which they happen to operate. It is interesting to observe, for example, that the previously cited Professor Gerber, although offering many other compelling arguments in support of his position, also raises the rhetorical question:

---

projections of D_t and Q_t. Most forecasts have treated R_t as a constant, implying either that D_t and Q_t also are constant over time or that they change at the same rate.

> Where will we find the plastic surgeons to handle the swelling tide
> of American women who are having their bosoms augmented and
> their faces dewrinkled upon reaching age 50? There are dozens of
> similar imponderables that make hazarding of predictions about
> future physician *requirements* a matter of Byzantine complexity
> [1973a, p. 14; emphasis added].

It is surely a matter of personal judgment whether a desire for augmented bos-
oms constitutes a requirement to be provided for under a public health manpower policy, or whether the demand and supply of face dewrinklers and bosom
augmenters can be safely entrusted to the workings of private market forces.
Without settling the question here it may merely be observed that the concept
of medical need seems to be a rather elastic one.

As was stated earlier, the practical solution to the problem of defining medical need has usually been to take the highest prevailing physician-
population ratio observed among states or regions as the culturally relevant
standard. This method of defining physician "requirements" runs through
virtually the entire historical series of health-manpower forecasts, except those
prepared by Fein [1967] and Monsma [1969]. Probably the most explicit
formation of this approach is found in Edward Yost's *The U.S. Health Industry:
The Costs of Acceptable Medical Care by 1975* [1969]. Yost preambles his
forecast with the question: "What is the cost of comprehensive health service
for all U.S. citizens equal to that currently supplied to middle-class geographic
areas?" [p. 100]. He then proceeds to answer that question by way of the basic
need equation:

$$Y = X + \Delta X \tag{2-3}$$

where Y is the ratio of physicians, or dentists, or nurses, or hospital beds, to the
population of Westchester County, New York (home of many executives and
professionals working in New York City); X is the corresponding ratio for the
United States as a whole; and Δ is the change in X required to bring the United
States up to Westchester County standards [pp. 100–1]. From the language of
Yost's analysis it appears that he considers ΔX as the difference in the level of
medical services available to families in Westchester County and in the United
States as a whole [p. 103]. There is also the clear implication that the health-
care consumption pattern in Westchester County furnishes an appropriate
national standard. Using equation (2–3), Yost estimates that a national aggregate
of 492,000 physicians (or 398,520 active physicians providing patient care)
would be required by 1975 to offer the nation as a whole the kinds of physician
services enjoyed in 1967 by middle-class American families. To achieve this target
within the eight-year period from 1967 (the year of his forecast) to 1975, he
suggests, would require 142 additional medical schools each producing the

national average of 87 graduates per school. It would be a program requiring a nonrecurring outlay of $11 billion in 1970 dollars and an additional $0.7 billion per year in recurring costs [p. 103]. Incidentally, there is no mention in his analysis that such a program, even if it were physically or fiscally feasible, might be the height of folly, as should become obvious upon contemplation of the long-run implications of such a program. (In this connection, see once again Figure 2-2.)

It is clear that the popular definition of acceptable health man-power endowments virtually guarantees one continued escalation in estimated future physician requirements, unless, of course, it could be assumed that increases in the aggregate supply of physicians will, over time, eliminate any interstate or interregional differences in physician endowments. As was argued at length in Chapter One, this assumption is hardly warranted in a country in which physicians are free to locate in accordance with their personal prefer-ences and in a market context in which suppliers exercise considerable control over the demand for their services and the fees that can be charged for them. As long as the physician endowment of the most favored state or region is taken as the relevant index of medical need, then, just so long will there be reports of a doctor shortage, even at the aggregate level. These reports will be all the more believable if the distribution of physicians is sufficiently uneven to leave truly acute shortages of medical personnel in at least some areas, or if there are acute shortages in one or the other particular specialty.

Assumptions Concerning Physician Productivity

Quite aside from the potential to exaggerate per capita require-ments of medical *services*, the use of physician-population ratios in highly endowed regions as national standards can lead to problems of yet another sort. It is obvious from the definition of R_t in equation 2-2 that a state or region may have a relatively high physician-population ratio either because its residents enjoy a relatively high per capita utilization of physician services (D) or because the average annual output per physician (Q) is relatively low, or because of a combination of both factors. In this connection the data in Tables 2-5 and 2-6 are illuminating. Table 2-5 presents, for three of the nine United States Census Divisions, data on relative physician-population ratios, data on the organization of and output from private medical practices, data on per capita utilization of physician services, and on physician fees and incomes. As far as relative endow-ment with medical manpower is concerned, the three Census Divisions in Table 2-5 represent the most highly endowed, a moderately well endowed, and the most poorly endowed divisions in the United States. Table 2-6 shows data similar to those exhibited in Table 2-5 except that the "regions" are metropolitan areas of different sizes. This table is added to corroborate the data in Table 2-5.

The pattern exhibited by Tables 2-5 and 2-6 is revealing. In regions or locations with relatively high physician-population ratios, the average physi-

Table 2-5. **Regional Differences in Certain Health-Care Statistics, United States, 1969-70 (figures in parentheses are indexes with New England set to 1.0)**

		Census Divisions		
	Year	*New England*	*East-North Central*	*East-South Central*
1. Number of Active M.D.'s involved in Patient Care as their Primary Activity, per 100,000 population	1970	161 (1.00)	115 (0.71)	95 (0.59)
2. Average Annual Number of Hours Worked per M.D.:[a]				
a) Total practice hours	1969	2,504	2,495	2,568
b) Hours of direct patient care	1969	2,128	2,151	2,303
3. Average Annual Number of Patient Visits per M.D.:				
a) Total patient visits	1969	4,808 (1.00)	6,611 (1.38)	8,408 (1.75)
b) Office visits only	1969	3,384 (1.00)	4,799 (1.42)	6,052 (1.79)
4. Total Visits per Hour[b]				
a) Total visits per practice hour	1969	1.92	2.65	3.27
b) Total visits per hour of patient care	1969	2.25	3.07	3.65
5. Average Number of Auxiliary Personnel Employed per Physician	1967	1.3	1.8	2.1
6. Percentage of Physicians in Group Practice	1969	9.3%	17.4%	19.4%
7. Average Fee for a Routine Follow-Up Office Visit:	1970			
a) General Practice		$6.79	$6.29	$5.21
b) Internal Medicine		9.40	8.05	7.20
c) Pediatrics		7.53	6.94	5.40
d) General Surgery		9.76	7.76	6.85
e) Obstetrics/Gynecology		9.77	9.32	7.60
8. Average Net Income (all specialties)	1970	$38,019.00	$47,000.00	$41,963.00
9. Reported Number of Physician-Patient Visits per Capita:				
a) Based on Survey of Physicians	1969			
−total patient visits		7.7	7.6	8.0
−office visits only		5.4	5.5	5.8
b) Based on Household Surveys[c]	1970	4.4	4.0	4.1
10. Infant Mortality Rate[d]	1968			
a) White		19.2	19.4	20.9
b) Nonwhite		31.8	35.4	40.5

Table 2-5 continued

	Year	Census Divisions		
		New England	*East-North Central*	*East-South Central*
11. Socioeconomic Indicators	1970			
a) Personal Per Capita Income		$4,469.00	$4,306.00	$3,146.00
b) Percentage of Population with Completion of:				
—no school years		1.5%	1.1%	2.5%
—less than 4 school years		3.9	4.0	12.5
—less than 6 school years		8.9	8.6	22.2
c) Percentage of All-Year-Round Housing That Has:	1970			
—no piped water		0.6	1.3	10.1
—no flush toilet		1.3	2.4	14.9
—no bathtub or shower		2.6	3.3	16.2
—more than 1 person/room		6.2	7.2	11.2

[a]Reported average number of hours worked per week, times reported average number of weeks worked per year.

[b]Line 3a divided by line 2a or 2b.

[c]These figures are not for the Census Divisions proper, but for the Northeastern, North-Central, and Southern Census Regions, and include only office visits.

[d]Number of deaths of infants under 1 year of age per 1,000 live births.

Sources: Lines 1 to 4, 8 and 9a calculated from raw data in Table C-1; line 5 calculated from *Medical Economics, Inc., Continuing Survey, 1967*; line 6 from Todd and McNamara [1971]; lines 7a to 7e from American Medical Association [1972], Table 43; line 9b from *United States Statistical Abstract 1971*, Table 93; line 10 from *United States Statistical Abstract 1972*, Table 82; line 11a from ibid., Table 519; line 11b from U.S. Department of Commerce, Bureau of the Census [1972b], Table 156; line 11c from U.S. Department of Commerce, Bureau of the Census [1971a], Tables 3 and 4.

cian appears to work relatively fewer weeks per year and appears to see relatively fewer patients per week, so that his value for Q is relatively low. The lower value of Q, however, does not reflect itself fully in physician income, for it is offset to a large extent by higher fees per patient visit. (As was argued in Chapter One, this is precisely what one would expect on the basis of theory alone.) Physicians in relatively poor regions do not appear to rely more heavily on support from hospital facilities than do their colleagues in more highly endowed regions; instead, physicians in the poorer regions tend to employ relatively more support personnel in their practices and tend to have a higher preference for group-medical practices (a setting sometimes thought to enhance the productivity of all types of health manpower).[1] Finally, it would appear from the data in Table 2-5 that the total number of patient visits per member of the resident population—one possible proxy for variable D in equation (2-2) above—is roughly the same in all three Census Divisions. One arrives at this con-

[1]In this connection, however, see also the discussion on group medical practices in Chapter Four.

Table 2-6   Physician-Population Ratios, Patient Loads, and Medical
Fees by Size of County, United States, 1970

Demographic County Classification[a]	Physician-Population Ratio[b]	Weekly Patient Visits		Fee for an Initial Office Visit
		Total	Office	
Nonmetropolitan:				
10,000–24,999	51	223	167	$ 7.15
25,000–49,999	64	217	164	7.13
50,000 or more	87	192	153	7.96
Metropolitan:				
50,000–499,999	107	194	150	8.65
500,000–999,999	141	167	140	9.33
1,000,000–4,999,999	150	138	114	9.00
5,000,000 or more	191	124	109	10.34

[a]Numbers refer to inhabitants.
[b]Number of nonfederal physicians in patient care per 100,000 resident population as of December 31, 1970.
Source: American Medical Association [1972], tables 55, 56 and 58.

clusion whether one bases it on visits as reported by physicians or on visits as reported by patients themselves. The conclusion is consistent also with a study of American pediatricians by Yankauer et al., in which it was found that southern pediatricians delegate substantially more routine medical and clerical tasks to auxiliary personnel than do pediatricians in the New York metropolitan region [1970, p. 36]. The analysis also revealed that pediatricians in the South tend to put in an average of 40 practice hours per week, compared to an average of 28.5 hours spent by their counterparts in New York.

One must hasten to add that "patient visits" are not a homogeneous commodity and that the data in the tables reflect more than meets the eye. On some health indexes—for example, the infant mortality rate—the New England and East North Central states fare better than the East South Central states. Thus, the argument could be made that the "quality" of care Southern physicians dispense per patient visit is inferior to that dispensed by their Northern colleagues. But here also great care must be exercised in the interpretation of the data, lest effects properly attributable to a superior socioeconomic environment be inadvertently credited to physicians. As is shown in lines 11–12 of Table 2–5, levels of education, of income, and particularly of housing conditions in the South are inferior to those found in the North. These factors may also be reflected in morbidity and mortality rates.

Proper measurement of the true value (health status) added by medical personnel in the various regions of the United States requires a rather more penetrating analysis than is intended here. Tables 2–5 and 2–6 have been presented mainly to raise the question: Just what is being proposed when the physician-population ratio of the most richly endowed region or state is proffered as the culturally relevant standard of physician density for the nation as a whole? Is it proposed that all Americans should enjoy the level of health care enjoyed by residents of the most highly endowed region? Or is it suggested that the comportment of physicians in the most highly endowed region be a standard for all American physicians? If the latter—and by proceeding in terms of physician-population ratios one inevitably offers that prescription—then Tables 2-5 and 2-6 warrant at least the suspicion that by aiming for the highest prevailing physician-population ratio one may inadvertently accept inefficiently organized and unnecessarily costly medical practice as a national standard. And that inefficiency receives official blessing if public health manpower policy responds passively though conscientiously to whatever dire predictions emerge from this forecasting methodology.

Few of the health manpower forecasts cited in this chapter have given the role of physician productivity—that is, the time path of variable Q_t in equation (2-2)—the attention it deserves. To be sure, passing reference to the desirability of greater efficiency in health care production was made in virtually all of the reports, and some of them even included recommendations to that effect. These recommendations, however, were typically vague and perfunctory. One has the impression that they were offered in roughly the same spirit and with roughly the same hope of success as are calls for greater honesty in government or for greater public decency. Furthermore, one senses in these reports the latent fear that any major improvement in the efficiency of health care production will inevitably be purchased at the price of lower quality.

The sensitivity of future physician requirements to assumptions about physician productivity can be made visible if equation (2-2) is rewritten as:

$$R_t = \left(\frac{D_o}{Q_o}\right) e^{-\sum_{s=1}^{s=t} (q_s - d_s)} \tag{2-4}$$

where q_s denotes the percentage increase in Q over the period from $t - 1$ to t; d_s is the growth of D similarly defined; and D_o/Q_o is the normative physician-population ratio for the year in which the forecast is made. (As noted earlier, this is typically the highest ratio observed in any of the nation's states or regions.) If one assumes, for the sake of illustration, that the growth rates q_s and d_s remain constant at levels q and d over the entire forecast horizon, then (2-4) becomes

$$R_t = \left(\frac{D_o}{Q_o}\right) e^{-(q-d)t} \tag{2-5}$$

and R_t can be plotted on the difference $(q - d)$ as is done in Figure 2-3.

In Figure 2-3, the base-year physician-population ratio (D_o/Q_o) is taken to be 185 active physicians per 100,000 population, a ratio broadly representative of some of the better-endowed New England states in 1970. The

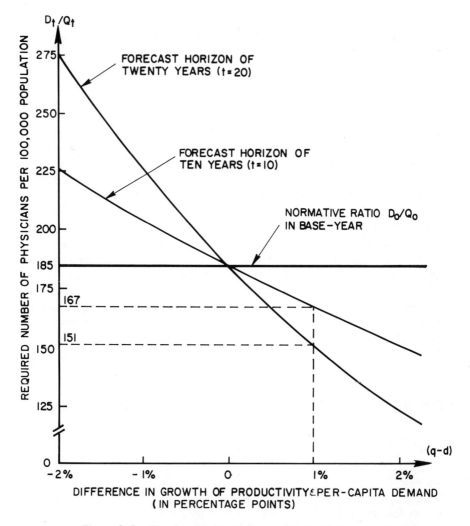

Figure 2-3. The Sensitivity of Future Physician Requirements to Growth in Physician Productivity

steeper of the two curves represents a forecast horizon of 20 years (1990), and the flatter a horizon of 10 years (1980). The slopes of the curves indicate the sensitivity of predicted physician requirements to assumptions about the relative values of q and d.

If q equalled d—an assumption often incorporated into health man-power forecasts—then the required M.D.-population ratio would, of course, remain at 185 per 100,000 during the entire forecast horizon. On the other hand, if in 1970 a set of policies could have been implemented such that average annual growth in physician productivity during the following two decades were one percentage point higher than the annual growth in the per capita utilization of physician services, then the required ratio at the end of the forecast horizon would have been only 151 physicians per 100,000 population. Relative to a forecast based on maintenance of the base-year ratio of 185 per 100,000 and for a population of roughly 250 million in 1990, this turn of events would have lead to a reduction of about 85,000 in the number of M.D.'s that would otherwise have been "required." The corresponding number for 1980, based on a projected population of 225 million, is 40,500. These figures must surely strike one as significant, especially if held up against the annual number of medical graduates (between 15,000 and 16,000) likely to be produced during the next several decades.

One may ask whether this illustration is at all empirically relevant, given the values d and q tend to take on in the real world. It may therefore be illuminating to explore what their values have been during the past two decades or so, and to speculate about their probable values in the future. The historical review is presented in Chapter Three, where an attempt is also made to identify probable sources of past growth in physician productivity. The potential for future productivity growth is assessed in Chapter Four.

NOTES

1. For a more extended review of health manpower forecasts to 1967, see Butter [1967].
2. In this connection, see Hansen [1970].
3. These details were furnished in testimony before the House Subcommittee on Public Health and Environment. See U.S. Congress, House [1971], Part 2, pp. 941–2.
4. This estimate is based on Series E of the current population projections prepared by the U.S. Bureau of the Census [1972a], Table 1, p. 12. The population figure is roughly 225 million.
5. Average class size in 1973 is the sum of the entering classes in academic years 1970–71 through 1973–74, divided by four. According to data conveyed to the author in private communication by the Division of Manpower Intelligence, Health Resources Administration, Department of Health, Education and Welfare, the enrollment figures were: 1970–71: 11,348 M.D.'s and 623 D.O.'s; 1971–72: 12,375 M.D.'s and 670 D.O.'s; 1972–73: 13,390 M.D.'s and 767 D.O.'s; 1973–74: 13,857 M.D.'s and 823 D.O.'s.
6. This projection was conveyed to the author in private communication by the Division of Manpower Intelligence, Bureau of Health Resources Development, Health Resources Administration, Department of Health, Education and Welfare.

7. In this connection, see also Gerber [1967].
8. Testimony before the House Subcommittee on Public Health and Environment. See U.S. Congress, House [1971], pp. 296–7.
9. See Fein [1967], Hansen [1964], Jones, Struve and Stefani [1967], and Rayack [1964].

Chapter Three

Recent Trends in Physician Productivity

Fundamental to any discussion of physician productivity is an operational definition of that term. On the surface, the definition of manpower productivity is straightforward enough: the average[a] productivity of any type of manpower is simply the output produced by one unit of that manpower during a given period. In the context of medical practice, however, the definition of output raises a number of conceptual problems. The first section of this chapter is addressed to these conceptual problems. In the second section the magnitude and potential sources of past growth in physician productivity are briefly explored.

I. PHYSICIAN PRODUCTIVITY: SOME CONCEPTUAL ISSUES

Alternative Definitions of Physician Output

It is sometimes held that, in the health-care industry, "output is what output does." Applied to physicians as producers of health care this is taken to mean that the physician's output should be measured strictly by his impact on his patient's health. At the conceptual level this strikes one as a sensible prescription, especially if health is understood to include mental health status. At the empirical level, however, this conception of physician output loses its appeal.

It is analytically useful to think of the generation of better health as a production-decision process—sketched out in rudimentary form in Figure 3-1—in which the patient plays the central role. After all, it is the patient who decides to purchase the intermediary products—physician services, hospital services, drugs—and who combines these commodities with other inputs such as

---

[a]The *average* productivity of an input is to be distinguished from its *marginal* productivity. The latter is defined as the additional output produced by adding one more unit of the input to a fixed bundle of other inputs.

housing, nutrition, and his or her own time and knowhow in the production of health.[b] The setting of this production process is the patient's entire socio-economic environment which, along with attitudes toward health matters may either enhance or counteract the potential benefits from the consumption of medical care. The latter, in short, is only one of many inputs in the production of health—and perhaps not the most crucial.

This conception of the health production process is not entirely popular in the health literature, for it appears to impute to patients a degree of sovereignty widely assumed to be absent in the traditional physician-patient relationship. In his *Professional Dominance* [1970], for example, Eliot Freidson makes much of the loss of basic civil rights suffered by hospital patients, and it is part of our folklore that doctors issue orders and patients dutifully follow them. It may be argued, however, that a large proportion of physician services are rendered under an arrangement in which the physician plays essentially the role of a management consultant, counselling his patients in the management of their health production process. (At the same time, the physician is, of course, also a provider who produces some of the health services used in the production of health.) The fact that some patients delegate considerable managerial reponsibility to their physician and that, by virtue of his superior technical competence, the latter has considerable influence over his patients is no reason to view patients simply as passive inputs into the production of their own health and to hold the physician wholly or even predominantly responsible for his patients' health status.

If it were practically feasible to specify the health production process (section C of Figure 3-1) accurately and to predict patients' future health status in the absence of intervention by a physician, then an outcome-based measure of physician output would certainly be compatible with the conceptual framework sketched out above. Indeed, such a measure would be preferred, as it automatically adjusts for the "quality" of the physician's managerial and medical services. Unfortunately, it has so far been impossible, at the empirical level, to control successfully for the vast array of inputs that go into the production of patients' health. In the absence of such control, it is analytically more appropriate to think of the physician's output simply as the intermediary product "physician services," and to base one's output measure on some index of the volume of physician services rendered per period. This approach is actually in keeping with the practice of measuring the output of, say, the consumer durables industry (the auto industry, for example) in terms of the durable (automobiles) produced rather than in terms of the consumer services (passenger miles) actually rendered by these durables. In this view, the physician is credited

---

[b]Models of this production process can be and have been rigorously specified. See, for example, Grossman (1972).

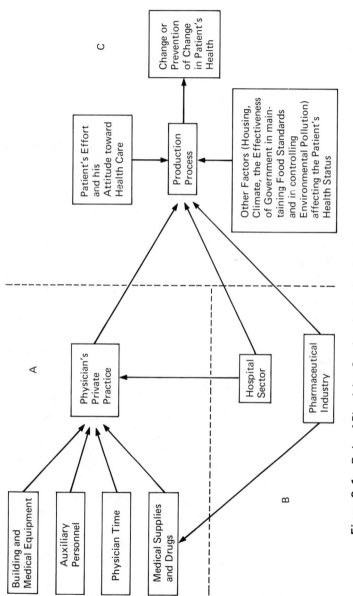

Figure 3-1.   Role of Physician Services in the Production of Health.

with output whether or not his services actually modify his patients' observable health status.[c]

Detailed information on the rates of individual services produced by physicians is rarely available to outside researchers. In the absence of such information, researchers have typically had to resort to cruder proxies. The more readily available and hence more popular among these have been (1) data on annual gross receipts by physicians, or annual expenditures on physician services; and (2) data on hourly, weekly, or annual physician-patient visits of various types. These indexes have been widely used in the health-economics literature, their obvious weaknesses notwithstanding.

Annual gross receipts by physicians, or annual expenditures on physician services, reflect the entire array of diagnostic, preventive and therapeutic services rendered by a physician's practice on an inpatient or ambulatory basis and included in his bill. The services covered by this definition of physician output range from those produced by the physician himself, to ancillary services such as x-rays, tests on body specimens, history-taking and record-keeping sometimes (though not always) produced by auxiliary personnel for whom the physician takes direct responsibility. If as a result of task delegation the physician's practice produces and sells more services per average patient visit while the number of weekly visits remains constant, then under this broad definition of physician output one would view this as an increase in physician productivity. The reasoning is that, had the physician produced these added services himself, he could clearly not have maintained the same rate of patient visits as before.

In empirical research the approximation of physician output by expenditure or gross income data can lead to some bias. For example, the official time series on "national expenditures of physician services" constructed and published by the Department of Health, Education and Welfare is developed from Internal Revenue Service data on annual gross receipts reported by physicians. If in one year physicians generally tended to have, say, x-rays or specimen tests performed by outside facilities that billed patients directly, while in some later year a larger proportion of physicians produced such services on their own premises or billed patients directly for services subcontracted to outside facilities, then the expenditure series would lead one to interpret as an increase in physician productivity what was really a mere shift in the locus of production or in billing practices.

A similar bias can arise in empirical production analyses based on cross-section samples of individual physicians, particularly in comparisons of

[c]Implicit in this approach is the assumption that the physician's choice of treatment will be dictated entirely by the patient's needs. There are some indications that, within the context of a fee-for-service system, this condition is not always met, that is, that some physicians prescribe medical treatment essentially in response to financial rewards they themselves stand to reap therefrom [Monsma, 1970]. The extent to which medical ethics are actually compromised in this way is not known at the present time.

solo with group practitioners. Quite aside from the problem of interphysician variation in professional fees, the gross income data one is likely to use as an output measure may reflect mere differences in the extent to which individual medical practices have internalized the production of ancillary services and the revenues therefrom. These and other problems associated with the expenditure- or income-measure are discussed more fully in a later part of the book. For the moment it suffices to note that results based on such data must be interpreted with caution.

The American Medical Association has suggested that the output of the medical care industry be defined as "the service consisting of the *control* or *management* of diseases or other physical or mental conditions, whether actual or potential" [1964, p. 10]. One can think of the management of a patient's medical condition—actual or potential, real or imagined—as a coordinated series of medical and nonmedical tasks. The tasks (including that of coordinating them) may be performed either by the patient, or by the physician who is the patient's primary contact with the health care system, or by the physician's staff, or by medical specialists to whom the patient is referred, or by specialized outside facilities, such as hospitals for inpatient care and laboratories for diagnostic tests. The performance of each of these tasks involves health manpower of various types. If it is possible somehow to reduce the input of physician time into tasks normally involving the physician's participation, or if such tasks can be wholly delegated to auxiliary personnel or capital equipment, then the physician can devote more of his time to tasks that truly require his participation. Other things being equal, he should then be able to render such services to an additional number of patients per unit of his time, and his productivity could be said to have increased. From the standpoint of health manpower policy this is an appealing definition of physician productivity, for productivity gains so defined would imply a reduction in the number of physicians required to manage a given set of medical conditions (or to care for a given population) as long as the vector of services rendered per condition remains constant.

One plausible index of the patient flow handled (or number of conditions managed) by physicians is their rate of patient visits per period. In using that output measure as an alternative to the broader expenditure measure, one tacitly assumes that, once a patient-physician contact has been established, the attending physician will see to it that the patient receives all medically necessary management counselling and medical services, whether these services are produced by the physician himself, by his staff, or by an outside practice or facility. Presumably on this logic, physicians' annual, weekly or hourly patient visits have long been taken as meaningful indexes of physician productivity. Much of the empirical analysis in Part II of this book will be based on this output measure as well.

Whatever the weekly patient load of a physician's practice may be, he could probably increase that load even further simply by reducing the time spent on tasks that require his participation. If physician output is measured by the rate of patient visits, such a development would naturally be interpreted as an increase in his productivity. Conversely, if the physician decided to reduce his weekly patient load in order to spend more time in face-to-face contact with each of his patients, such a move would be interpreted as a decrease in his productivity. These implications of the visit measure are often found trouble-some, for by increasing his hourly patient flow the physician may simply be trading off the quality of his services for the sake of quantity, and vice versa. For the moment we leave that problem aside. We will return to it at the end of Chapter Seven, after the various ways of increasing the physician's patient load have been more fully explored.

Output per Physician vs. Output per Dollar of Input

Some unnecessary confusion appears to exist even over the denom-inator of the definition of physician productivity. In his widely quoted *Economics of American Medicine,* for example, economist Seymour Harris begins his chapter on the "Productivity of Doctors" with the quite reasonable observa-tion that "a rise of [physician] productivity means that a given number of doctors working X hours can produce more (yield increased services) than with unchanged productivity" [1964, p. 130]. Curiously enough, he then goes on to argue:

> Earlier we noted that the Bane Committee was the authority for the statement that each physician in a given period of time sees twice as many patients as he did a generation ago. Does this mean that he is twice as productive as he was a generation ago?
> Not at all. First, he uses more of other factors of production—hospital facilities, office equipment, increased numbers of comple-mentary workers, for example, nurses, pharmacists, other tech-nicians, researchers... [p. 132].

Here the author appears to suggest that an increase in the rate of output per unit of some input rate ought not to be taken as an increase in the productivity of that input if the increase was brought about through more intensive use of other inputs. That there is something wrong with this conception of input pro-ductivity is soon recognized by the author himself when he states, "Produc-tivity increases . . . when the high cost factor [the physician] is economized through increased numbers of personnel and greater use of plant and equipment" [p. 134]. This conception of physician productivity would be more nearly acceptable, were it not for the fact that the relative costs of inputs are brought into the definition. The fact is, of course, that the average productivity of any input X can be increased through greater use of even a relatively more expensive input as long as the rate of output per unit of X is thereby increased. That this kind of productivity gain may not be economically attractive—because it may drive up the average costs per unit of output—is an entirely different matter, and one that should not be confused with the concept of input productivity as such. This confusion, however, is fairly common in discussions on physician productivity, especially in connection with the effect of group medical practice on physician productivity. The intended focus of such discussions is, by definition, the rate of output per unit of physician time; the argumentation, on the other hand, is all too often developed on "the rate of output per dollar spent on all medical inputs collectively." The latter ratio is certainly not without interest, but it is not an index of physician productivity at all.

In this book two distinct concepts of physician productivity are used. The first of these may be referred to as average *hourly* physician productivity, defined as the volume of physician output per hour of physician time spent in active practice. The second is the average *annual* physician productivity; it is defined as the annual rate of physician output per physician, and was referred to earlier as variable Q. The second index is obviously the product of the annual number of hours worked per physician and the average hourly physician productivity. The index may be of interest if one's concern is primarily about the availability of physician services to consumers, and one is relatively less interested in the particular sources (hours worked or hourly productivity) of any increase in the index. Physicians, on the other hand, are more likely to be interested in their average hourly productivity because it strongly determines the rate at which their own time can be translated into income. If one suspects that the number of hours worked per physician will not rise in the future, or perhaps that it will or should decline, then the hourly productivity index will be of main interest also to the formulators of health manpower policy.

II. LONG-RUN GROWTH IN PHYSICIAN PRODUCTIVITY

At the end of Chapter Two it was shown that the number of physicians required to service future populations of given sizes can be sensitive to the relative values of two parameters: one, the average annual growth rate in the per capita utilization of physician services (denoted by d), and the other the annual growth in output of such services per physician (denoted by q). It was seen that for a forecast horizon as short as one decade a mere one percentage-point difference between these parameters could easily turn a projected physician shortage into a surplus, and vice versa. The relative values these parameters are likely to take on in the future are therefore of crucial importance in the formulation of health manpower policy.

Although past values of any variable are not necessarily indicative of its future values, a look at the recent past may nevertheless furnish a good starting point for speculation about the future. In the remainder of this chapter we therefore examine recent trends in per capita utilization and physician productivity.

Most prior evidence on the secular growth of the use and the supply of physician services has been developed from expenditure data, an emphasis inevitably carried over into this chapter as well. In later chapters, however, relatively greater emphasis will be placed on patient visits, particularly in comparisons of individual medical practices. Which of these output measures is preferable depends to some extent on the context of the analysis and, more importantly, on one's assessment of the relative accuracy of the available data. The important point is that one be consistent, that is, that both per capita demand and output per physician be measured in the same units. The objective is, after all, to compare growth rates in these two variables.

Recent Trends in the Demand for
Physician Services

Table 3-1 presents average annual growth rates in real per capita expenditures on physician services during the period 1950–70. One set of estimates is based on deflation of the expenditure series by the physician-fee

Table 3-1. **Historical Values of Parameter** d**—the Annual Growth in Per Capita Utilization of Physician Services, 1950–70**

	1950	*1960*	*1968*	*1970*
1. Per Capita Expenditures on Physician Services in Current Dollars (E_t)	$17.76	$30.92	$54.36	$65.28
2. Deflators:				
a) Physician-Fee Component of the CPI (1967 = 100) (CPI_t)	55.2	77.0	105.6	121.4
b) Fuchs-Kramer Index of "Average Price Received" (1956 = 100) (FKI_t)	76.6	117.4	173.7	–
3. Estimated Values of d:[a]	Based on CPI		Based on FKI	
1950–60	2.2%		1.3%	
1960–68	3.2		2.2	
1968–70	2.2		–	
1950–68	2.6		1.7	
1950–70	2.6		–	

[a]Calculated as:

$$d_{t,t-n} = \frac{100}{n} \log_e \left(\frac{E_t}{E_{t-n}} \cdot \frac{I_{t-n}}{I_t} \right)$$

where I_t is either CPI_t or FKI_t, and subscripts t and n denote years.
Sources: Line 1–*Statistical Abstract of the United States 1972*, Table 92; line 2a–ibid., Table 90; line 3a–Fuchs and Kramer [1972], Table 3, p. 9.

component of the Consumer Price Index (*CPI*). The alternative set is based on a price deflator developed by Fuchs and Kramer (1972).

The physician-fee component of the *CPI* is estimated by the Bureau of Labor Statistics as a weighted average of reported customary fees for a small set of standard medical procedures, such as office and home visits, appendectomies, deliveries, and so on. The expenditure series, on the other hand, is essentially an aggregate of the annual gross receipts reported by self-employed physicians to the Internal Revenue Service. These gross receipts reflect the quantity of services supplied by physicians times the "average price" received per service. The latter may deviate from "customary" fees because of secular changes in the percentage of patient billings actually collected or because physicians may charge some patients (such as poor patients) fees other than customary ones. Fuchs and Kramer's index of "average price received" is an attempt to take these factors into account. During the period under consideration that index appears to have risen faster than the CPI^d, so that growth rates calculated with the Fuchs-Kramer index will be lower than those obtained on deflation by the *CPI*. For reasons indicated, the former are likely to yield a more accurate picture of past growth in real per capita expenditures on physician services.[e]

Table 3-1 suggests that, on the broad conception of physician output, the per capita consumption of physician services has grown at annual average rates between 1.3 and 2.2 percent during the last two decades. The higher values are characteristic of more recent years and probably reflect the phasing in of the Medicare and Medicaid programs during the late 1960s. Table 3-2, on the other hand, suggests that the growth in per capita expenditures on physician services has not been paralleled by growth in per capita utilization of physician-patient visits. In fact, according to the utilization data gathered by the National Center of Health Statistics (NCHS), nonhospital patient visits per capita appear to have remained virtually constant during the 1960s and were slightly lower in 1970 than they were in 1957-59.

The NCHS series, however, appears to understate the actual number of nonhospital physician visits per capita. In one study of this bias, it was found that consumers enrolled in a group health plan reported to the interviewers only about two-thirds of the visits they were known to have made.[1] Whether this finding is representative of the U.S. population as a whole is not clear; nor is it known whether the percentage of under-reporting has changed

[d]The index rose faster than the *CPI* because, by virtue of more extensive insurance coverage, the average collection ratio rose during the period, and patients who previously were charged fees below the physician's customary level were increasingly charged the latter.

[e]An earlier attempt to construct an "average price index" for physician services can be found in Feldstein [1970], pp. 122-123. Since Feldstein's price series is not included in his published paper, the Fuchs-Kramer index is used throughout this chapter.

Table 3-2. Number of Nonhospital Physician Visits Per Capita, United States, 1957-70

Year	Number of Nonhospital Physician Visits Per Capita[a]
1957–59	5.0
1963–64	4.5
1966–67	4.3
1968	4.2
1969	4.3
1970	4.6

[a]Defined for the civilian, noninstitutional population of the United States. Visits exclude inpatient hospital visits, but include visits to hospital outpatient departments and telephone consultations.

Sources: For 1957–59: *United States Statistical Abstract 1962,* Table 85; for 1963–69: U.S. Department of Health, Education and Welfare, National Center for Health Statistics, *Vital and Health Statistics,* Series 10, No. 11, Table 14; No. 43, Table 16; No. 60, Table 19; No. 63, Table 20; for 1970: *United States Statistical Abstract, 1972,* Table 100.

over time. The data in Table 3-2 also exclude physician visits to patients in hospitals. There is evidence that the proportion of hospital visits in total patient visits has increased over time. According to information published by the American Medical Association, for example, hospital visits were 26 percent of total patient visits in 1969 [1971, p. 57] and about 28 percent in 1971 [1973, p. 62]. The per capita demand of patient visits of all types may therefore have increased at least somewhat during the period under consideration, although surely not as rapidly as expenditures on physician services. Thus one concludes from Tables 3-1 and 3-2 that the bulk of the observed increase in per capita expenditures represents an increase in the number of services rendered per patient visit.

In their previously cited analysis of expenditures on physician services, Fuchs and Kramer come to the same conslusion. According to the authors a good part of the observed increase in services per visit reflects the growth of specialization during that period. Relative to a general practitioner, the authors argue, a medical specialist tends to charge more for his time, spend more of his time per patient visit, and prescribe and supply more ancillary services (such as x-rays, electrocardiograms, and tests of body specimens) per visit, all of which tend to increase real expenditures per visit. Fuchs and Kramer estimate that, over the period 1948-68, the quantity of services per patient visit increased at an annual rate of 2.8 percent. Of this increase, roughly 0.9 percentage points (or 32 percent) are estimated to reflect the growing trend toward medical specialization. The remaining 1.9 percentage points appear to reflect an increase in services per visit, even for general practices [1972, p. 17]. This increased service-intensity obviously need not spell a concomitant increase in the use of physician time per visit. Most of the added services can be, and probably are being, produced by auxiliary personnel working with specialized medical equipment.

Whether these historical values of d furnish a reliable clue to the future is another matter. One could imagine a set of very generous policies under which per capita utilization of physician services might grow at an annual rate exceeding perhaps even 3 percent. Such policies might include a universal and publicly financed health insurance scheme with low or zero co-payments on the part of patients, with fee-for-service reimbursement for physicians, without measures to control the utilization of health services, and accompanied by a manpower policy committed to meet any demand that becomes manifest under that insurance scheme. Such a development, however, seems improbable in the United States, at least in the foreseeable future. A more plausible assumption would be that for $(q - d)$ in equation (2-5) to exceed one percentage point, the average annual output per physician would have to increase at a rate of somewhere between 2.5 and 3 percent per year (if output is defined by expenditures on physician services) and at most 1 percent per year (if one measures output by number of patient visits).

Recent Growth in Physician Productivity

During the period 1950-1970, the long-run average growth rate in output per man-hour for the United States private sector as a whole has been about 3 percent per year, although due to a decline in hours worked the output per employee—the analog of variable Q in equation (2-2)—has grown at a somewhat lower rate. Estimates of growth in physician productivity during the postwar period have fallen on either side of this figure. Almost without exception these estimates have been based on time series on physician incomes or on national expenditures on physician services.

At the low end of the spectrum are estimates by Joseph Garbarino, who calculated annual average productivity gains of 2.4 percent for the period 1946-51 and of 1.9 percent for 1949-54.[2] Fuchs and Kramer, in their previously cited study, arrive at an estimate of 2.1 percent per year for the entire period 1948-68 [1972, p. 17]. These figures are consistent with Jeffrey Weiss' assertion that "if the 1950 production function for health services had been utilized to produce the 1960 output of health services the nation would have needed an additional 46,286 physicians" [1966, p. 212].

Weiss does not appear to have translated this conclusion into an estimate of annual productivity growth. Such a translation can easily be made with the aid of the simple forecasting model defined in equations (2-1) and (2-2). According to Weiss, maintenance of the 1950 "job coefficient for [physician] manpower" in 1960 would have required a total of 268,943 physicians to produce the 1960 output of physician services. In equation (2-2) the "job coefficient" referred to by Weiss is given by $1/Q$. If g denotes the average annual growth rate in the annual output per physician during the 1950's, then

$$Q_{60} = Q_{50}e^{10(g)} \tag{3-1}$$

where subscripts denote years. Furthermore, if the 1960 output of physician services is denoted by $D_{60}P_{60}$, then Weiss' conclusion is tantamount to the two algebraic statements

$$268{,}943 = \frac{D_{60}P_{60}}{Q_{50}} \tag{3-2}$$

$$222{,}657 = \frac{D_{60}P_{60}}{Q_{50}e^{10g}} \tag{3-3}$$

From these equations the value of g implicit in Weiss' conclusion can be calculated as 1.9 percent.

Weiss has elsewhere presented much higher estimates of productivity growth. For the period 1947–55, he has estimated annual productivity gains of 3.6 percent; for 1955–59, 4.0 percent; for 1959–64, 2.7 percent, and for the entire period 1947–64 3.4 percent.[3] It appears that Weiss derived these estimates from the time path of median gross incomes of physicians, deflated by the physician-fee component of the Consumer Price Index, and adjusted for increases in collection ratios over time.[4] In principle, Weiss' deflator should be an approximation to the "average price" deflator used by Fuchs and Kramer. His estimate of physician productivity, however, exceeds these authors' estimate for roughly the same period by about 1.3 percentage points.

Weiss' higher estimates are in line with those calculated by the National Advisory Commission on Health Manpower [1967, p. 238]. The commission's estimates are reproduced in Table 3–3, primarily in order to display the methodology on which they are based. The commission deflated the time series of national expenditures on physician services by the physician-fee component of the Consumer Price Index. As already mentioned, this method is known to exaggerate the growth in real output per physician during these years. Furthermore, the commission used the total number of *active and inactive* physicians as the denominator in "output per physician." Since the expenditure series is constructed from Internal Revenue Service records on gross receipts of active self-employed practitioners, the more appropriate denominator would be *active physicians in private practice.* The number of private practitioners as a percentage of total active physicians has decreased during the past several decades. Productivity estimates based on these two series, even if derived from the same real expenditure series, will therefore differ, as may be seen by comparing columns 2 and 3 of Table 3–5.[f]

----

[f]Unfortunately, a series on physicians in private practice is available only up to 1968, at which time the American Medical Association reclassified its statistics and eliminated the series on private practitioners. Table 3–4 has therefore been extended only to 1968.

Table 3-3. Estimated Growth in Physician Productivity as Calculated by the National Advisory Commission on Health Manpower

	National Expenditures on Physicians' Services (millions)[1]	*Price Index*[2] *(1955-57 = 100)*	*Total Number of Physicians Active and Inactive (thousands)*	*Average*[3] *Annual Increase in Productivity (percent)*
Period From:				
1955	$3,680	90.0	255.2	—
To:				
1960	5,684	106.0	274.8	4.0
1963	6,891	114.4	289.2	3.3
1964	8,065	117.3	297.1	4.2
1965	9,003[a]	121.5	305.1	4.2

1. Productivity has been computed using the following formula:

$$\text{Prod}_t = \left[\frac{E_t}{E_o} \div \frac{P_o}{P_t} \div \frac{D_o}{D_t} \right] \ [\text{sic}]^b$$

where E represents expenditures, P the price index, and D the number of physicians. t represents the number of years from the base year, in this case 1955.

2. Social Security Administration, Social Security Bulletin, February 1967.

3. Bureau of Labor Statistics, *Consumer Price Index,* Physician Fee Component.

[a]The revised figure is $8,745.

[b]The formula really should be

$$\text{Prod}_t = \frac{100}{t} \log_e \left[\frac{E_t P_o D_o}{E_o P_t D_t} \right]$$

Source: Except for notes a and b, taken from National Advisory Commission on Health Manpower [1967], Table 6, p. 238.

The growth rates shown in Table 3-5 have been calculated from the raw data presented in Table 3-4. The first column in Table 3-5 is essentially a replication of the commission's estimates, albeit for different years and with expenditures in 1965 equal to $8,745 rather than $9,003.[5] The growth rates in the second column are based on real expenditures derived with the Fuchs-Kramer index on "average price received," but divided, once again, by the total number of physicians, active and inactive. Finally, the third column reflects real expenditures obtained with the Fuchs-Kramer index, divided by the number of active private practitioners only. For reasons already indicated, the estimates in column 3 represent the theoretically most defensible estimates of productivity gains based on expenditure data. The fact that these estimates are not too different from the commission's original estimates is not a vindication of the commission's method; it is pure happenstance.

Table 3–4. Time Series on National Expenditures on Physician Services, the Supply of Physicians, and Indexes of Physician Fees

Year (1)	National Expenditures on Physicians' Services (millions) (2)	Total Number of Physicians (thousands)		Indexes of Physician Fees[a]	
		Active and Inactive (3)	Active in Private Practice (4)	CPI (5)	Fuchs-Kramer (6)
1955	$3,689	255.2	169.9	65.4	96.1
1960	5,684	274.8	179.2	77.0	117.4
1965	8,745	305.1	190.7	88.3	137.8
1968	11,099	330.7	194.1	105.6	173.7
1970	13,600	348.3	N/A	121.4	N/A

[a]Column 5 is the physician-fee component of the Consumer Price Index (1967 = 100); for the Fuchs-Kramer Index, 1956 = 100.

Sources: Columns 2, 3 and 5: *Statistical Abstract of the United States 1972,* tables 91, 101 and 90, respectively; column 4: U.S. Department of Health, Education, and Welfare, Public Health Service, *Health Manpower Source Book* [1969], table 33, and Theodore et al. [1971], table E; column 6: Fuchs and Kramer [1972], Table 3.

Table 3–5. Alternative Estimates of the Productivity Parameter q, 1955–1970

	Estimated Average Annual Percentage Increase in Real Output per Physician, Based on:[a]		
Period	Consumer Price Index and Active and Inactive Physicians (1)	Fuchs-Kramer Index and Active and Inactive Physicians (2)	Fuchs-Kramer Index and Active Physicians in Private Practice (3)
1955–60	4.0%	3.2%	3.6%
1960–65	3.8	3.3	4.0
1965–68	–0.7	–2.5	–0.4
1968–70	0.5	–	–
1955–65	3.9	3.2	3.9
1960–68	2.1	1.2	2.5
1965–70	–0.2	–	–

[a]Calculated, on the basis of the raw data in Table 3–3, with the following expression:

$$g_{t,t-n} = \frac{100}{n} \log_e \left[\frac{NE_t P_{t-n} M_{t-n}}{NE_{t-n} P_t M_t} \right]$$

where NE = national expenditures on physician services, P = fee index, M = number of physicians, subscript t identifies the end of the period over which the growth rate as averaged and $(t - n)$ identifies the beginning of that period.

Source: Column 1 is based on columns 2, 3 and 5 of Table 3–4, column 2 on columns 2, 3 and 6, and column 3 on columns 2, 4 and 6.

Reliable data on the number of *patient visits* produced per physician are unfortunately not available for years prior to the mid-1960s. In their previously cited study, Fuchs and Kramer estimate that the annual number of patient visits per physician actually decreased at a long-run average annual rate of 0.7 percent over the period 1948-68 [1972, p. 17]. That estimate, however, is based on the visits reported by consumers to the National Center for Health Statistics. As indicated earlier, these data may be subject to some bias. Data from the *Medical Economics* surveys of self-employed physicians indicate a secular increase in weekly patient visits per physician, at least during the period 1965-70. As is shown in column 6 of Table 3-6, the average number of weekly patient visits per physician—adjusted for changes in the mix of medical specialties—seems to have increased at an overall average rate of 1.5 percent per year during 1965-70. This result stands in sharp contrast to the estimated growth in expenditures per physician during the same period. Table 3-5 suggests that, on the expenditure measure, physician productivity appears not to have grown at all during 1965-70, and that it even declined somewhat during 1965-68.

If the *Medical Economics* data on patient visits are reliable indicators of actual developments in the United States as a whole, then one is led to conclude either that the number of services rendered per patient visit has declined somewhat during 1965-70 or that there may be defects in the expenditure series on which the growth rates in Table 3-5 are based. It is interesting to observe, for example, that the official expenditure series developed from Internal Revenue Service records seems to be inconsistent also with the income statistics reported by self-employed physicians in the annual *Medical Economics* surveys.

Table 3-7 presents the average annual growth rate in real median net income per physician during 1965-68. It is seen that even after deflation by the Fuchs-Kramer index, the estimated growth appears to have been about 1 percent per year. This figure may be contrasted with the estimate of -0.4 percent shown in Table 3-5. It is true, of course, that the figures in Table 3-7 are directly comparable to those in Table 3-5 only if it can be assumed that the ratio of median to average net income and the ratio of average net income to average gross receipts per physician did not change significantly during 1965-68, and one has no assurance that this is so.[g] The actual time path of real expenditures on physician services per physician during the 1965-70 therefore remains a matter of conjecture.

Probable Sources of Past Productivity Gains

The conclusion from the preceding discussion is that while the actual magnitude of postwar growth in the per capita utilization of physician services

[g]Unfortunately, data on average gross income are not available for the period under consideration. In interpreting the results obtained from the median net income statistics, it should be kept in mind that the overall distribution of physician incomes tends to be skewed and that the average of that distribution tends to exceed the median.

Table 3–6. Estimated Annual Growth in Average Weekly Visits per Physician, United States, 1965–70

	General Practice	*Pediatrics*	*Obstetrics/ Gynecology*	*Internal Medicine*	*General Surgery*	*Weighted Average*
Office Visits:						
1965	140.5	123.4	89.7	83.7	70.5	114.6
1970[a]	150.0	143.0	109.8	88.5	84.0	122.4
Annual Growth	1.4%	3.0%	4.0%	1.2%	3.5%	1.4%[c]
Hospital Visits:						
1965	26.7	17.4	24.9	36.0	44.7	29.9
1970[a]	33.0	22.6	31.4	39.5	41.8	34.5
Annual Growth	4.3%	5.1%	4.6%	1.9%	-1.3%	2.8%[c]
Total Visits[b]						
1965	174.7	144.9	113.6	118.0	115.2	148.2
1970	188.0	166.4	142.3	132.6	128.0	160.5
Annual Growth	1.5%	2.8%	4.5%	2.3%	2.1%	1.5%[c]
Weights ($W_{i,t}$)						
1965	0.511	0.077	0.098	0.177	0.137	1.000
1970	0.441	0.089	0.118	0.197	0.155	1.000

[a]Calculated by multiplying the visits reported in American Medical Association [1972, p. 62], by the ratio: "average *total* visits reported by Medical Economics, Inc. for 1970 ÷ average *total* visits reported by the AMA for 1970" [1972, p. 60]. The Medical Economics data exclude active physicians over the age of 65 and hence the reported averages tend to be about 5 percent to 6 percent higher than those reported by the AMA, which reflect all active physicians.

[b]Includes home visits.

[c]Calculated as

$$ g = \frac{100}{5} \log_e \left[\frac{\sum_{i=1}^{i=5} (V_{i,70}\, W_{i,70})}{\sum_{i=1}^{i=5} (V_{i,65}\, W_{i,65})} \right] $$

where $V_{i,t}$ denotes the average number of weekly visits per physician in specialty i in year t, and $W_{i,t}$ denotes the proportion of physicians in specialty i in year t.

Sources: Data for 1965 and for total visits for 1970—private communication from Medical Economics, Inc.; office and hospital visits for 1970—American Medical Association [1972], Table 27, page 62.

and in the output of such services per physician remain a matter of debate, productivity growth does appear to have kept more or less in step with growth in per capita utilization. This conclusion is reached whether one measures physician output by gross receipts or by patient visits. The question is, once again, what, if anything, this historical pattern foretells about the future. Here opinions differ sharply.

Some students of the health care sector doubt that one can bank on sustained future growth in physician productivity. As early as 1959, for

Table 3-7. Apparent Growth in Real Median Net Income Per Physician, United States, 1965-1970

Year	Median Net Income[a] per Physician	Price Indexes		Annual Percentage Growth in Real Median Income	
		CPI (1967 = 100)	Fuchs-Kramer (1956 = 100)	Based on CPI	Based on Fuchs-Kramer Index
1965	$28,960	88.3	137.8	} 2.8%	} 1%
1968	37,620	100.6	173.8		

[a]As reported by Medical Economics, Inc., and presented in the *Statistical Abstract of the United States, 1972*, Table 97.

example, the previously cited Bane Committee had concluded that "there seems to be little room for increases in the already heavy patient load carried by the individual practitioner" [p. 22], an argument that was subsequently reiterated by Peterson and Pennell—two well-known health manpower specialists —who wrote in early 1963:

> Now [in 1963] a physician shortage faces this country as its major health problem. . . . It is safe to assume . . . that better utilization of physicians' services can effect only modest savings in professional time [p. 171].

Perhaps on the strength of such statements, Dr. Terry Luther, Surgeon General during the Kennedy Administration, flatly asserted during the congressional hearings on the Health Professional Assistance Act of 1963 that

> to expect physicians to provide increased amounts of service simply by treating more patients in a day—seeing each patient for a shorter time and delegating more tasks to less highly trained assistants— would be unrealistic [U.S. Congress, House, 1963, p. 87].

Given this pessimism on the part of health manpower specialists and public health authorities it is not really surprising that federal health manpower policy has concentrated almost wholly, and perhaps unduly, on efforts to provide the "appropriate" *numbers* of physicians, and has tended to brush aside as impractical any suggestion to enhance the efficiency with which physicians are used. In fact, during the congressional hearings on the 1971 Health Professions Educational Assistance Amendment the term physician productivity was hardly ever mentioned.

The pessimists on the productivity question do not deny that there have been such gains in past decades (although they may question the accuracy of the estimates presented earlier in this chapter). Rather, they seem to argue that the sources of these gains were of a sort that can either not be stimulated through public policy or that have been almost fully exploited by now. It has been observed, for example, that since the 1930s there has been a marked shift from the relatively more time-consuming home visits to less time-consuming office visits or even telephone consultations. In 1930, home visits amounted to roughly 40 percent of all out-of-hospital physician visits, a figure that had shrunk to 8 percent by 1957 [Somers & Somers 1961, p. 49] and to about 4 percent by 1965. This shift, it is argued, can explain a considerable part of observed productivity gains over this period, but it is a source that has obviously been fully exhausted by now.

The impact solely of a change in the mix of office, hospital and home visits on hourly physician productivity can be approximated in rough-and-ready fashion by the two expressions

$$V_{to} = \frac{a_o + hb_o + m(1 - a_o - b_o)}{a_t + hb_t + m(1 - a_t - b_t)} \tag{3-4}$$

$$R_{to} = V_{to} \left(\frac{a_t + hb_t x + m(1 - a_t - b_t)z}{a_o + hb_o x + m(1 - a_o - b_o)z} \right) \tag{3-5}$$

where

V_{to} = total visits per hour of patient care in year t/total visits per hour of patient care in base-year o.

R_{to} = revenue per hour of patient care in year t/revenue per hour of patient care in year o.

a_t = office visits as a proportion of total visits in year t ($t = t$ or $t = o$).

b_t = hospital visits as a proportion of total visits in year t.

h = the average time used per hospital visit/the average time used per office visit.

m = the average time used per home visit/the average time used per office visit

x = average revenue earned per unit of time spent on a hospital visit/average revenue per unit of time spent on an office visit.

z = average revenue earned per unit of time spent on a home visit/average revenue per unit of time spent on an office visit.

The approximate annual contribution (in percentage points) the shift has made to the growth in hourly physician productivity over the period from $t = o$ to $t = t$ can be obtained from these expressions as the growth rates

$$g_V = \frac{100}{t} \log_e(V_{to}) \tag{3-6}$$

$$g_R = \frac{100}{t} \log_e(R_{to}) \tag{3-7}$$

where g_V denotes the growth rate in visits per hour, and g_R that in hourly revenues.

      If fees per visit always varied in direct proportion with physician time spent per visit, then variables x and z in equation (3-5) would be equal to unity, and any secular increase in total patient visits per hour would be precisely offset by a fall in average revenue per visit. The growth rate g_R would therefore be equal to zero regardless of the value of g_V. On the other hand, if office, hospital, and home visits all fetched the same fee, then the average revenue per hour of patient care would rise at precisely the same rate as total visits per hour, that is, g_R would equal g_V. The actual values of h, m, x and z are likely to be such that g_R will be positive but smaller than g_V.

      Tables 3-8 and 3-9 may be of some assistance in the selection of plausible values of parameters h, m, x and z. Thus, as a very rough approximation it may be assumed that the average hospital visit tends to absorb about 1.4 times as much physician time as an average office visit, and that the corresponding figure for home visits is about 2.5 (and probably not as much as 3). Table 3-9 suggests that the average fee for hospital visits may not compensate fully for the higher time intensity of such visits. The fee data in that table, however, cover only routine follow-up visits and may not be indicative of the relative remuneration for all types of office and hospital visits. Indeed, a study of fees paid under the Medicare program has indicated that for the nation as a whole the average charge per hospital inpatient visit of all types (initial visits, consultations, and rounds) was 1.7 times as high as the average charge for office visits of all kinds.[6] This value is probably a more reliable index of relative remuneration and is used in Table 3-7 below. Finally, from frequency distributions of fees published in *Medical Economics* [7] it appears that the average fee for a routine daytime home visit in 1970 was $11 for general practitioners and $13 for pediatricians. It may therefore not be unreasonable to assume that the average charge for a home visit tends to be roughly 1.7 times as high as that for an office visit (see Table 3-9 for fees on routine office visits). These values suggest values of $x = 1.2$ and $z = 0.7$ as plausible first approximations. Since the aim is to isolate solely the effect of a change in the mix of visits on observed productivity growth, these values of h, m, x and z are held constant over the period from $t = o$ to $t = t$.

      Unfortunately, the previously cited data on the secular change in visit-mix exclude hospital visits, presumably because hard data on this type of visit are not available for the 1930s. One way to overcome this difficulty is to

Table 3–8. Estimated Time Intensity of Office, Hospital and Home Visits[a]

Medical Specialty	Average Number of Minutes Reportedly Spent Per			Implied Value of Variables	
	Office Visit	*Hospital Visit*	*Home Visit*	*h*	*m*
General Practitioners	16	23	42	1.4	2.6
Pediatricians	18	28	44	1.6	2.4
Obstetricians/					
Gynecologists	20	23	48	1.2	2.4
Internists	25	24	44	1.0	1.8

[a]Sample averages of 60 times average number of hours individual physicians reported to have spent on visits in a given category divided by the reported number of weekly visits in that category.

Source: Data from *Medical Economics,* Continuing Survey, 1964.

apply equations (3–4) and (3–5) solely to out-of-hospital activities of physicians, that is, to exclude time spent in the hospital from "hours of patient care." This is done under Item I in Table 3–10. An alternative is to make a plausible assumption about the proportion of hospital in total visits during the 1930s. The figures under item II in Table 3–10, for example, are based on the assumption that hospital visits were about 15 percent of total visits in 1930, 20 percent in 1957, and 25 percent in 1965. These assumptions are not implausible in the light of recent data on physician visits,[8] on trends in patient days per capita, and on physician-population ratios.[9]

In view of the series of somewhat arbitrary assumptions underlying Table 3–9, one would certainly not wish to defend the accuracy of these estimates with great vigor. Both the relative time requirements and fees for the three types of visits may have changed over the period considered, and so has the mix of medical specialists. Even so, as very rough approximations these esti-

Table 3–9. Relative Fees for Routine Follow-Up Visits in the Office and in the Hospital, 1970

Medical Specialty	Average Fee for a Routine Follow-Up		Fee for Hospital Visit Relative to Fee for Office Visit
	Office Visit	*Hospital Visit*	
General Practitioner	$6.35	$7.87	1.24
Pediatrician	7.17	8.75	1.22
Obstetrician/			
Gynecologist	8.89	7.61	.86
Internists	9.30	10.52	1.13

Source: American Medical Association [1972], Tables 44 and 45.

Table 3-10   Illustrative Estimates of Annual Growth in Observed "Physician Productivity" Attributable to Changes in the Mix of Patient Visits, 1930-1965

	Average Annual Compound Growth in:	
	Visits per Hour[a] *of Patient Care* g_v	*Revenue per Hour*[a] *of Patient Care* g_r
I. Out-of-Hospital Visits (Hours) Only:[b]		
1930–1957	2.0%	0.8%
1957–1965	0.7	0.3
II. Total Patient Visits and Hours of Care[c]		
1930–1957	1.6	0.8
1957–1965	0.3	0.4

[a]Calculated from equations (3-4) and 3-5) above, with $h = 1.4$, $m = 2.5$, $x = 1.2$ and $z = 0.7$.

[b]It is assumed that $a_{30} = 0.40$, $a_{57} = 0.92$, and $a_{65} = 0.96$, where subscripts denote year.

[c]It is assumed that $b_{30} = 0.15$, $b_{57} = 0.20$, and $b_{65} = 0.25$, so that $a_{30} = 0.4(1 - 0.15) = 0.34$, and similarly, $a_{57} = 0.74$ and $a_{65} = 0.72$.

mates are of some interest. They suggest, first of all, that the observed shift in the visit mix has indeed made a substantial contribution to the long-run growth in hourly patient visits of all types. Second, it is clear that the bulk of that contribution was made prior to the mid-1950s. But since physician fees do appear to compensate at least partially for the higher time intensity of home visits, the impact of the observed change in the visit mix on gross receipts per physician hour has been smaller than that on patient visits. In short, while the change in visit mix does appear to have made some contribution to observed productivity growth expressed in "expenditures on physician services," a good part of that growth appears to have originated in other factors.

Prominent candidates among these other factors are certain break-throughs in medical technology—new drugs or sophisticated medical equipment—and increasing reliance by physicians on support personnel and hospital facilities. Some care must be used, however, in assessing the relative contribution of these factors to physician productivity as that concept has been defined earlier. There can be no doubt, for example, that the widespread use of Penicillin, Streptomycin, and other antibiotics during the past few decades has been very effective against hitherto common diseases such as influenza, tuberculosis, syphilis, and polio.[10] Similarly important contributions to the health status of individuals or groups of people have been made by new capital-supported medical procedures in the treatment of kidney and heart disease. By themselves, however, these developments may not have contributed much to the rate of *medical services* produced per unit of physician time, and they would therefore not be reflected in productivity indexes expressed in terms of *medical services* rather than patients' *health status.* Technical breakthroughs of this sort will have contributed to productivity as measured in Tables 3-5 and 3-6 only to the extent that they enable physicians to treat more patients (or to generate more real gross receipts) per unit of physician time, regardless of the patients' medical condition. The development of disposable syringes and gloves, for example, may act as a breakthrough of this type.

Increasing reliance by physicians on auxiliary personnel is more likely to have contributed to the productivity gains noted earlier. In his previously cited study on the job structure of health manpower, for example, Weiss found that during the period from 1940 to 1960 the number of health workers with relatively high formal training (mainly physicians) increased at a much lower rate than did the number of health workers in jobs requiring less formal training [1966, Ch. 3]. Unfortunately, one can only speculate on how much these trends in the mix of health manpower have contributed to physician productivity as conventionally measured. Since Weiss' analysis is at the aggregate level, it merely suggests that the average physician is supported, directly or indirectly, by ever-increasing numbers of paramedical personnel. It is not clear whether this trend reflects the substitution of paramedical for medical manpower in the production of services that had traditionally been produced by physicians, or whether it reflects primarily the emergence of new services that have been rendered by paramedical personnel right from the start. Furthermore, it is not known how many of the latter services were billed through physicians' offices and hence were reflected in the time series on physicians' gross receipts—one of the series on which productivity estimates are based. Finally, in the absence of time series on the number of patient visits per physician and on the number of aides physicians employ in their own practices, it is impossible to assess the impact of the overall manpower trends on physician productivity measured by rates of patient visits.

These uncertainties notwithstanding, a number of analysts see a direct causal relationship between past changes in the overall mix of health manpower and past gains in physician productivity, and they view that relationship as a significant potential for sustained productivity growth in the future. In their study on behalf of the National Advisory Commission on Health Manpower, for example, Jones, Struve and Stefani concluded that

> despite the increases in productivity that were obtained in the past decade, significant opportunities still appear open to exploitation for the next decade. For example, in 1964 almost one-fourth of the physicians in private practice employed four or more auxiliary workers. Almost half of all physicians in private practice, however, employed less than two auxiliary workers. Increasing grouping of practice [sic] offers still other opportunities. By and large, the

projected 4 percent per year increase in productivity appears to be within reach [1967, p. 244].

This sanguine view—one that has gained increasing currency in recent years—stands in stark contrast to the pessimistic conclusions cited a few pages ago. As was illustrated in Figure 2–3, such differences of opinion are of no small importance to health manpower policy, for they can translate themselves into rather substantial differences of views concerning future physician requirements. The commonly mentioned potential sources of future gains in physician productivity and the controversy still surrounding that topic therefore warrant a closer look.

NOTES

1. The study was undertaken by the National Center for Health Statistics and covered members of group health plans where the actual number of visits by individual patients was known. In this connection, see the *Report of the National Advisory Commission on Health Manpower* [1967], Vol. II, Appendix IV, p. 224.
2. Quoted in Klarman [1969b], Table 3, p. 371.
3. Ibid.
4. In this connection, see the U.S. Department of Health, Education and Welfare, Office of the Secretary [1967], p. 21, where the methodology is described. See also Gorham [1967].
5. The lower figure is given in the *Statistical Abstract of the United States, 1972,* Table 91, p. 66.
6. Quoted in Fuchs and Kramer [1972], p. 54.
7. See Arthur Owens [1971b], p. 196.
8. American Medical Association [1971], Table 21, p. 57.
9. Donabedian, Axelrod and Agard [1970], pp. 48 and 104.
10. Fuchs and Kramer [1972], p. 13.

Chapter Four

The Potential for Future Gains in Physician Productivity: A Broad Overview

As already indicated, the optimists on the productivity issue tend to cite two major reforms of medical practice as potential sources for future gains in physician productivity: (1) the formation of group medical practices; and (2) the substitution of paramedical and clerical personnel for the physician, and the substitution of capital equipment and medical supplies for all types of health manpower. This chapter will review in broad overview the *a priori* reasoning and the empirical evidence on which these proposals rest. In the first part of the chapter the focus is on the potential contribution of group medical practice to physician productivity. In the second part the potential of input substitution is examined.

On the surface it may appear that any argument over the feasibility of the above proposals revolves strictly about the technology of physician-care production, that is, about their *technical feasibility*. For the most part this is undoubtedly true. Mere technical feasibility, however, reveals nothing about physicians' probable *economic behavior* and hence about the probable future time path of annual output per physician (Q). To project the latter one needs to know not only what is technically feasible, but also (a) what particular practice mode or configuration of medical inputs physicians are likely to choose in future years, and (b) to what extent physicians will actually attempt to maximize (or succeed in maximizing) the rate of output technically attainable with the particular combination of inputs they have chosen. It follows that disagreements over the future time path of physician productivity may reflect differences of views concerning either the technology of physician-care production, or the economic behavior of physicians, or both.

I. PHYSICIAN PRODUCTIVITY IN GROUP MEDICAL PRACTICE

The distinction between the *technical* properties of a production process and the *economic* behavior of those managing that process is an important one, and failure to observe it has led to much confusion in the literature on physician productivity. Nowhere has this confusion been more persistent than in discussions concerning the merits and demerits of group medical practice. In advancing the case for that mode of practice its proponents commonly cite studies in which the experience of *prepaid group medical practice plans*—such as the Kaiser Foundation Medical Plans in California or the Health Insurance Plan of Greater New York (HIP)—is compared with that of insurance plans offering roughly similar coverage, but on a fee-for-service basis and through private practitioners of the patients' choice. (See, for example, Fein [1967], pp. 104-4, and Boan [1966].) In such comparisons the prepaid group practice plans are usually shown to report lower per capita utilization of services—particularly of surgery and hospital days—and hence lower annual costs per enrollee at risk than do the fee-for-service plans. Table 4-1 is an example of the data typically emerging from such studies.[1]

Comparisons of this sort may be relevant to an evaluation of alternative health insurance systems. Their bearing on the relative merits of group medical practice *per se* is at best indirect. The distinction that needs to be made in this connection is between the cost savings generated by the purely *economic*

Table 4-1. Comparative Statistics for Kaiser and California—1965

	Kaiser		California	Ratio of Kaiser to California	
	Northern California	*Southern California*		*North*	*South*
1. Hospital beds/1,000	1.73	1.66	3.39	0.51	0.49
1a. Age Adjusted	1.99		3.39	.59	—
2. Hospital days/1,000	532	520	891	.60	.58
2a. Age Adjusted	612	—	891	.69	—
3. Average Daily Cost of Hospitalization	$56.06	—	$63.48	.88	—
4. Average Length of Stay	6.6	6.0	6.5	1.02	.92
5. Annual Hospital Cost per Person	$29.82	—	$56.06	.53	—
5a. Age Adjusted	$34.30	—	$56.06	.61	—
6. Physicians/1,000	.925	.906	1.26	.73	.72
7. Physician Visits per Person	4.63	—	4.91[a]	.94	—
8. Per Capita Cost of Physician Services	$44.32	—	{ $67.	.66	—
			{ $88.	.50	—
9. Other Related Expenses per Capita	$ 7.69	—	$ 8.76	.88	—
10. Total Per Capita Expenses	$81.83	$83.87	{ 131.82	.62	.64
			{ 152.82	.54	.55

[a]Western United States: July 1963–June 1964.

Source: National Advisory Commission on Health Manpower [1967], p. 209.

incentives inherent in prepayment and the essentially *technical* properties of production in a group practice setting.

At the broadest level, a group medical practice may be defined as the rendering of medical services by three or more physicians organized to provide medical care through the joint use of equipment and personnel, with the income from the practice distributed according to a predetermined scheme, and with services being rendered either on a fee-for-service basis or under some prepayment plan.[a] Group practice arrangements are widely believed to yield so-called *economies of scale.* Precisely defined, the latter are said to exist if the unit cost of producing a commodity decreases as its rate of output increases.

Prepayment in health care delivery, on the other hand, is best thought of as a purely financial arrangement between potential consumers of health services and some organization—not necessarily controlled by physicians— that obligates itself to render to enrolled consumers a comprehensive set of medically necessary health services against prepayment of an annual capitation fee. It is essentially a form of health insurance. The ambulatory care system coupled with this financial arrangement may be either a single group practice, a network of group practices, or a network of solo practices, or, conceivably, a mixture of both group and solo practices. Inpatient care may be rendered either in facilities owned by the organization or under a contractual arrange-ment with legally independent inpatient facilities.

Prepayment and Health Manpower Utilization

Prepayment for comprehensive medical care is the essential charac-teristic of the so-called Health Maintenance Organization (HMO) that has received so much attention in recent years.[b] The arrangement is thought to

[a]This definition corresponds to the official characterization of group practices adopted by the Council on Medical Service of the American Medical Association [Todd and McNamara, 1971, p. 2]. It embraces both single- and multispecialty groups. In 1969, there were 6,371 such groups in the United States whose physician members totalled 40,093 or 17.6 percent of all active nonfederal physicians in the country. Two-thirds of these groups were in the 3 to 4 physician size-category. Some authors (e.g., Roemer [1965, p. 1156]), prefer to confine the term group practice to multispecialty groups. In 1969, there were 2,418 such groups in the United States having a total membership of 24,439 physicians, or about 10.5 percent of all active nonfederal physicians. Most American group practices, it may be noted, render their services on a fee-for-service basis. In 1969 only 396 groups rendered some care on a prepaid basis, and only 85 of these rendered 50 percent or more of their services on that basis.

[b]Some authors consider the group practice setting as an integral part of any Health Maintenance Organization. It is a view apparently also taken by President Nixon in his message to Congress on a "National Health Strategy" [1971, pp. 3016–7]. In his message the President ascribed to an HMO "two essential attributes"—(a) the prepayment feature, and (b) the multispecialty group practice mode, a delivery system he likened to the super-market in retailing. However, as Paul Ellwood (one of the chief proponents of the HMO concept) has pointed out, there is no reason why the HMO concept need be wedded to the group practice setting [1971].

engender greater efficiency in both the production of health and the production of health services.[c] That expectation is based on the theory that an organization obligated to render comprehensive health care against prepaid premiums will, in the first instance, persuade its subscribers to make do with the least expensive, medically adequate configuration of health *services*—hence the frequently observed substitution of ambulatory for inpatient care in prepaid group practices. To the extent that the organization, through its medical practitioners, is sufficiently persuasive, prepayment can thus induce patients to manage their own health production process (segment C in Figure 3-1) more efficiently. There is of course the possibility that the insurer or his agents might succumb to an economic conflict of interest and persuade the insured to make do with inadequate amounts of health care. If the prepayment plan enjoys a regional monopoly, its health maintenance program would therefore have to be monitored by some regulatory agency. On the other hand, if the plan competes for subscribers with other prepayment plans or alternative delivery systems, then market forces would presumably prevent the individual plan from withholding necessary services and regulation might not be required.

In addition to inducing efficiency in the production of health, prepayment can also provide the insurer with a powerful economic incentive to produce or to procure those services actually delivered to subscribers in as efficient a manner as possible. Together, the economies achieved in the production of health and those achieved in the production of health services may well mean a significant reduction in the medical manpower required for a given population at risk.

The hypothesized effect of prepayment on health manpower utilization seems to find empirical support in the record of the major prepaid group practice plans. Some relevant statistics are presented in tables 4–2 and 4–3. The data suggest that the prepaid plans appear to get by with significantly fewer physicians per 100,000 population at risk than does the health care sector as a whole. Furthermore, the prepaid plans seem to employ relatively more physicians in the primary-care specialties than does the health-care sector as a whole.

Although the data in Tables 4–2 and 4–3 are highly suggestive, some care in their interpretation is nevertheless in order. First, the population covered by the prepaid plans tends to be younger and of relatively lower health risk than the United States population as a whole; in particular, the U.S. figures reflect a higher proportion of the chronically ill. As two spokesmen for the Kaiser Plan put it in a recent symposium on the operation of that plan: "Our members cannot be described, in a statistical sense, as representative of our general [U.S.] population. As compared with the latter, we are younger, and relatively under-represented in certain population groupings, for example, the

[c]In this connection the reader may wish to refer back to Figure 3–1 where the distinction between health- and health services-production is made graphic.

Table 4-2. Number of Physicians per 100,000 Population at Risk: Kaiser Foundation Health Plans and State Health-Care Sectors as a Whole, 1969[a]

Region	Kaiser Foundation Health Plans (Prepaid Group Practice Plans)	Health-Care Sector as a Whole	Prepaid Plans as a Percent of Health-Care Sector
Northern California	102	161	63%
Southern California	90	161	56
Oregon	67	128	52
Hawaii	83	133	62

[a]Includes only nonfederal physicians in patient care.
Source: Ellwood et al. [1971], p. II-3.

Table 4-3. Number of Physicians per 100,000 Population at Risk: Prepaid Group Practices and the United States Health-Care Sector as a Whole, 1967[a]

Medical Specialty	Prepaid Group Practice Plans[b]	U.S. Health Care Sector as a Whole	Prepaid Plans as a Percentage of U.S. Health Care Sector
General Practice and Internal Medicine	45.2	44.4	102%
Pediatrics	18.0	7.6	236
Obstetrics/Gynecology	8.1	8.5	95
General Surgery	6.5	13.4	49
Opthalmology	3.7	4.5	82
Anesthesiology	1.5	4.8	31
Pathology	1.8	3.7	49

[a]Includes only nonfederal physicians in patient care.
[b]Data for prepaid plans in the United States as a whole represent six large plans in various parts of the country. In this connection, see U.S. Department of Health, Education and Welfare, Public Health Service (1967), Table 6 in the Appendix.
Source: Adapted from data presented in Ellwood et al. [1971], p. II-4.

unemployed, the indigent, the wealthy, the self-employed and people living in rural and other non-metropolitan areas." [2] There also is evidence that members of the prepaid plans tend to obtain about 10 to 15 percent of their physician care from practitioners outside their plan.[3] This tendency by itself narrows considerably the manpower-utilization gap in Table 4-2. Finally, it may be the case that the physicians practicing under the few existing prepaid plans are not representative of the practice style that would be adopted by American physicians in general, were all of them practicing under prepaid schemes. Before the experience of existing prepaid plans can be generalized to the U.S. population as a whole, there has to be a clearer understanding of the manner in which the behavior of the individual practitioners would be brought into line with the objectives of the prepaid plans under which they would practice.

While mose of the empirical evidence on prepaid plans has been drawn from plans delivering their services through group medical practices, it is not legitimate to attribute the observed economies under these plans mainly or even partially to the group practice mode per se. Indeed, after examining the operation of the Kaiser Foundation Health Plan, the National Advisory Commission on Health Manpower came to the conclusion that, in spite of the greater efficiency widely attributed to group medical practice, the Kaiser groups were actually not able to do much about the cost per unit of service (relative to that experienced by the health care sector as a whole), and that almost all of the cost savings observed under the Kaiser Plan reflected reductions in the number of units of services required per person, that is, a reaction to the prepayment system [1967, p. 213]. To make the case for the economic superiority of group practice per se, one has to adduce evidence on economies of scale in medical practice.

Group Medical Practice and Health
Manpower Utilization

It is a widely held belief that the production of virtually any commodity is characterized by economies of scale and that the production of health services is no exception. In his *The Doctor Shortage,* for example, Rashi Fein argues that

> it would, after all, be quite unusual if there were no economies of scale in the provision of physician services. It is difficult to think of any area of activity in which economies of scale are nonexistent. While this observation cannot be considered proof that economies do exist, this writer would conclude that the "burden of proof" should be on those who deny their existence rather than on others to demonstrate that they are present [1967, p. 98].

Economies of scale in medical practice may have several sources. First, some inputs into the production process—for example, x-ray machines or autoclaves—are indivisible in the sense that they are highly specialized and can be used to capacity only for very large patient loads. Second, increases in the scale of production make possible ever finer division of tasks among inputs and thus permit specialization among even those inputs—paramedical personnel and primary-care physicians for example—that are not inherently specialized to perform only one or a narrow range of tasks. Such specialization increases the productivity of the inputs involved. Third, the precision with which the daily mix of cases coming to a medical practice can be predicted is apt to increase with the average daily rate of patient flow. Greater accuracy in this prediction, in turn, tends to permit superior scheduling of all types of health personnel and may thus increase manpower productivity. Finally, large-scale production runs usually permit bulk purchasing of at least some inputs and thus permit the purchaser to reap scale economies generated elsewhere. Large group practices, for example, have been found to enjoy economies in the procurement of drugs and medical supplies. Such economies, however, have no direct effect on manpower productivity.

The *a priori* case for the economic superiority of group medical practice has a certain intuitive appeal. The empirical evidence on the issue, however, is far less convincing and has left the matter surrounded with controversy. In examining this evidence, it is well to keep in mind the focus of our discussion: the productivity of *medical manpower*. There are, after all, at least two distinct ways in which group practices may be thought to be economically superior to solo practices, namely: (1) they may enhance the average productivity of physicians, or (2) even if they do not enhance the average productivity of physicians, they may still permit greater efficiency in the use of other medical inputs (such as equipment, floor space, or auxiliary personnel) and thereby lower the unit costs of medical services.[d] If one's concern is solely with the unit cost of medical services, this distinction would, of course, be sheer pedantry. If one is concerned with future requirements of physician manpower, on the other hand, the distinction clearly is not trivial.

One of the earliest studies on the economics of group medical practice is an analysis of Canadian group and solo practices by J.A. Boan [1966]. In that study, Boan comes to the conclusion that "according to the evidence available it appears that productivity per physician is higher in a group setting, other things being equal, than in solo practice" [p. 5]. Since Boan's study is still widely quoted [4] and at least parts of his argumentation are representative of the case generally made for group practice, his study furnishes a convenient anchor for a critical examination of the group practice concept.

Boan begins his analysis with the proposition that group practice permits the division of labor to be carried further than is possible in solo practice. "If specialization and division of labor is more easily accomplished in a group practice setting," he argues, "then there is a strong *prima facie* case that productivity is higher" [p. 23], for some of the effects of specialization will be of a sort that permit "the physician to spend more of his working day on purely medical matters while someone else takes care of the remainder of the work" [p. 24]. This hypothesis is eminently plausible *a priori*. Yet Boan's test of the hypothesis is highly suspect.

[d]Consider the hypothetical case in which task delegation to the technically or legally feasible limit leaves the physician with a patient flow that employs him fully but employs his aide only two-thirds of a full-time equivalent. (It may, of course, still pay him to employ the aide.) If three physicians, each in precisely this situation, formed a group practice, their own productivity would not thereby be increased, but they might get by with only two aides nearly fully employed.

The most glaring shortcoming of Boan's empirical analysis is that it is developed without resort to some measure of output, presumably because such a measure was not available at the time. To circumvent this difficulty, Boan proposes an indirect test based on the theory of factor (input) markets. If one assumes that the "[medical care] market mechanism allocates resources roughly in line with their contribution to production" [pp. 24–25], he argues, then it may be concluded that interpractice differences in the number of aides employed per physician reflect primarily interpractice differences in the contribution aides make to the output from the practices, other things being equal. In plainer English, if medical practitioners behaved like competitive businessmen, then they could be assumed to hire additional aides up to the point at which the value of the additional practice output generated by the aides just ceases to cover the additional outlays on salaries and fringe benefits. Since physicians pay aides roughly the same salary regardless of their mode of practice, one could then assume that in a practice mode (e.g., group practice) found to employ relatively more aides per physician, the productivity of aides must be correspondingly higher. If this were not so (in other words, "if there [were] no difference in productivity when physicians are assisted by nurses, technicians and clerical personnel in the provision of medical services") Boan goes on, then "those who employ fewer aides should have higher incomes, on the average, than those who employ more. In this case those who employ more helpers would be doing so [merely] because they find it convenient to make use of such assistance"; they would be trading some income for greater ease of practice [p. 25]. According to Boan, his hypothesis is therefore maintained if, relative to solo practitioners, group practitioners employ more aides per physician *and* enjoy higher incomes. It is a line of argument frequently followed by those who favor the group practice concept.

Table 4–4, taken directly from Boan's study, indicates the staffing pattern in Canadian solo and group practices revealed by a survey of medical

Table 4–4. Reported Number of Nurses, Technicians, and Clerical Personnel Employed per Doctor, in Group Practice and in Solo Practice, Canada, 1960[a]

Categories of Employees	Group Practice	Solo Practice	
		General	Specialist
Nurses	0.5	0.3	0.3
Technicians	0.4	0.05	0.07
Clerical and Other	1.0	0.4	0.5
Total Employees	1.9	0.8	0.9

[a]Based on data from the Questionnaire on the Economics of Medical Practice, administered by the Royal Commission on Health Services to all physicians and surgeons in Canada, March 1962.

Source: J.A. Boan [1966], Table 3–2.

practices in 1962. It is seen that group practitioners in that year appeared to employ roughly twice as many aides per physician as did solo practitioners. At the same time, Boan points out, the average income of group practitioners was significantly higher than that of solo practitioners [p. 25]. "From this it follows," Boan concludes, "that medical productivity is higher in group practice, since otherwise it would not be possible to employ so much assistance and have net incomes that are higher than solo practitioners [sic]" [p. 28].

To further buttress his case, Boan develops a statistic defined by him as "the average cost per physician of employing nurses, technicians and other non-medical staff, on a per employee basis" [p. 30]. His estimates of this statistic for solo and group practices are reproduced in Table 4–5. These estimates lead Boan to assert, once again, that "on the basis of these figures [column 3 of Table 4–5] it would seem that doctors in group practice can make more efficient use of paramedical and nonmedical personnel than can doctors in solo practice" [p. 30].

Although Boan's first test—a test quite commonly applied in support of group practice—does have the appearance of plausibility, his second test is puzzling indeed. It can be seen from Table 4–5 that Boan arrived at his "average cost of employing aides per doctor per employee" by dividing the "average cost per doctor" by the "number [of aides] employed per doctor." From the discussion surrounding the table it is not clear precisely how the "average cost per doctor" is defined. Since the cost of "medical and office equipment" is broken out as a separate category, however, one must assume that the cost data in Table 4–5 reflect essentially the salaries and fringe benefits of aides and exclude the cost of equipment. If so, then the data in the table are disturbing, for on the reasonable assumption that the salaries received by auxiliary personnel do not vary systematically and strongly with the physician's mode of practice, one would have expected the figures in column 3 to be roughly the same for all practice modes and close to the average salary and fringe benefits paid aides

Table 4–5. Average Annual Cost per Physician of Employing Nurses, Technicians, and Other Nonmedical Staff, on a per Employee Basis, in Group Practice and in Solo Practice, Canada, 1960, and in Six Groups, 1962

	Number Employed per Doctor	Average Cost per Doctor	Average Cost per Doctor per Employee
Six Private Group Practices	2.17	$6,272	$2,890
Group Practice	1.9	5,800	3,052
Solo General	0.8	5,900	7,375
Solo Specialist	0.9	6,840	7,600

Source: J.A. Boan [1966], Table 3–6. For notes to the table, the reader is referred to the original source.

during the year of the underlying survey. In that case, Boan's data raise the interesting question why solo practitioners seem to pay their aides more than do group practitioners,[e] but the data shed no light on the relative productivity of health manpower in group and solo practice. (In fairness to the advocates of group practice, it must be added that this part of Boan's analysis is not typical of the general argument made for that practice mode.)

But even Boan's first test is open to question, its plausibility notwithstanding. There is evidence (to be presented in Chapter Five) that the typical physician does *not* optimize his staffing pattern in the hypothesized manner; instead, both solo and group practitioners appear to fall short of the optimal staff size competitive businessmen would hire. Since Boan's empirical analysis is only as valid as the assumptions on which it rests, his indirect test therefore loses much of its power. Boan's conclusions, however, may be questioned also on at least two other grounds. The first of these has to do with the composition of the auxiliary staff in solo and group practices. The second centers on the composition of output in solo and group practice and on the effect of differences in the output mix on observed physician income.

Boan's data suggest that one type of manpower of which group practices seem to make particularly heavy use (relative to solo practices) is the category of "clerical and other personnel." Furthermore, his data also reveal that within his sample of group practices, the number of clerical aides per physician increases with the size of the group while the number of nurses or technicians per physician tends to decrease with practice size [p. 27]. A strikingly similar pattern can be detected also in data from Douglas Egan's analysis of member clinics in the U.S. Medical Group Management Association [1969, p. III-2]. These results permit two alternative interpretations. The proponents of group practice—Boan among them [p. 28]—regard the results as support for the hypothesis that group practitioners devote a greater proportion of their time to purely medical tasks, leaving the business side of their practice in the hands of administrative and clerical personnel. But one may also take the phenomenon as evidence for the hypothesis that group practices tend to be relatively less efficient than solo practices in their use of personnel, or that the problem simply of coordinating large groups of professionals generates added red tape and other diseconomies of scale.

[e]From private communication with the author it appears that the "total cost [of aides] per doctor" is the sample average of the reported amounts paid by physicians for auxiliary personnel, and the "number employed per doctor" is the sample average of the number of aides employed. Column 3 of Table 4-5 probably reflects the fact that the cost per doctor was obtained by averaging reported outlays on aides over only those physicians who reported actually having had such outlays, while the number of aides per doctor was obtained by averaging over all physicians in the sample, whether or not they employed aides. Since many solo practitioners do not employ any aides (while practically all group practitioners do), this statistical error could easily account for the fact that "average cost per doctor per employee" in solo practice is more than twice as high as that reported for group practices. In fact, the group practice figures in column 3 of Table 4-5 do seem close to the average annual salaries of Canadian paramedical personnel in 1962, the year of the underlying survey.

In his analysis of private solo practices, single-specialty group practices and several large-scale outpatient hospital clinics, Joseph Newhouse [1973] sees support for the latter hypothesis. Newhouse preambles his empirical analysis with the so-called "theory of groups," according to which individual members of any partnership lose their economic incentive to work for the welfare of the group as its size increases. The theory is based on the plausible assumption that individuals ultimately pursue their own economic interest. Since in a partnership the good or bad consequences of any individual act will be shared by all members of the group, the individual's incentive to contribute positively or to prevent negative effects (such as unnecessary costs) is correspondingly lessened.

Newhouse finds the theory of groups confirmed in a comparison of the "total overhead cost per patient visit" observed in the hospital outpatient clinics with that observed in the private solo or group practices. In that comparison, overhead costs are defined as all nonphysician costs except the cost of space and of ancillary services such as x-rays, EKG tests, and so on. The activities covered by this overhead figure thus include billing and cashiering costs, medical record-keeping, administration, registration, household and property, and institutional overhead charged by the hospital to its clinics, and so on. The data indicate overhead cost per visit of $14.24 for the clinics and of $4.54 for the private solo and single-specialty group practices. The billings and cashiering costs per visit were $2.07 in the clinics and $0.46 in the private practice, the corresponding figures for medical record-keeping were $1.13 and $0.35., respectively. Newhouse views these results as "extremely strong confirmation" of the hypothesis that clinics tend to be relatively more inefficient in their use of medical inputs and that there may be "simply too many warm bodies at clinics" [p. 43].

Newhouse may be entirely correct in asserting that the typical hospital outpatient clinic in this country is highly inefficient in its use of medical resources. In 1970, for example, the average cost per patient visit in the outpatient departments of New York City hospitals was $33.15, and between $50 and $60 for a good many of these hospitals.[5] The data referred to above, however (Newhouse's Table 1), do not by themselves justify that conclusion. *A priori*, one has no assurance that the higher *nonphysician* costs per visit in the clinics are not more than offset by lower *physician* costs per visit. Suppose, for example, that one compared two types of medical practitioners: one type employing an average of two aides per physician, the other not employing any aides at all. A comparison simply of non-physician overhead costs per visit would obviously indicate a much higher figure for the first type of practitioner than for the second. But one could surely not infer from this comparison that physicians of the second type are relatively more efficient in their use of medical resources. On the contrary, if one compared these practices on the cost of *physician time* per visit spent on billing, record-keeping, and so on, one would almost certainly have to conclude that physicians without aides, by failing to delegate these clerical chores to less expensive clerical personnel, are wholly inefficient in the use of their own time. The failure to employ the technically permissible least-cost mix of personnel is just as serious a source of inefficiency as is the failure to use personnel, once hired, to maximum effect.[f]

In the particular case under discussion, there is also the question of whether individual cost components of hospital outpatient clinics can be meaningfully compared with those of private solo or single-specialty groups. First, the clinics are by nature multispecialty groups who presumably maintain comprehensive medical records on the whole patient. From the article it is not clear how a visit to the clinic is defined, but conceivably such a visit may lead to a patient-physician contact with more than one medical specialist. If so, a comparison of costs per visit is suspect. Furthermore, the outpatient clinics of hospitals typically serve members of the lower income classes whose processing simply requires much paperwork. One would suppose, for example, that the billing and cashiering function in private practices is an intrinsically simpler task than it is in hospital outpatient departments.

As a further test of his hypothesis, Newhouse estimates a statistical relationship between total office salary costs per visit (excluding the personnel cost of producing ancillary services), on the one hand, and the monthly number of office visits and the mode of practice, on the other. This analysis appears to be confined solely to the sample of private solo and single-specialty group practitioners. The results indicate that, *for given visit rates*, medical practice with cost-sharing arrangements tends to increase the salary costs as defined above—precisely what the theory of groups would predict. The same result is observed also for each of the individual components of the total cost figure (that is, the salary costs of record-keeping, billings, and appointments).

This finding is decidedly contrary to the popular notion that "economies are to be had if ten to a hundred physicians practice together rather than one, through the economic use of space, of secretarial help, of equipment, and so on" [Harris 1964, p. 140] , for it must be remembered that this part of Newhouse's analysis is confined solely to private practitioners in solo and single specialty group practices. To be sure, even this part of Newhouse's analysis is open to criticism. The sample included only 20 practitioners and the results appear to have been dominated by one extreme observation [p. 47] . There is no control for the possible effects of medical specialty on costs, or for possible interpractice variation in the nature of the output produced. It might, for example, be argued once again that the higher clerical costs per visits observed under cost-sharing simply means that cost-sharing physicians delegate a higher

---

[f]Economists refer to inefficient use of inputs actually hired and at the producer's disposition as "technical inefficiency" or "X-inefficiency." A failure to employ the least-cost from among alternative, technically feasible input combinations is referred to as "economic inefficiency" or "Y-inefficiency." In the evaluation of his Table 1, Newhouse concentrates solely on X-inefficiency without considering the possibility that clinics may conceivably be characterized by higher Y-inefficiency.

proportion of their clerical and administrative chores to assistants and are hence able to devote more time per visit to purely medical matters. In that case, the observed cost differential may actually reflect a highly efficient form of task delegation. Even so, Newhouse's study does at least entitle one to question the prevailing orthodoxy on group medical practice. It is entirely conceivable that, while economies in the use of some types of manpower are *technically* feasible in a group practice setting, the *economic behavior* of professionals in groups engenders inefficiencies that more than offset the technical economies potentially available.

The contention by Boan and other advocates of group practice that the typically higher incomes of group practitioners document the economic superiority of that practice mode also is open to question. The argument over-looks the fact that the mix of services rendered by large group practices tends to differ substantially from that produced in solo practices. In his by now well-known study of solo and group internists in the San Francisco Bay area, for example, Richard Bailey found that while the group practitioners in his sample did enjoy higher gross and net incomes than did their colleagues in solo prac-tice, the extra income represented for the most part revenues from the sale of ancillary services. Specifically, the percentage of gross revenues earned through the sale of ancillary services was 15, 34, and 48 percent, respectively, for solo internists, internists in small single-specialty groups, and internists in large multispecialty groups. Bailey also suggests that by virtue of their higher income from ancillary services, internists in the larger groups could apparently afford to work 20 to 25 hours fewer per month than solo practitioners and 10 hours fewer per month than internists in small single-specialty groups.

Finally, Bailey observed that internists in group practices do not seem to push task delegation any further than do solo internists, and that the latter actually handled a larger volume of patient visits per month and per hour than did group internists. This observation is consistent with the pre-viously cited study by Yankauer et al. who found that "patient care task dele-gation by 394 pediatricians in [multispecialty] groups was distinctly less common than task delegation by 739 solo practitioners, 277 two-man, 287 three-man and 130 four-man pediatric [single] specialty groupings" [1970, p. 45]. In its analysis of the Kaiser Foundation medical groups, the National Advisory Commission on Health Manpower also had mentioned that

> the study group [did not] find evidence of major innovations in the practice of medicine; Kaiser physicians use standard medical practices and procedures during their contacts with patients and there does not appear to be unusual substitution of auxiliary per-sonnel for physicians [1967, Vol. II, p. 207].

It may be suggested that, if one adopts the broad definition of physician services proposed in Chapter Three, then the higher rate of ancillary services rendered by group internists ought to be viewed as a bona fide increase in physician productivity. Such an argument would overlook the fact that the phenomenon observed by Bailey is likely to reflect merely a shift in the locus of production of these services: the solo practitioners in his sample simply sent their patients to outside facilities for such services. This shift in the locus of production will clearly not add to physician productivity, unless the shift itself causes certain necessary services to be produced that were not rendered prior to the shift.

It can even be argued that a shift in the production of ancillary services from specialized outside facilities to the physician's practice will not only fail to enhance physician productivity in the aggregate, but may also serve to *increase* the average cost of these services. In view of the specialized and indivisible equipment typically used in the production of ancillary services, their production is undoubtedly subject to significant scale economies. If one assumes that physicians who do not own the necessary equipment subcontract such services to large, specialized producers—such as hospitals or laboratories—that can in fact realize these economies, then it may very well be that the internalization of the production process in a group practice will involve production at a scale that is suboptimal and unnecessarily costly.[g]

In a later paper growing directly out of his earlier work cited above, Bailey proposes a model of medical practice in which the latter is viewed as a multiproduct firm whose product line becomes ever more extensive as the scale of the firm increases [1970]. To examine the effect of practice mode (or scale) on the productivity of individual inputs, Bailey argues, it is first necessary to disaggregate the overall output from medical practices into distinct product (service) lines, each characterized by a separate and unique production process. In Bailey's view, it is then analytically appropriate to divide the entire set of products into subsets whose elements are technically related to one another through sharing some "dominant input." Thus elements of the subset of "physician products" share physician time as their dominant input; the elements of the subset "ancillary services" share medical technicians as their dominant input, and so on. The point Bailey seeks to make is that no product in one subset is necessarily a joint product with any other product in a different subset. Consequently, their production processes may be treated as technically independent, and the addition of products in one subset need have no effect whatsoever on the production process for services in other subsets. The model considerably weakens the *a priori* case for economies of scale in medical practice.

[g]In fact, one need not be excessively cynical to suggest that the presence of, say, an x-ray machine on the premises of a medical practice will encourage its use beyond the absolutely necessary or even the medically safe. There is, after all, the pressure to amortize such equipment. It may therefore be that well-equipped group practices, particularly those selling their services on a fee-for-service basis, will over-supply their patients with ancillary services, thus driving up the cost of medical treatment even further.

Bailey's model is a plausible specification and capable of resolving the apparent paradox that, on the one hand, large group practices are typically observed to employ more auxiliary personnel per physician than do smaller practices, while, on the other, the physicians in large group practices are not observed to treat more patients per hour or to push the delegation of medical tasks to assistants any further than do their colleagues in solo practice or small partnerships. According to the theory, the number of aides per physician increases with practice size not because of more extensive substitution of paramedical for physician time, but simply because large practices offer a more extensive product line and the added products require additional paramedical personnel for their production. This model and the empirical foundation on which it rests are, of course, a complete invalidation of the thesis that higher ratios of paramedical-to-medical personnel and higher physician incomes in group practice are *prima facie* evidence of enhanced physician productivity in that setting.

Although one is inclined to accept Bailey's interpretation of the data on group practices, his paper does contian some subtle flaws. Bailey, it will be recalled, found that in the production of strictly "physician products," group practitioners did not push task delegation any further than did solo practitioners. According to him, this suggests that the possibility of increasing physician productivity through task delegation is, in general, quite limited [1970, pp. 270-1]. That inference ought not to be drawn from the data. As is shown later in this chapter (Tables 4-7 to 4-9), there appears to be considerable room for augmenting physician productivity (in the production of what Bailey calls "physician services") through health manpower substitution. The fact that physicians have so far failed to take advantage of this potential seems to reflect not the technical infeasibility of task delegation but, first, a lack of economic pressure on physicians to conduct their practice efficiently, and second, a penchant for traditional patterns of practice or perhaps even a fear of malpractice suits.

It should also be recognized that even if, as Bailey suggests, the *technology* of health-care production as such is essentially invariant to scale or practice mode—that is, even if the production processes for distinct medical services tend to be characterized by so-called "constant returns to scale"[h] and these processes are intrinsically unrelated to one another—the technology of any production process is but one part of a much wider economic decision framework. Intrinsically independent production processes do become related to one another if they are managed by a single decisionmaker within the confines of a single practice where they can be made to share certain inputs that need not be

[h]A production process is characterized by *constant returns to scale* if an increase of the same proportion in all rates of input increases output by the same proportion as well. Increasing returns to scale would prevail if output were to increase more than proportionately.

shared on purely technical grounds. Physician-support personnel, for example, is normally hired on the basis of 40 or so hours per week, rather than on an hourly basis. Large group practices may be able to spread these blocks of paramedical-aide time over several intrinsically independent production processes and thus find it economically attractive to delegate some of the physicians' workload to aides, while a solo practitioner, facing precisely the same *technical* opportunity for task delegation, might find that task delegation *economically* unattractive because the delegatable tasks do not fill an aide's entire workweek. (This economic interdependence among technically independent processes is easiest brought out in the context of a so-called activity-analysis model, described briefly in Chapter Five and at greater length in Golladay et al. [1974], Reinhardt [1973b] and Smith et al. [1972].) It is in this indirect way that group practice may permit the realization of some gains in physician productivity not economically justifiable in solo practice. This is quite obviously an aspect of the hypothesis Boan sought, but failed, to support with his data.

Some advocates of group practice find the economist's preoccupation with manpower productivity or scale economies entirely misplaced. From the writing of the Somers' [1961], for example, it is clear that they see the main benefits of that practice mode not so much as a reduction in the unit cost of its services as in their superior quality [p. 507]. The more important sources of higher quality are seen to be the continuity of care made possible in an organization in which comprehensive patient files can easily be transferred from specialist to specialist, and the formal and informal peer review group practice is thought to engender.

It may be argued that these quality gains, while not reducing the physician input per unit of service, should nevertheless lead to a reduction in the medical manpower required to maintain given populations at a given overall health level. Such an argument would be compelling. As the Somers' warn, however,

> it does not follow that this form of organization provides automatic quality control. As already noted, group practice—especially in large urban clinics—is liable to certain abuses, not unlike those in other large corporations, which may reflect themselves in the quality of care—impersonality, factionalism, and favoritism in financial affairs. Overemphasis on business at the expense of patient care appears to be the chief complaint of doctors who have left group practice [p. 116].

The late Richard Weinerman, widely recognized as an authority on health-care delivery systems, has offered similarly sobering observations on the group practice mode. According to Weinerman, "Group conferences, medical audits, and informal office consultations . . . [are] common in the descriptive literature but infrequent in daily practice." [6] Weinerman was further persuaded to the view that multi-specialty groups are in danger of becoming mere assemblies of medical specialists whose individualist practice style seems to be "increasingly irrelevant to the health needs of unselected populations." [7] In this respect, Weinerman is echoed by sociologist Eliot Freidson who, from a slightly different perspective, has offered the caveat:

> When men work together in the same place, on the same terms, and with common work problems, they will develop a set of standards and procedures by which to judge and manage those problems, and they will discourage deviation from those standards. . . . [But merely] the fact of participating together in the same organized setting provides no assurance that the actual standards colleagues do agree upon and enforce will be either technically or socially adequate: the only assurance is that there will be standards of some kind and that they are likely to be narrower and better enforced than if the same men were scattered through a variety of settings [1970, pp. 220–222].

Why or how the chosen standard of quality will deviate from "socially adequate" norms is not made clear, but presumably the author has in mind an undue emphasis on intellectually interesting medicine at the expense of the more routine health-care needs of patients.

One is left, then, with the following conclusions concerning the economic merits of group medical practice *per se*: There is reason to believe that group practice may, on balance, enhance the quality of health services, particularly if different specialties are brought together under one roof. It is equally reasonable to suppose that treatment of illness in multispecialty groups can yield substantial savings in patients' time, a valuable resource that is all too often treated as a free good by physicians and economists alike. It was argued above that under certain circumstances the group practice mode can effectively resolve the problem of input indivisibility, thus enhancing somewhat the productivity of at least some inputs, including perhaps the productivity of physicians. Finally, the group practice mode affords physicians the luxury of a relatively more regular, predictable work schedule. Since the solo practitioner's unpredictable work schedule is often cited as a justification for high physician income, this particular attribute of group medical practice represents no small benefit. From the narrower viewpoint of health manpower policy adopted in this book, however, the formation of group practices is not likely to constitute a significant development. This is not to say that such a practice mode is not to be preferred to solo practice on any of the other grounds enumerated above. It merely means that there is no reason, *a priori*, to expect significant economies in the use of physician time from group practice per se, and that there is no empirical evidence to suggest otherwise.

II. INPUT SUBSTITUTION AND
PHYSICIAN PRODUCTIVITY

The Substitution of Equipment and Supplies
for Medical Manpower

Americans are almost unrivaled in their ingenuity of substituting labor-saving devices for manpower. In industries whose output is fairly standard—for example, in agriculture or automobile manufacture—that type of input substitution has typically enabled a given pool of manpower to service ever-increasing populations. In the health-care sector, however, the infusion of capital tends to alter the nature of the product and frequently renders existing services or procedures obsolete. Consequently, greater capital-intensity in the production of health services does not automatically generate economies in the use of health manpower.

There can be no doubt that sophisticated medical equipment has significantly improved physicians' ability to maintain or restore their patients' health. Devices rendering cardiac assist or capable of filtering human blood to remove toxic substances (renal dialysis) are only the more dramatic examples of such equipment. It is now possible to examine patients with internal probes that transmit diagnostic information to an external receiver via telemetry. New machinery enables surgeons to maintain and repair a kidney outside the patient's body and to reimplant it hours later. And a computer-based x-ray system recently developed at Georgetown University enables physicians to obtain cross-sectional profiles of any part of the human body with unprecedented accuracy, thus eliminating much of the need for exploratory surgery.[8] If one defines the output of the health-care sector in terms of some unchanged concept of health status (e.g., age-specific morbidity and mortality of patients treated), then these and similar technical breakthroughs must surely be viewed as sources of increased physician productivity. In assessing the economic impact of these productivity gains, however, a distinction must be made between those gains likely to result in a reduction in the overall physician requirement for given populations at risk, and those almost automatically offset by technology-induced increases in the demand for physician time.

There are a number of areas in which more intensive use of capital does enable physicians to serve a larger population. At the very basic level, it should be possible to enhance the physician's hourly patient load simply by placing at his disposition two or more examination rooms so that little of his time is wasted while patients prepare themselves for examination. A spacious and well-designed floor plan may also enhance the average productivity of the physician's auxiliary staff. (For empirical evidence on the effect of examination rooms on health manpower productivity, see Table 4–8.) Similarly, while the bulk of the medical supplies and instruments in medical practice are complements of the physician and his aides, significant productivity gains can undoubtedly be achieved by substituting disposable medical and surgical kits for some activities of health manpower.

Some time in the future, picture-phones, telemetry, and two-way television will probably be used to monitor chronically ill patients in extended care facilities—or convalescent patients in their homes—without requiring frequent direct physician-patient contact. Furthermore, with the aid of high-resolution two-way television and a network of centrally located computers and remote terminals, it should one day be possible to introduce in the United States a latter-day version of the Russian feldsher system. Under such a system, the primary entry point for patients in areas short of medical manpower (remote rural locations or depressed urban centers) would be a paramedical assistant linked via a two-way television system to medical specialists in some hospital or clinic. Guidance on when and when not to consult the specialists could be given the paramedic through direct access to decision algorithms stored in a centrally located computer. The link to the computer could also be used to transmit to the physician results from any diagnostic tests the paramedic may have performed (perhaps with the aid of automated test devices) and the patient's medical history. Such a system, which is already technically feasible, may well turn out to be the only practical answer to the seemingly chronic maldistribution of medical manpower in this country. Finally, two way communication via high-resolution television and the computer may permit some economies also in the staffing of regional hospital networks. Through such a communications system physicians in different locations can maintain audio-visual contact with one another, and one specialist (such as a radiologist) may be able to service several small hospitals from one location. The implementation of that kind of system does, of course, presuppose a serious commitment to regional planning.

In principle, computers could also be used as a partial substitute for the physician's skill in face-to-face contacts with patients. Until now, the health industry has used computers mainly for certain housekeeping chores such as scheduling and accounting. The true potential of the computer, however, lies in its ability to act as an "intellectual" and "deductive" instrument, that is, as a consultant to which the individual physician can turn during his examination of patients. William B. Schwartz, one of the few physicians who has actually experimented with this use of computers, has suggested that

> it seems probable that in the not too distant future the physician and the computer will engage in frequent dialogue, the computer continuously taking note of history, physical findings, laboratory data, and the like, alerting the physician to the most probable diagnoses and suggesting the appropriate, safest course of action. ... One may thus project a revolution in the health-care system in which the importance of remembering facts is sharply reduced, the decision-making process is aided and abetted by computers, and

many tasks formerly in the domain of the physician are taken over
by a consortium of computers and paramedical personnel [1970,
p. 1258].

The development projected by Schwartz strikes one as input substitution in the classical sense. But it is difficult to predict its impact on future
physician requirements. If recourse to the computer's logic and memory substantially enhances the accuracy of the physician's diagnosis—and hence the
effectiveness of his intervention—then greater use of the computer may well
reduce the amount of physician time required to manage given medical conditions. Under these circumstances a given population could be adequately cared
for by a smaller number of physicians than are currently required.

Yet it is conceivable that diagnostic-assist devices of the sort contemplated by Schwartz will inevitably inflate the patient's conception of what constitutes "quality care." Physicians who are sensitive to their patients' preferences
may then feel compelled to engage in time-consuming consultation with the
computer even in cases where that improves little on the physician's initial diagnosis. If that pattern of care were to become popular, the physician and his
computer would gradually come to be viewed as complements. It would then be
entirely possible that the introduction of computers into medical practice would,
on balance, add to the number of physicians required to serve a given population
"adequately." The beneficial side effects of that development would, of course,
be a standardization of the quality of physician care, and an overall elevation of
acceptable standards of quality. The question remains, however, whether the
added quality would be worth the added cost in medical manpower and equipment.

The preceding considerations can probably be generalized to the
bulk of modern equipment used in patient care. For the most part, the availability of such equipment permits physicians to perform otherwise impossible
procedures, to restore health in otherwise untreatable cases, and to maintain
life in otherwise hopeless cases. As was suggested earlier, the availability of this
wider range of services unquestionably enhances the physician's contribution
to the health-production process. But the introduction of sophisticated medical
equipment also tends to increase the demand for physician services. First,
patients with hitherto untreatable conditions will demand treatment if it
becomes feasible, and such treatment may be highly physician-intensive. Second,
those patients whose life is prolonged with the aid of modern equipment often
place a continued and heavy additional demand on the physician's time. Finally,
consumers in general tend to adjust rather quickly to technical progress in
medicine and expect the application of new technology even if it is both capital
and manpower intensive.

As noted earlier, in principle it should be possible to substitute
capital for health manpower in the production of a given set of health services,

and in some instances such capital-labor substitution undoubtedly takes place. The point developed in this section is that, in practice, the infusion of capital into the production of health care also facilitates the production of new types of services for which a demand is created by the mere existence of the new, capital-using technologies. If one can judge from past experience in this area, a realistic prognosis seems to be that any future health manpower savings achieved through bona fide capital-labor substitution in the health care sector is likely to be offset—and perhaps even more than offset—by capital-induced increases in the demand for health care, and hence in the demand for all types of health manpower. Such an outcome obviously does not make greater capital intensity in health care production an unattractive proposition. One merely should not expect the infusion of capital into the health care sector to permit reductions in the aggregate physician-population ratio in future years.

The Substitution of Paramedical for Medical Manpower

In Chapter Three it was suggested that the management of a patient's medical condition—an acute or potential illness, real or imagined— is best thought of as a series of tasks coordinated by one or more physicians acting as the patient's "management consultants." A number of these tasks—inpatient care, for example—can be performed only by specialized facilities and fall outside the range of tasks normally considered "physician services." Some of the latter—x-rays or laboratory tests, for example—may be performed by outside facilities as well; but they also can be and often are performed on the premises of a physician's practice, either by him or by his staff.

The set of "physician services" may be further divided into "clerical," "data gathering," "diagnostic," and "therapeutic" tasks. The first of these categories includes the purely clerical chore of running a medical practice. By data gathering is meant the retrieval of diagnostic information from patients (either through physical examination, the drawing of body specimens, or the taking of patient histories) and the processing of that information (in laboratory related tasks) for subsequent diagnosis—the third category. Finally, the category of therapeutic tasks includes the administration of medications or immunizations, the suturing and dressing of wounds, minor and major surgery, the counselling of patients concerning diets and drug regimens, and so on. Together, the data gathering, diagnostic, and therapeutic tasks constitute the so-called "patient-care" tasks.

Within categories, tasks may be arrayed according to the degree of technical competence and medical judgment they require. For practical purposes it is reasonable to assume that if the physician chose to do so, he could perform all of the tasks within each of the four categories. With the exception of some administrative and entrepreneurial tasks, however, virtually all of the clerical chores can be delegated to nonmedical personnel working either in the physician's practice or in outside billing and bookkeeping services. Many of the patient-care tasks also require only modest skill and can safely be delegated to so-called allied or lower-level health workers who, incidentally, could also perform most of the clerical chores. Typical examples of low-skill patient-care tasks are the weighing and measuring of patients, the taking of blood pressure or temperature, the administration of screening tests for vision and hearing, the drawing of body specimens or the taking of a basic history, simple types of therapy, and direct assistance to physicians in the performance of specific medical procedures and minor surgery. None of these tasks involves medical judgment.

In principle, the low-skill patient-care tasks could be delegated also to intermediate-level health workers, commonly referred to as physician extenders. This category of manpower includes the newly emerging Physician Assistants or Medex, pediatric nurse practitioners or child health associates, midwives, family nurse practitioners, and experienced registered nurses. Unless input indivisibility dictates otherwise,[k] the delegation of low-skill tasks to physician extenders is clearly wasteful, for the latter are competent enough to perform higher-skill tasks (such as complete well-child care, the diagnosis and treatment of moderately ill patients, the suturing and dressing of uncomplicated wounds, the application of more complex therapies, the counselling of patients regarding their diet and drug regimens, and last but by no means least, the rendering of comfort and psychological support to patients). Physician extenders could also function as the patient's primary contact in under-doctored areas. Finally, some bold visionaries would entrust to them even tasks now thought to lie solely within the physician's province. In testimony before the U.S. Senate Health Committee, for example, William Schwartz argued that

> there seems little question that physician's assistants, taking patient histories, carrying out physical examinations, and administering intravenous fluids, can greatly augment the efficiency of the doctor and thus contribute to the relief of the physician shortage. I would like to suggest, however, that this approach to the use of non-physicians is much too limited. It is conceivable that by going further we can produce a revolution in the use of health manpower in which the physician's efforts are truly reserved for those tasks which require his high level of skill, education and intellect. I am suggesting, in other words, that if we undertake a rigorous analysis of what the doctor does, we will almost certainly find that a substantial number of his tasks, now considered sacrosanct, could be done instead by skilled technicians who could be quickly trained for single specialized tasks: for example, to diagnose and treat simple fractures, remove an appendix, strip varicose veins, carry out thera-

[k]Input indivisibility in this context refers to the fact that health manpower can be hired only in discrete units; for example, in blocks of 40 hours per week.

peutic abortions, or perform needle biopsies of the kidney and liver. Such new uses of manpower could well free a significant additional fraction of the physician's time [1971, p. 448].

Figure 4-1 represents a hypothetical division of the overall set of tasks performed by a medical practice into those that are performed by a physician, those that are delegated to physician extenders, those that are delegated to allied health workers, and those performed by nonmedical personnel. It is worth emphasizing that the diagram is a purely hypothetical illustration and is not meant to reflect the economically most desirable allocation of tasks. The point is that, given a set of medical conditions to be treated and the set of required tasks implicit therein, any development or action that moves the demarcation line between the unshaded and the lightly shaded areas to the left is apt to increase the productivity of the physicians, other things (including the quality of the overall management of the conditions) being equal. It may well be that, because of the need for supervision of physician extenders, the delegation of a task normally requiring 10 minutes of physician time to a physician extender may actually free only 8 minutes of physician time (and may require 20 minutes of the physician extender's time).[1] Even so, as long as some physician time is freed at all, task delegation will enable the physician to treat more cases per unit of time and hence increase his hourly productivity. The same argument can be made concerning the productivity of physician extenders. Any development or action that shifts the demarcation line between the lightly and darkly shaded areas to the left should, other things being equal, enhance the extenders' productivity. Finally, since health manpower in general has no comparative advantage in the performance of clerical tasks, it is self-evident that the productivity of any type of health manpower can be increased by delegating those tasks to clerical and administrative personnel, unless the problem of input indivisibility renders that delegation uneconomic.

The catch in the previous paragraph may be thought to lie in the qualifier "other things being equal." First, some students of healthcare deem it virtually impossible to delegate tasks from higher to lower level health manpower without diminishing the quality of the care being rendered. That point is addressed at the end of the book. In the meantime, we proceed on the assumption that task delegation will not be pushed to a point at which the medical soundness of the treatment is being impaired.

A second problem is that the set of tasks performed in the management of given medical conditions may not be invariant to the staffing pattern

[1]In their analysis of pediatric practices, for example, Charney and Kitsman [1971] discovered that physicians spend an average of 12.8 minutes per visit with a well child, while a pediatric nurse practitioner spends an average of 21 minutes on such a visit. In an unrelated study, Zeckhauser and Eliastam [1972] found that a pediatric nurse practitioner spending eight hours per day on well child care can replace only about four hours of a pediatrician's time.

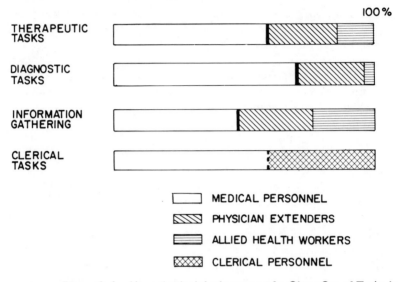

Figure 4-1. Hypothetical Assignment of a Given Set of Tasks in a Medical Practice.

(and hence the nature of task delegation) in physicians' practices. To explore this problem further, it is useful to categorize the entire set of tasks corresponding to a medical condition in yet a different manner, namely into the following.

  I. Those tasks that will always be prescribed by the physician but that will be produced on his premises only if he has the appropriate staff, failing which they will be produced by outside facilities.
 II. Those tasks the physician prescribes only if he employs sufficient staff to perform them, failing which they will not be performed at all in the management of the condition.
III. Those tasks that will always be prescribed by the physician and performed in his practice either by him (in the absence of support personnel) or by him and any staff he employs.

    If an increase in the physician's auxiliary staff merely causes him to internalize the production of type I services previously produced elsewhere, then his hourly productivity is obviously not increased, even though the gross receipts of his practice may increase substantially. Actually, it is conceivable that such a development would decrease the physician's hourly productivity in treating patients if the added personnel requires additional supervision on his part.
    Matters are more complicated if an increase in the physician's auxiliary staff results simply in additional output of type II services. One possibility is that these services may not be necessary from a strictly medical point of

view, in which case the added personnel will not enhance the physician's hourly productivity in treating patients, and may in fact lower it if the additional personnel must be closely supervised by him. But it is also conceivable that the added services so enhance the quality of the treatment that the physician can manage given medical conditions with greater dispatch (say, with fewer physician-patient encounters). In that case, the additional personnel may indirectly enhance the physician's productivity in treating patients.

It is in the performance of type III tasks that the employment of additional aides can make the greatest contribution to physician productivity. Careful task analysis of medical practices with a variety of staffing patterns, and in a variety of medical specialties, has indicated that far too many physicians still routinely perform tasks that could just as safely be performed by intermediate- and lower-level health workers or by clerical personnel.[9] There is also evidence that where intermediate-level health workers are employed, they are usually burdened with tasks that should really be delegated to lower-level assistants.[10] In other words, neither physicians nor physician extenders seem to be used to maximum effectiveness.

One of the classic studies of this sort is an analysis of task delegation in pediatric practices by Yankauer et al. [1969, 1970] . The analysis was based on information from a mail survey of all members of the American Academy of Pediatrics residing in the United States, including roughly 90 percent of all board certified pediatricians in this country. The survey was undertaken in 1967 and achieved the unusually high response rate of 90 percent. Table 4–6, taken directly from one of the papers coming out of the study, indicates with great clarity the relationship between task delegation and the number of aides employed per pediatrician. Although it may well be that some of the aides' time was spent in the performance of type I and II tasks—see, for example, the footnote identified by an asterisk in the table—it is also clear that by increasing his staff the pediatrician is relieved of many low-skill tasks he would otherwise have performed himself. From our discussion in Chapter Two it will be recalled that the survey also showed pediatricians in the South (where the physician-population ratio is very low) to delegate a far greater number of routine tasks to auxiliary personnel than do pediatricians in New York (having one of the highest physician-population ratios in the country).

The effect of task delegation on physician productivity may be inferred from Table 4–7, also taken directly from Yankauer et al. The productivity index in that table is the median rate of weekly patient visits, a rate that may be taken as a proxy for the number of medical conditions treated and whose use as a productivity index has already been defended earlier. Several interesting conclusions emerge from this table. First, it is obvious that the number of aides per pediatrician and the degree of task delegation tends to be highly positively correlated with the number of patients seen by the pediatrician per hour or per week. Second, the presence of an intermediate-level

Table 4-6. Percentage of Times Selected Tasks Were Performed by
Pediatricians, by Total Number of Health Workers Employed in
Practice Setting[a]

	Total Number of Health Workers Employed				
	1-1.5 (N:647)	2-2.5 (N:807)	3-3.5 (N:522)	4-4.5 (N:351)	5 or more (N:1086)
Technical Tasks					
Weighing	32	9	8	1	2
Body Measurements	46	19	17	13	10
Immunizations	75	42	35	27	18
Parenteral Drugs	81	50	41	32	25
Vision Screening*	44	24	16	13	8
Hearing Screening*	54	44	39	34	22
Developmental					
Screening†	73	70	69	61	65
Laboratory Tasks					
Hemoglobin/					
Hematocrit*	44	22	18	13	4
Urinalysis	38	36	18	16	7
Blood Count/Smear*	21	17	15	9	4
Clerical Tasks					
Inventory/Supply	11	3	3	2	2
Growth Charting	49	42	42	51	44
Insurance Forms	22	10	8	8	6

*Percentage of respondents reporting task "not done" in office decreased significantly in
direct relationship to total number of health workers employed.

†Percentage of times task reported as "not done" is between 12–20 percent with no
appreciable variation by total number of health workers employed.

[a]The data for this table were derived from tabulations that excluded 567 practitioner respondents (13 percent of the total) who fell into one or more of the following categories:
graduation from medical school prior to 1925; maintaining two offices with practice
equally divided between the two; spending less than 20 hours per week in office practice;
conducting only a consultation or subspecialty practice.

Source: Yankauer et al. [1969], p. 1108.

health worker (registered nurse) among the aides permits a more extensive
range of tasks to be delegated and, as would be expected, tends to enhance
physician productivity, other things being equal. Third, for a given number of
aides per pediatrician, physician productivity tends to be somewhat higher in
small partnerships than in solo practice. And finally, the median number of
hours pediatricians spend in their office tends to increase slightly with the
number of aides they employ and with physician productivity. This finding
requires added comment.

It has been suggested that, while input substitution is technically
feasible and certainly capable of increasing the physician's hourly productivity,
the ability to earn a higher net income per hour enables physicians to work
fewer hours per week without loss in income. As a consequence, it is argued, the

Table 4-7.   Office Hours, Office Visits and Patient Care Task Delegation in Specified Pediatric Practice Arrangements Employing Different Numbers and Types of Health Workers

Practice Arrangement	Number (1)	Median Hours* in Office (2)	Median Total Visits* (3)	Col (3) / Col (2) (4)	Percent Respondents Delegating 10 or More Tasks (5)
Solo Practice					
1 worker (RN absent)	392	31.0	81.5	2.60	6.1
2 workers (RN absent)	263	34.8	105.1	3.03	11.4
3 workers (RN absent)	59	37.2	110.8	2.98	13.6
1 worker (RN present)	94	33.4	93.1	2.78	10.8
2 workers (RN present)	239	35.0	108.5	3.10	16.5
3 workers (RN present)	84	36.7	131.1	3.57	27.4
Two-Man Practice					
2 workers (RN absent)	91	33.3	91.0	2.73	1.1
3 workers (RN absent)	86	36.3	113.4	3.12	8.1
2 workers (RN present)	69	34.7	112.7	3.25	8.6
3 workers (RN present)	115	36.4	116.6	3.20	12.2
4 workers (RN present)	79	36.5	123.9	3.39	19.0
5+ workers (RN present)	83	38.7	127.9	3.31	20.4
Three-Man Practice					
4 workers (RN present)	61	35.2	108.6	3.09	13.1
5+ workers (RN present)	215	38.4	126.1	3.28	13.4
Four-Man Practice					
5+ workers (RN present)	130	38.5	115.9	3.01	19.9
Five or More (Multispecialty)					
5+ workers (RN present)	395	37.3	105.1	2.82	7.5

*Per week. "Total visits" includes only visits for health supervision and acute illness. "Special appointment" visits (about one per week, averaging ½ hour per visit nationally) and visits for "shots only" (primarily allergy shots, averaging about 10 per week nationally) are excluded from the figures on visits.
Source: Yankauer et al. [1970], p. 39.

bulk of any gains in hourly productivity is likely to be converted by physicians into added leisure rather than added medical services [Garbarino, 1959]. This prognosis is consistent with any reasonable economic theory of physician behavior; but so is the hypothesis that increases in hourly productivity will either not affect or even increase the number of hours worked.[m] In short, the quantitative impact of this so-called "income effect" of productivity gains on hours worked cannot be predicted *a priori*; it is a purely empirical question on which conclusive evidence is still lacking.

The data in Table 4-7 neither support nor contradict the hypothe-

[m]For a formal model of this sort, see Appendix B.

sis of a negative income effect of productivity gains on hours worked. These data might be observed even if, other things being equal, there were indeed a tendency among physicians to convert increases in hourly net income partially or wholly into added leisure. Factors other than hourly income influence the number of hours physicians choose to work, and over a nationwide cross-section of physicians these other factors may swamp any latent negative income effect of productivity gains. One possibility, for example, is that physicians do respond positively to a perceived excess demand for their services, and that they engage in task delegation not so much in order to increase their hourly income and their hours of leisure, but mainly to meet a perceived excess demand without having to increase the length of their workweek. The afore-mentioned fact that pediatricians in the southern states push task delegation further than do their colleagues in New York lends support to this interpre-tation of Table 4-7.

The findings presented in Tables 4-6 and 4-7 are corroborated by virtually any other study of medical practices. Table 4-8, for example, suggests the joint and separate effects of paramedical aides and of the number of exam-ination rooms on the gross income, net income, and weekly rate of patient visits reported by a nationwide sample of physicians. The sample represents the responses to a survey of self-employed physicians undertaken in 1970 by Medical Economics, Co., publisher of the fortnightly *Medical Economics.* In Table 4-8 all medical specialties are combined. Roughly similar data, broken down by medical specialty and based on an earlier survey, are shown in Table 4-9. Both tables

Table 4-8. Apparent Effect of Auxiliary Personnel and the Number of Examination Rooms on Physician Productivity

Number of Examining Rooms per Solo M.D.	Number of Full-Time Office Aides	Physician's Total Professional Hours per Week	Office Visits per Week	Practice Gross	Practice Net
5 or more	3	66	164	$96,200	$51,380
4	2	63	154	79,810	44,460
3	2	63	115	64,610	37,470
2	1	62	87	58,500	35,900
1	0	58	45	45,800	32,560

Note: Examining rooms include all those available for the respondent's individual use in his principal office, whether or not they are shared with other physicians. Full-time aides are office assistants (nurses, secretaries, Girl Fridays, receptionists, bookkeepers, office mana-gers, etc.) employed 35 or more hours per week. Two part-time aides have been counted as one full-timer. Office visits are limited to those during which the doctor personally saw the patient. All data apply to self-employed M.D.s under age 65. Anesthesiologists, pathologists, and radiologists have been excluded from the patient-visit tabulations. Income figures apply to 1969; all other data are for 1970. Numbers of aides, hours, patient-visit rates, and income figures are medians.

Source: Owens [1971], p. 93.

Table 4–9. Relationship between Number of Aides per M.D. and Practice Hours, Hourly Patient Visits and Expenditures on Medical Supplies per Visit

	Number of Aides per M.D.[a]				
	0 to 0.51	0.5 to 1.00	1.0 to 2.00	2.01 to 3.00	More Than 3.00
Total Practice Hours/Week:[b]					
General Practitioners (N = 371)	54	55	59	60	62
Pediatricians (N = 133)	49	50	50	56	55
Obstetricians/Gynecologists (N = 101)	49	51	55	53	61
Total Patient Visits/ Practice Hour[c]					
General Practitioners	2.2	2.6	3.2	3.8	4.0
Pediatricians	1.8	2.6	3.3	3.8	3.9
Obstetricians/Gynecologists	1.7	1.9	2.5	2.8	3.2
Medical Supplies/Office Visit[d]					
General Practitioners	$0.55	$0.45	$0.56	$0.55	$0.66
Pediatricians	.56	.33	.49	.50	.66
Obstetricians/Gynecologists	.41	.48	.43	.62	.78

[a]Includes solo practitioners only. N denotes number of respondents.

[b]Excludes time spent on reading, research, and teaching.

[c]Patient visits include visits to patients in the home or in hospitals.

[d]Reported expenditures on medical supplies and drugs and small instruments per visit at the physician's office.

Source: Averages based on data from Medical Economics, *Continuing Survey*, 1967.

show, once again, that over a cross-section of physicians hourly productivity is positively correlated with hours worked per week. Table 4-9 also indicates that the physician's average expenditure on medical supplies, drugs, and small instruments per office visit is not strongly influenced by the number of aides he employs and increases substantially only when the staff exceeds three persons. If the employment of aides reflected itself solely in tasks of type I or Type II, one would expect that particular expenditure figure to rise more steeply with the size of the staff than it does. Combined with the data on hourly patient visits, the data on medical supplies suggest that there is considerable delegation of type III tasks to the aides and that their employment does enable the physician to treat more patients per unit of time. Incidentally, the average number of aides per physician for the sample underlying Table 4-9 was 1.9 for general practitioners, 1.7 for pediatricians, and 1.6 for obstetricians and gynecologists.

One of the drawbacks of tabular displays of any variable is that it is difficult to control for more than a few of its determinants at one time. Tables 4-8 and 4-9, for example, suggest at best only the approximate effect of task delegation on physician productivity, and they may do so in a biased fashion if other determinants of weekly patient visits vary systematically with the number of aides per physician. Furthermore, information presented in tabular form cannot be conveniently incorporated into forecasting models such as equation(2–2). These problems can be overcome by summarizing empirical observations on medical inputs and output in a statistically estimated "production function" capable of controlling for all determinants of output—and for any interaction among those determinants—simultaneously. The production function itself is a purely technical relationship indicating the rates of output that are technically attainable with alternative combinations of input. If the function is known, however, it may be used to determine the degree of task delegation (or the size of the auxiliary staff) that is most desirable from an economic viewpoint. This optimum may be either the least cost combination of inputs capable of producing a given rate of output or, from the perspective of a private practitioner, the combination of inputs that maximizes his net income for a given number of hours of his own time.

Statistical estimates of the sort just described are presented and evaluated in Chapters Five and Six. The unit of analysis throughout these chapters is the individual physician in private medical practice, and for the most part the focus is solely on the office-based part of the physician's practice. The empirical part of the analysis is based on a nationwide cross-section sample of general practitioners, pediatricians, obstetrician-gynecologists, and internists in solo practice or in two- to four-man single-specialty groups. This mix of specialties and practice modes represents the vast majority of primary-care physicians in the United States, a category said to be plagued by the most acute shortage of medical manpower.

Unfortunately an adequate description of statistical production-function estimation involves a fair amount of technical detail. Although the discussion in the next two chapters is developed at an internally consistent level of technical difficulty, these chapters necessarily deviate somewhat from the much less technical overall tenor of the book. Readers unfamiliar with economic theory or statistical analysis may therefore wish to go lightly on the next two chapters or perhaps even proceed directly to Chapter Seven, where the salient conclusions from the analysis are summarized and their implications for health manpower policy are explored.

NOTES

1. For classic examples of the studies referred to in the text, see Anderson and Sheatsley [1959]; Densen, Jones, Balamuth and Shapiro [1960]; Densen, Shapiro, Jones and Baldinger [1962]; Perrott [1966]; Roemer [1962]; and Roemer et al. [1972].
2. See Anne R. Somers, ed. [1971], p. 42, and Weinerman [1964], p. 884.
3. Anne R. Somers, ed. [1971], p. 48.

4. See, for example, Donabedian [1969]; Fein [1967], pp. 102, 109, 110; Bailey [1968]; Klarman [1971]; and Newhouse [1973].
5. In this connection, see Epple and Reinhardt [1972]. The costs of outpatient departments do, of course, include also certain administrative overhead passed down from the hospital to the departments. Even so, the study cited here suggests that manpower is used inefficiently in the hospital clinics studied.
6. Quoted in Glasgow [1972], p. 8.
7. Quoted in Ibid., p. 8.
8. Reported in *The New York Times* (October 10, 1973), p.8.
9. See, for example, Bergman et al. [1966, 1967]; Drui [1973]; Duncan et al. [1971]; Feldman [1972]; Riddick et al. [1971]; Smith et al. [1972]; Yankauer, Connelly and Feldman [1969, 1970]; Yankauer, Schneider, Jones, Hellman and Feldman [1972].
10. Yankauer, Jones, Schneider and Hellman [1971], p. 1551.

Part Two

A Production Function for Physician Services

Chapter Five

Technical and Economic Determinants of Physician Productivity: A Basic Analytic Framework[1]

In the abstract, the annual, monthly or weekly rate of output produced by a physician's practice may be thought of as the dependent variable in the technical production relationship

$$Q = f(H, \mathbf{L}, \mathbf{K}; \mathbf{A}) \tag{5-1}$$

In this expression, Q is some index of output (measured, perhaps, by annual, monthly or weekly patient visits, or by gross billings to patients); H denotes the number of hours the physician works per year, month or week; vector $\mathbf{L} = (L_1, L_2, \ldots, L_m)$ denotes his use of various types of auxiliary personnel (measured either by hours worked or simply by the number of each type of aide more or less permanently employed by the physician); and vector $\mathbf{K} = (K_1, K_2, \ldots, K_n)$ reflects the services of various types of equipment, instruments, and supplies— hereafter referred to simply by the generic term capital—used by the physician and/or his aides.

Vector $\mathbf{A} = (A_1, A_2, \ldots, A_z)$ denotes still other factors potentially affecting the productivity of the inputs used in the physician's practice. For example, some elements of vector $\mathbf{A}$ may describe the setting (group or solo practice) in which the physician works; others may characterize his access to hospital or laboratory facilities; still others may characterize the patients typically treated by the physician's practice, and so on. Variables H, $\mathbf{L}$ and $\mathbf{K}$ are productive inputs hired, acquired or contributed by the physician. Factors subsumed under $\mathbf{A}$ are not viewed as productive inputs as such; in fact, many of them are exogenous to the physician's production decision process.

The productive inputs H, $\mathbf{L}$ and $\mathbf{K}$ may act either as *complements* of or *substitutes* for one another. Strictly speaking, complementary inputs are those that must be used in roughly fixed proportion to one another. They are productive only if coupled with the appropriate amounts of their complements. Less than the appropriate amount renders them unproductive altogether; more than the appropriate amount adds nothing further to their productivity.

Inputs that can perform roughly similar functions are substitutes for one another as far as these functions are concerned. Their average productivity depends on the relative proportions in which they are used. For given rates of output, the productivity of the first input can usually be increased by using less of that input and appropriately more of the second, and vice versa. There may of course be technical limits to this type of substitution, and even before that limit is reached the savings in the use of the first input may not justify the cost of the additional amounts required of the substitute. How soon the technical limit to input substitution is reached depends on the degree of similarity of the two inputs in the performance of the function (or task) under consideration. In technical parlance, it depends on the elasticity of substitution between the two inputs, which is a property of the underlying production function.[a] How soon the economic limit to input substitution is reached depends, in the first instance, on the underlying elasticity of substitution and, secondly, on the relative unit costs of the two substitutes.

Some students of medical practice are inclined to view certain types of lower-level health workers (for example, clerical or low-skilled medical assistants) strictly as complements of medical manpower. On this approach, only bona fide physician extenders (physician assistants, Medex, pediatric nurse practitioners, and so on) are treated as potential substitutes for the physician. That dichotomy between types of auxiliary personnel strikes this author as invalid.

In Chapter Four the point was made that, in principle, the physician could perform the entire range of medical and clerical tasks associated with the treatment of a medical condition, save those that can only be provided by outside specialists or specialized facilities. Indeed, it is the case that quite a few physicians do not directly employ any aides at all and hence perform many routine and low-skill tasks that could be delegated to auxiliary personnel. That the employment of even lower-level allied health workers effectively frees the physician from the performance of such tasks and thus enhances his hourly productivity may be inferred from Tables 4-6 and 4-7 of the preceding chapter. In view of these data, it would seem more natural to treat all types of paramedical and clerical personnel as potential substitutes for medical manpower, and for one another. The present analysis is based on that view.

---

[a]If the elasticity of substitution between two factors is zero, they are not substitutes for one another. If the elasticity is infinite they are perfect substitutes for one another and, for all intents and purposes, indistinguishable as far as the production process is concerned. If the elasticity is greater than zero but less than infinite, the two inputs can be substituted for one another, but they are not perfect substitutes, and to maintain a given output rate successive reductions of equal amount in one input must be compensated by ever increasing increments of the other input.

As was suggested in Chapter Four, probably the bulk of capital inputs used in medical practice—and especially small instruments and medical supplies—act as complements rather than as substitutes for health manpower, although some instances were noted in which added floor space or superior office equipment might be used to enhance the productivity of the physician and/or his aides. If one views the production function as a descriptive tool setting forth the entire array of inputs that go into the production of some output, then capital inputs that are complementary to health manpower should nevertheless be included as separate inputs in one's production function specification. On the other hand, if the production function is to be used solely as an indicator of technically feasible substitution among inputs—as is the intention of this book—then little information is lost by including among the arguments of the production function only one input for each pair of complementary inputs. In assessing the economic merit of input substitution, the cost of the excluded complement is then simply added to the cost of the one included in the function. On this approach, for example, the annual cost of additional floor space minimally required by an additional aide would be added to the annual salary and fringe benefits paid the aide. Additional outlays on instruments or medical supplies would be handled in similar fashion. The production-function specifications under discussion in this and following chapters are thought to be of this second variety.

Empirical estimation of physician-care production functions—such as equation (5-1) above—is obviously a useful first step in the analysis of physician productivity. The bulk of this and following chapters will be devoted to that task. The present chapter proceeds mainly at the conceptual level. The first section develops a suitable algebraic specification of the production function for the context of medical practice and examines some problems of estimating the parameters of that function from nonexperimental data. Section II illustrates the use of empirical production functions in the estimation of optimal manpower employment in medical practice and in forecasting future physician requirements. The estimated functions themselves are presented and evaluated in Chapter Six.

Estimated production functions indicate, of course, only to what extent it has been found *technically* feasible to increase hourly physician productivity (Q/H) through greater use of auxiliary personnel (L) or capital (K). As noted in the introduction to Chapter Four, to predict the probable future time path of hourly or annual physician productivity $(Q/H$ and Q, respectively) one must be able also to explain how physicians choose the input rates $H,$ L and K and predict what rates will actually be chosen in the future. In other words one must posit a theory of physician behavior and estimate its structural parameters empirically. To date such a model has not been estimated, and that task cannot be attempted in this book for want of the requisite data. Even so, there is some merit in exploring such a model at the conceptual level, and this is done in Appendix B. The subject matter is relegated to an appendix because consid-

eration of it within this chapter would deflect the discussion unduly from its
primary focus: the technical feasibility of health manpower substitution. Later
parts of that discussion, however, will draw heavily on Appendix B. It should
therefore be viewed as an appendix to this chapter.

I. ESTIMATION OF PRODUCTION FUNCTIONS FROM NONEXPERIMENTAL DATA

The Algebraic Form of the Function

Properly defined, a production function is a mathematical relationship—or a set of mathematical relationships—describing the technology under
which the inputs into a production process are transformed into output. If it is
possible to measure the rate of output by a scalar, the underlying technology can
typically be captured in a single equation, usually nonlinear. Widely used
examples of single-equation production functions are the so-called Cobb-Douglas
function

$$Q = A\Pi_j(X_j^{a_j}), \quad A, a_j > 0 \text{ for } j = 1, 2, \ldots, k \tag{5-2}$$

the constant-elasticity-of-substitution (CES) production function of the general
form

$$Q = A[\Sigma_j(a_j X_j^b{}_j)]^{1/c}, \quad b_j, c < 0$$

$$A, a_j > 0 \quad j = 1, 2, \ldots, k$$

$$\Sigma_j a_j = 1 \tag{5-3}$$

or polynomials of various degrees, such as the quadratic

$$Q = A + \Sigma_j(a_j X_j) + \Sigma_j(b_j X_j^2) + \sum_{i<j}(c_{ij} X_i X_j) \quad j = 1, 2, \ldots, k. \tag{5-4}$$

In these expressions, Q denotes as before a rate of output, X_j is the corresponding
rate of use of the jth input, and the remaining symbols denote the parameters
to be estimated.

If the output from a productive activity can be measured only in
terms of vectors, the algebraic specification of the production function consists
of an entire set of (usually) linear or (occasionally) non-linear equations, each
describing one of many technically feasible alternative processes with which a
given type of output in the overall output vector can be produced. For example,
if Q_i^r is defined as the rate at which the ith type of output is produced by using
the rth of k possible processes that could be used to produce that type of output,

then that production process might be characterized as

$$Q_i^r = \min \left[\frac{X_1}{a_{1i}^r}, \frac{X_2}{a_{2i}^r}, \ldots, \frac{X_m}{a_{mi}^r} \right], \quad \begin{array}{l} r = 1, 2, \ldots, k \\ i = 1, 2, \ldots, n \end{array} \tag{5-5}$$

where X_j denotes the rate of the jth input available for production, and the input coefficient a_{ji}^r represents the minimum amount of the jth input required to produce one unit of the ith output via the rth process. This specification implies that within a production process, inputs must be used in fixed proportions and cannot be substituted for one another. However, processes distinguish themselves from one another by calling for different input proportions. It follows that input substitution can be effected by switching partly or wholly from one process to another (or others). If Q_i denotes the aggregate rate of the ith output produced by whatever mix of processes is used to produce that output, and $p_i^r = Q_i^r / Q_i$ is the proportion of Q_i produced with the rth process, then the production function characterizing the aggregate output rate Q_i may be written as

$$Q_i = \min \left[\frac{X_1}{z_{1i}}, \frac{X_2}{z_{2i}}, \ldots, \frac{X_m}{z_{mi}} \right], \quad i = 1, 2, \ldots, n \tag{5-6}$$

where z_{ji} is a weighted average of the input coefficient a_{ji}^r, that is

$$z_{ji} = \sum_{r=1}^{k} (p_i^r a_{ji}^r) \tag{5-7}$$

The set of equations (5-6) is a complete specification of the general production function (5-1), with output being measured by an n-dimensional vector. Since the individual production processes are also known as "activities," this characterization of the entire production technology is referred to as "activity analysis." If the parameters a_{ji}^r of the activity model are known, linear-programming techniques can be used to select that set of proportions p_i^r that minimizes the resource costs of producing a given vector of outputs Q^O. Implicit in that solution is, of course, an optimal pattern of input substitution.[2]

On the surface, activity analyses of production processes have much to recommend themselves; they penetrate to the very fine detail of these processes. It is not all that easy, however, to apply such analyses properly to medical practice. First, the reduction of medical practice to a finite set of nonstochastic, fixed-coefficient, linear production functions, and the derivation of optimal input combinations from this set of "activities" through linear programming techniques is in itself rather mechanistic and quite a bold analytical step. Unless great caution is used in applying the method and interpreting the results therefrom, the approach may easily endow one's estimates with a semblance of precision that belies the amorphism typical of the production of professional services. As this author has suggested elsewhere, for example, there is the danger that the optimal input combinations—and the implicit practice costs—one derives in this way are overly optimistic estimates of the typical input combinations required to produce given sets of services even in a relatively efficient practice (see Reinhardt, 1973b, pp. 215–18). One wonders whether the bulk of medical practitioners and their aides will be capable of living up to the exacting norms so derived. If not, the indicated optima may actually serve to mislead policy-makers in the health manpower area.[b]

In addition to these rather fundamental problems, it is also clear that the implementation of activity analysis presupposes fairly detailed information on alternative feasible production processes for each distinct medical service, and reliable estimates of the input coefficients a^r_{ji} characterizing each process. Such information could be developed by panels of experienced and imaginative medical practitioners or, alternatively, by painstaking time-and-motion studies of medical practices in operation. The latter approach in particular is enormously expensive. It is true, of course, that one should not abandon the idea of procuring empirical information in this way just because it is expensive. Yet it is pertinent to ask here, as well as in any other empirical research, whether the added information so gained justifies its high opportunity costs.

The present analysis proceeds on more aggregate data on medical practices and is based on production-function specifications of the single-equation variety. The empirical estimates of these functions indicate the increases in physician output that have, on average, been experienced by practitioners in a large cross-section sample of physicians in response to increases in the number of aides per physician. Built into this average is the slack time that is an integral part of organized human effort—for example, breakages in manpower-time that may result from unexpected changes in patient scheduling or from the fact that human beings generally cannot perform for any length of time on the stringent and rather mechanistic formulas that might be suggested by a formal activity analysis—and also the physicians' varying ability to use a given number of aides per physician. Since health manpower policy in this country must be implemented through the good offices of the typical American physician, it is hoped that these estimated averages will be of use in the formulation of that policy.

In presenting their specifications of single-equation production functions, a good many authors tend to dispense with a justification for the chosen algebraic form altogether. This omission seems to be based on the notion that over the empirically relevant range of inputs, any one of the more popular functions is a good approximation to the production surface being investigated, so that one's choice of a function can be dictated essentially by mathematical con-

[b]I am indebted to Mark Pauly of Northwestern University for enlightening me on this point.

venience. It must never be forgotten however, that one single equation is expected to capture the entire technology under study. That circumstance alone dictates that one's *a priori* specification of the function be made with extreme care, lest the purely mathematical properties of one's specification predetermine the economic implications one infers from one's estimate.[3]

The present analysis seeks to estimate the relationship between medical inputs and the physician's rate of output (to be measured either by rates of patient visits or by gross billings to patients). Since a physician can operate his practice without any auxiliary personnel whatsoever, the *a priori* specification of the production function should permit positive rates of output to occur even when the input of auxiliary personnel is zero. On the other hand, it is reasonable to postulate that positive rates of output in medical practice always do presuppose positive input rates of some capital and of physician time. Finally, it is desirable that one's a priori specification permit both increasing and decreasing marginal productivity ($\partial Q/\partial X_j$, for all $j = 1, 2, \ldots, k$) over the empirically relevant range of inputs.

The requirements set forth above effectively rule out the use of the popular Cobb-Douglas function in its conventional form. That function presupposes positive rates of all inputs at positive rates of output; it dictates that the marginal productivity of inputs diminishes throughout the entire range of inputs but never reaches zero or negative values; and it implies that the elasticity of substitution between any two inputs is unity anywhere on the production surface. The Cobb-Douglas function, however, can easily be made more flexible if it is modified as in equation

$$Q = A \prod_{j=1}^{m} (X_j^{a_j} e^{-b_j X_j}) e^{g(X,Y;c)} \qquad (5\text{-}8)$$

In this specification, the elements of vector $X = (X_1, X_2, \ldots, X_m)$ represent essential inputs that must be used at positive rates for positive rates of output to occur, and those of vector $Y = (Y_1, Y_2, \ldots, Y_n)$ represent inputs (such as auxiliary personnel) that are not necessarily required at positive rates of output. Function $g(X,Y;c)$ should be specified as nonlinear in the nonessential inputs to permit both increasing and decreasing marginal products of these inputs. Furthermore, if the use rates of essential inputs vary considerably over one's sample, it is desirable that $g(X,Y;c)$ also contain cross products of the essential and nonessential inputs so that the use rates Y_j at which the marginal products of the nonessential inputs reach either a maximum or zero vary as a function of the essential inputs. If the elements of X do not vary sufficiently over one's sample, however, then the cross-products are apt to generate problems of multicollinearity, and one may have to forego that refinement.

Connoisseurs in these matters will recognize equation (5–8) as a marriage between a so-called transcendental production function [4] and some exponential function. The marginal products of the inputs and the rates of change in these marginal products are given by the expressions:

$$\frac{\partial Q}{\partial X_j} = \left[\frac{a_j}{X_j} - b_j + \frac{\partial g(\cdot)}{\partial X_j} \right] \cdot Q \tag{5-9}$$

$$\frac{\partial^2 Q}{\partial X_j^2} = \left[(\frac{a_j}{X_j} - b_j + \frac{\partial g(\cdot)}{\partial X_j})^2 + \frac{\partial^2 g(\cdot)}{\partial X_j^2} - \frac{a_j}{X_j^2} \right] \cdot Q \tag{5-10}$$

$$\frac{\partial Q}{\partial Y_j} = \frac{\partial g(\cdot)}{\partial Y_j} \cdot Q \tag{5-11}$$

$$\frac{\partial^2 Q}{\partial Y_j^2} = \left[\frac{\partial^2 g(\cdot)}{\partial Y_j^2} + (\frac{\partial g(\cdot)}{\partial Y_j})^2 \right] \cdot Q \tag{5-12}$$

where $g(\cdot)$ denotes $g(\mathbf{X}, \mathbf{Y}; c)$. The degree of returns to scale implicit in function (5-8) varies over the production surface, as may be seen from the elasticity of output with respect to scale. The latter is defined as:

$$E(\mathbf{X},\mathbf{Y},p) = \frac{\partial f[(p\mathbf{X}), (p\mathbf{Y})]}{\partial p} \cdot \frac{p}{f[(p\mathbf{X}), (p\mathbf{Y})]}$$

$$= \sum_{j=1}^{m} (a_j - pb_jX_j) + p \left(\frac{\partial g(\cdot)}{\partial p} \right) \tag{5-13}$$

In that expression $f[(p\mathbf{X}), (p\mathbf{Y})] = Q$ denotes the production function (5-8) with each input rate multiplied by scalar p. Finally, using Allen's definition of the partial elasticity of substitution for pairs of inputs [Allen, 1938, p. 504] it can also be shown that function (5-8) is a variable-elasticity-of-substitution production function. Thus the function imposes even fewer restrictions on one's estimate than does the CES production function. If $g(\mathbf{X},\mathbf{Y};c)$ is specified in a form that is linear in parameters c (e.g., a simple polynomial), then the entire production function can easily be transformed into a linear function on conversion into logarithms, and its parameters can be estimated by linear regression techniques.

The production function estimates to be presented in the next chapter are based on a specific version of equation (5-8). These estimates are developed from the input-output rates reported by a cross-section of self-employed physicians. The estimates therefore constitute essentially a compact statistical summary of these physicians' experience; they indicate the rates of output that have, *on average,* been obtained by the physicians in the sample with alternative combinations of inputs. Empirical averages of this sort may, of course, be precisely what one is looking for; they can suggest what may be expected, on average, from an overall change in the mix of health manpower, and they can serve as benchmarks against which to assess individual provider facilities.[5] The problem with such averages is that they may be inherently biased and hence generate misleading conclusions. Since this potential short-coming is often pointed out in connection with empirical production functions, and since the estimates to be presented further on are, in fact, open to such criticism, the nature of this estimation bias warrants extended examination here. A simple example will serve to illustrate the problem.

Potential Problems in the Estimation of Production Functions

Consider a set of hypothetical producers—not necessarily physicians—each transforming two inputs into some type of output that can be measured by a scalar. It is assumed that these producers use a common technology and, to keep the illustration simple, that this technology is properly described by the production function

$$Q_i = C \cdot X_{1i}^A \cdot X_{2i}^B \cdot M_i \tag{5-14}$$

where subscript i denotes the ith producer, X_{ji} his use-rate of the jth input, Q_i his rate of output, C is a constant, and M_i is an index characterizing the ith pro-ducer's *technical efficiency*.[c] Index M may be thought of as an *unobservable* in-put loosely defined as the "management factor." To simplify matters further it is useful to assume that all producers use identical rates of the first input, and thus to think of the common value X_1^A as part of the constant term C. Equation (5–14) therefore reduces to the logarithmic equivalent

$$q_i = c + Bx_{2i} + m_i \tag{5-15}$$

where lower-case letters denote the logarithms of the corresponding upper-case variables. Since the management factor M_i is, by assumption, unobservable, m_i in equation (5-15) acts essentially as an error term.

The most straightforward (and most commonly used) method of estimating parameters c and B of a production function such as (5–15) would be to obtain a cross-section sample of observations on Q_i and X_{2i} and to regress the logarithm of the former onto the logarithm of the latter. This general approach

---

[c]By *technical efficiency* in this context is meant the ability to obtain the maximum rate of output attainable with a given combination of inputs. Technical efficiency must be distinguished from *economic efficiency*, which reflects the ability to select the least-cost combination of inputs for a given rate of output. In this connection see also foot-note f in Chapter Four.

was, in fact, adopted in obtaining the production-function estimates reported in Chapter Six. Unfortunately this very convenient formulation of the regression model may violate the fundamental assumption that the error term in one's production-function specification—a term that contains the unobservable management factor M_i—is uncorrelated with the regressors (in this example x_{2i}). It is well known that this lack of independence generally results in biased parameter estimates, a possibility that has led many authors to question the usefulness of single-equation production-function estimates.[6] It turns out, however, that the presumed severity of the single-equation bias actually rests on a rather stylized model of the production-decision process. In particular it rests on the assumption that producers invariably choose their input and output rates so as to maximize profits. The economic context in which physicians make their input-output decisions differs substantially from this stylized model, and the estimation bias one is likely to encounter in that context may not nearly be as serious as is sometimes alleged.

To elaborate on the preceding assertion we will proceed with our example on the assumption that the producers in the hypothetical sample actually have chosen their input-output rates Q_i and X_{2i} in an attempt to maximize their net income or, equivalently, the net income per unit of X_1. The words "in an attempt" are chosen deliberately here, because not every producer may actually achieve what he attempts to do. For the ith producer, net income may be defined as

$$Y_i = P_i Q_i - W_i X_{2i} - F_i \qquad\qquad (5\text{-}16)$$

In equation (5-16) F_i denotes the ith producer's fixed costs (the cost of the first input), and it is assumed that he can hire additional units of the second input at a constant price W_i and sell additional units of output at a constant price P_i.

On the preceding assumptions the observed rates Q_i and X_{2i} must be presumed to have satisfied the technical constraint

$$Q_i = C X_{2i}^B M_i \qquad\qquad (5\text{-}17)$$

as well as the profit-maximizing condition $\partial Y_i / \partial X_{2i} = 0$, which in turn implies the equality

$$X_{2i} = \left[\frac{CBP_i M_i}{W_i V_i} \right]^{1/(1-B)} \qquad\qquad (5\text{-}18)$$

The multiplicative term V_i in equation (5-18) may be viewed as an index of the ith producer's relative *economic efficiency*. Inclusion of that term in the input-decision equation for X_2 makes allowance for the fact that, try as he might, relative to a truly income-maximizing use rate X_{2i}, the ith producer may have been economically inefficient by hiring either too much ($V_i < 1$) or too little ($V_i > 1$) of the second input. In the context of medical practice, if X_{2i} denotes auxiliary personnel, V_i may also represent certain psychic costs (or benefits) the physician associates with the employment of auxiliary personnel, costs that he adds to the objective salary costs W_i when choosing his input rate X_{2i}. (For a more detailed explanation of the latter point, see Appendix B, especially equation [B-7b]).

Equation (5-18) indicates that, under the assumptions made above, the management factor, M_i, is fully transmitted to decisions concerning the use rate X_{2i}: other things being equal, technically efficient producers (those with relatively high indices M_i) hire more of the second input than do technically inefficient ones. The regressor x_{2i} in equation (5-15) is thus clearly correlated with the error term m_i. The consequences of this fact for the least-squares estimate of B (the coefficient of x_{2i} in (5-15) can be assessed by the expression

$$\gamma = \operatorname*{plim}_{N \to \infty} \left[\frac{\displaystyle\sum_{i=1}^{i=N} (q_i - \bar{q})(x_{2i} - \bar{x}_2)}{\displaystyle\sum_{i=1}^{i=N} (x_{2i} - \bar{x}_2)^2} - B \right] \tag{5-19}$$

In that expression, the first term within the square brackets will be recognized as the conventional least-squares estimator of parameter B, obtained from regression equation (5-15), and γ as the *asymptotic bias* of that estimator. Now from equations (5-17) and (5-18) above, the observed values of q_i and x_{2i} satisfying these equations can be derived as in

$$q_i = (1 - B)^{-1} [c + B(b + p_i - w_i - v_i) + m_i] \tag{5-20}$$

$$x_{2i} = (1 - B)^{-1} [c + b + p_i - w_i - v_i + m_i] \tag{5-21}$$

(with lower-case letters once again denoting logarithms of the corresponding upper-case variables). If one inserts these expressions into equation (5-19) and makes the reasonable assumption that all covariances save that between p_i and w_i are essentially zero, then the asymptotic bias of the estimator for B can be reduced to

$$\gamma = \frac{(1 - B)\, \sigma_{mm}}{\sigma_{pp} + \sigma_{ww} + \sigma_{vv} + \sigma_{mm} - 2\sigma_{wp}} \tag{5-22}$$

where, in general, σ_{rs} denotes the covariance between variables denoted by r and s. (For a derivation of (5-22) see Reinhardt [1970, Appendix B].)

Equation (5-22) may be viewed as a rough-and-ready guide in an assessment of the single-equation bias likely to be encountered in the estimation of production functions from cross-sections of producers. The equation suggests that, other things being equal, the greater the interproducer differences in technical efficiency over one's sample of producers, the larger the estimation bias inherent in the estimator of parameter B. Conversely, other things (σ_{mm}) being equal, the more widely the prices (P and W) faced by producers vary over one's sample, or the more widely the producers in one's sample differ in their ability or willingness to maximize profits (that is, the more V varies over the sample) the smaller will the bias in the estimator of B tend to be.

It may appear that the preceding argument is tied to a specific example and hence not very illuminating. But the argument can easily be generalized to more than one input [7] and to other production-function specifications. The latter assertion may perhaps be more obvious if the argument is rendered graphically.[8] Thus in Figure 5-1 the curved lines are graphs of production function (5-17) for three alternative values of the management factor M_i. The vertical lines represent the input-decision equation (5-18), a function

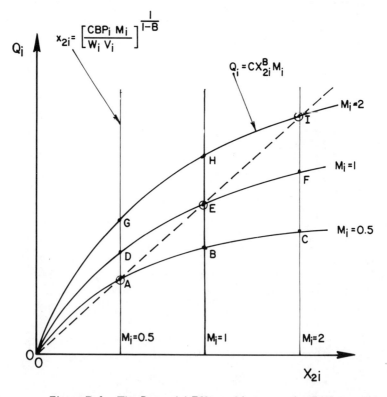

Figure 5-1. The Potential Effect of Interpractice Differences in Technical Efficiency on Statistical Estimates of the Production Function

whose position also is partially fixed by the value of M_i. In Figure 5-1, it has been assumed that all producers face common values for variables C, B, P, W and V, so that M_i is the only variable altering the position of their input-decision equation.

Suppose now that each producer in one's sample can be identified with one of the three values of M_i, shown in Figure 5-1, and consider first the case where all producers face the same input and output prices and are all characterized by the same index of economic efficiency ($\sigma_{vv} = 0$). In that case all observations on Q_i and X_{2i} must fall onto either point A or E or I in Figure 5-1. The estimated function obtained from this sample—line AEI—clearly overstates the effect of changes in X_2 on the rate of output Q. This is the estimation bias referred to above.

At the other extreme one can imagine a case in which all producers in one's sample are equally efficient technically ($M_i = M$ for all i so that σ_{mm} = 0), but face different prices ($\sigma_{pp} \neq 0$ and $\sigma_{ww} \neq 0$) and differ substantially in their ability or willingness to select economically efficient input combinations (that is, σ_{vv} is relatively large). In that case one's scatter of observed input-output combinations would obviously have to lie on the common production function and would hence trace out the exact shape of the latter. The least-square bias defined by equation (5-22) would be zero.

Finally, the most probable case is one in which all of the variances in equation (5-22) are positive. The vertical input-decision lines in Figure 5-1 might then be situated anywhere in the diagram, and one's observations might fall anywhere onto the three production functions. Even in this case, however, one may be able to identify the *approximate* shape of the true production function through single-equation estimation. For example, if it can reasonably be assumed that the producers in one's cross-section sample faced markedly different product and factor prices (σ_{ww} and σ_{pp} large), and if it can further be assumed that these producers differ much more markedly in their ability (or willingness) to maximize profits than they do in their technical ability to transform inputs, *once hired*, into output ($\sigma_{vv} > \sigma_{ee}$), then one may expect the scatter of observed input-output combinations to be much more widely dispersed *along* the true production surface than vertical to it, and the estimated function—for example, line DEF in Figure 5-1—to deviate only slightly from the true production function. Certain characteristics of medical practice in this country persuade one that a nationwide cross-section sample of physicians is likely to meet these conditions, and that the single-equation bias of a production function estimated from such a sample is not likely to be intolerably biased.

First, many physicians in this country are probably not at all constrained by market forces in their input-output decisions. Under these circumstances it is not clear that physicians who are potentially more efficient in a technical sense will automatically employ more aides and supporting capital than do physicians who are inherently less efficient, technically. But even if many physicians in one's sample were market constrained, they certainly do not face common fee schedules and input prices. As Tables 5-1 and 5-2 suggest, the price variances over a nationwide sample of physicians tend to be fairly large. Furthermore, the price of at least one input—the physician's own time—is wholly subjective and must be assumed to vary from physician to physician. (In this connection see Appendix B, especially equation (B-6b).)

It may also be doubted that all physicians in one's cross-section sample exhibit the same degree of ability or willingness to choose inputs so as to maximize income per hour of their own time. In some localities they may be constrained by law from doing so, and, as was suggested earlier and is set forth more fully in Appendix B, some physicians may even associate psychic costs with the employment of auxiliary personnel. Variance σ_{vv} over one's sample is therefore likely to be rather large.

Finally, in view of their fairly standard formal training, one wonders whether physicians actually do differ significantly in their ability to use auxiliary personnel effectively—that is, how much the management index M actually does vary over a random sample of physicians. In general, physicians use standard and well-advertised medical equipment, and their aides also receive fairly standard training. This uniformity of training may explain why Richard Bailey, in his previously cited study, found that "there was no discernible difference in the way in which group or solo internists [in his sample] used their paramedical personnel [1968, p. 1297]. From Chapter Four it will be recalled that the National Advisory Commission on Health Manpower also had found no difference in the manner in which Kaiser physicians and solo practitioners used their

Table 5-1. Typical Fees Charged for Common Medical Procedures, General Practitioners,[a] 1965

	Sample Average	Standard Deviation	Coefficient of Variation
Comprehensive diagnostic history and physical examination	$15.44	10.53	0.74
Initial visit (noncomprehensive)	5.19	2.13	0.41
Follow-up visits, usual or routine	4.30	1.12	0.26
House call, one person	7.48	2.29	0.31
Follow-up examination and evaluation per day	5.51	1.63	0.29
Appendectomy	160.89	31.97	0.20
D&C, diagnostic	62.11	20.67	0.33
Complete obstetrical care	137.71	33.71	0.24
T&A child	65.66	15.32	0.23
Urinalysis	1.81	0.75	0.41

[a]The data summarized in this table are based on physician responses to the question "Please state the fee you most frequently charge for each of the following services. . . ." It should be noted that the corresponding statistics for internists, OBG specialists and pediatricians exhibit a quite similar pattern.

Source: Data from *Medical Economics,* Continuing Survey, 1965.

Table 5-2. Average Salaries of Paramedical Aides Paid by General Practitioners, 1965

	Sample Average	*Standard Deviation*
Registered Nurses	$4,200	850
Technicians	4,000	1,160
Office Aides	3,300	850

Source: Data from *Medical Economics,* Continuing Survey, 1965.

auxiliary personnel [1967, Vol. II, p. 207]. In short, there is reason to suppose that σ_{mm} may not be all that large over a sample of American physicians. This is, however, a question on which further research is clearly in order before one can come to any firm conclusion.

In principle, an alternative to single-equation estimation of the production function would be the specification of a complete production-decision model for private medical practitioners (as is done in Appendix B), and to estimate the entire model by a simultaneous-equations method. In the context of medical practice this approach is not promising. First, the requisite data would be very hard to come by. More importantly, the economic behavior of self-employed physicians is not well understood at this time. As is argued in Appendix B, this problem has marred a number of attempts to estimate models of physician behavior in the past. In view of the serious specification errors that could creep into at least some equations of such a full-blown model, the production function one would estimate as part of that model would probably suffer from even more serious bias than is likely to be encountered in single-equation estimation.

Attempts to estimate the parameters of the production function by estimating a reduced form of the model (for example, the cost function) or relationships derived from the first-order conditions of such a model (for example, the input-decision equations labeled (B-6b) and (B-7b) in Appendix B) also are not likely to be successful in the context of medical practice. To treat the cost function as a reduced form one would have to assume that the physician's rate of output is exogenous to his decisions and that the same is true of the input prices he faces (including that of his own time). These assumptions are patently unwarranted. Inference of the production-function parameters from estimates of the input-decision equations is equally risky. First, input-decision equations such as (B-6b) and (B-7b) in Appendix B are themselves subject to the very bias one seeks to eliminate in the production-function estimate. To convert the input-decision equations into proper reduced forms (that is, equations expressing rates of inputs solely as a function of *exogenous* variables) requires one to solve the set of equations consisting of the production function and the first-order conditions simultaneously for the rate of output and the rates of input. The resulting equations for the inputs are then functions primarily of stochastic error terms and of the unobservable parameters of the physician's trade-off function between income and leisure. In short, this so-called "indirect approach" to production-function estimation is likely to yield coefficient estimates that are either inherently implausible or are marred by intolerably high variances.[9]

A potentially more promising approach would be to estimate the production function via two-stage-least-squares (TSLS), with the instruments for the (presumably endogenous) inputs in the production function drawn from a wider production-decision model for physicians. An attempt was made to follow that approach with the data that were available to this study [Reinhardt, 1970, pp. 81–5]. Unfortunately, the estimates obtained in the first-stage equations were extremely poor, so that the estimated regressors inserted into the (second-stage) estimation of the production function were generally nowhere near their observed values. It is therefore not surprising that the production-function estimates obtained in this way were by and large implausible. These disappointing results undoubtedly reflect the fact that the instruments available to the analysis were not really suited for the purpose at hand. Many of these instruments (for example, the wages for auxiliary personnel or the per capita income in the physician's locality) were actually statewide rather than local observations, and some of the variables assumed to be exogenous (for example, the physician's fees) were probably not truly exogenous in the first place. Unless adequate data for the TSLS approach are at hand, the superiority of that approach over single-equation estimation ought not to be taken for granted (as it so often seems to be in the literature).

In view of the implausible results obtained with TSLS estimation, the production-function estimates presented in the next chapter were ultimately obtained via single-equation estimation. Although no pretense is made that these estimates are completely free of bias, it is nevertheless assumed that whatever bias there may be is probably not very serious. This assumption in turn rests on the arguments developed earlier in this section, a line of reasoning, incidentally, that appears to have persuaded quite a few economists—among them Griliches [1963, 1967], Konijn [1959] and Walters [1963]—to advocate or adopt single-equation estimation of production functions in full awareness of the possibility that some bias may thereby creep into one's estimates. For, as Walters has observed on this point, given the alternatives open to researchers, it would actually be "dangerous to be pedantic about the superiority of simultaneous-equations over single-equation methods" of estimating production functions [1963, p. 17].

II. APPLICATIONS OF PRODUCTION FUNCTIONS TO HEALTH MANPOWER RESEARCH

Empirical production functions—whether specified as single equations or sets of linear activities—offer one considerable analytic flexibility. They can be used as benchmarks against which to rank individual provider facilities in terms of their technical and economic efficiency.[10] Using expressions such as equation (5-13) they can be used to test for the presence or absence of returns to scale. If the prices of all inputs are known, one can use the production function to derive the producer's cost function, rather than estimating the latter directly from observed data on costs and output.[11] Implicit in this derivation is of course a least-cost combination of inputs for each rate of output. Given the focus of the present analysis, this optimum is of prime interest to us. Finally, estimates of the production function can be incorporated directly into health manpower forecasts and enable one to assess the effect of health manpower substitution on future physician requirements.

Optimal Staffing Patterns in Medical Practice
For the sake of illustration, suppose that the technology of health-care production in individual medical practices can be reasonably well described by a three-input production function

$$Q = f(H, L, K) \qquad\qquad (5\text{-}23)$$

where H denotes, as before, the number of hours the physician works per period, L denotes the number of assistants (or the number of assistant-hours per period) he employs, and K is an index of the capital equipment and floor space he uses. For the moment there is no need to specify the algebraic form of this function precisely.

In representing the input of auxiliary personnel by a single variable we proceed on the simplifying assumption that there is only one type of such personnel, or that all ostensibly distinct types of personnel are effectively treated as perfect substitutes within the physician's practice. It is also well to recall that, given the focus of our analysis, our production function specification is thought to include only one of each pair of complementary inputs. Reasons for this procedure were given in the introduction to this chapter.

Given a specific version of production function (5-23) above, the optimum staffing pattern is implicit in the optimal input combination (H, L, K). The question is how that optimum should be defined. To make any headway in this direction, it is best to proceed initially on the notion that the optimal combination (H, L, K) is one that maximizes the satisfaction the individual practitioner derives from the conduct of his practice.[d] As is shown in Appendix B, this implies that H, L and K would be chosen so as to satisfy the technical constraint defined by the production function, as well as the first-order conditions

[d]This optimum may not coincide with one defined on society's perspective. The social optimum would be a staffing pattern that minimizes the real social resource costs of producing the rate of medical services demanded. We return to this distinction in the final chapter of the book. In the meantime, our interest centers on the physician's perspective.

$$(P^* - S^*)f_H(H, L, K) = P_H \tag{5-24}$$

$$(P^* - S^*)f_L(H, L, K) = W^* + E^* + P_L \tag{5-25}$$

$$(P^* - S^*)f_K(H, L, K) = R^* \tag{5-26}$$

In these expressions, P^* denotes the marginal revenue received from the sale of the marginal unit of output (with output measured, say, by patient visits); S^* denotes the outlays on drugs and supplies on the marginal unit of output; P_H is the shadow price the physician attaches to the marginal hour of leisure (defined as $U_X/U_Y(1 - t^*)$ in Appendix B); W^* is the marginal outlay on salary and fringe benefits occasioned by the employment of the marginal aide; E^* is the outlay on complementary floor space and equipment necessitated by the employment of the marginal aide (converted to an equivalent rate per period); P_L is the psychic cost or benefit the physician may associate with the employment of the marginal aide (defined as $U_L/U_Y(1 - t^*)$ in Appendix B); and R^* is the marginal cost per unit of capital (K), also converted to a rate per period. Finally, $f_H(H, L, K)$ denotes $\partial f(H, L, K)/\partial H$, and $f_L(H, L, K)$ and $f_K(H, L, K)$ are similarly defined.

In principle, equations (5-23) to (5-26) could be solved simultaneously for the optimal input combination $(\hat{H}, \hat{L}, \hat{K})$ and the associated optimum output rate $\hat{Q}$. In practice that solution would be hard to come by, if for no other reason than that some of these equations contain unobservable "shadow prices" $(P_H$ and $P_L)$ perceived only by the physician. Something useful can nevertheless be learned from this general framework.

Suppose, for example, that the production function faced by the physician, as well as P^*, S^*, W^*, E^* and R^* are known. Suppose further that the physician does not associate any psychic costs or benefits with the employment of aides as such (that is, $P_L = 0$), and that he has decided to work H_o hours per period. On these assumptions, L and K are the only unknowns in equations (5-25) and (5-26), and can hence be obtained from these equations. Since P_L is assumed to be zero, the solution values of L and K will maximize the physician's hourly income for given values of the remaining variables in the two equations. For auxiliary personnel the solution value $\hat{L}$ may be written as some function

$$\hat{L} = L(H_o; P_o^*, S_o^*, W_o^*, E_o^*, R_o^*) \tag{5-27}$$

where subscript o denotes given values of the subscripted variables. For purposes of the present analysis, $\hat{L}$ is viewed as the optimal staffing pattern we wish to determine. Unless the physician has a distinct aversion (or is peculiarly attracted) to the employment of auxiliary personnel, he should indeed view $\hat{L}$ as optimal, and failure to attain it would reflect *economic inefficiency* on his part. From society's perspective, employment of at least $\hat{L}$ aides per physician would be deemed desirable as well.[e]

   If one continues with the assumption that $P_L = 0$, that the production function is known, and that values for P^*, S^*, W^* and E^* are given, one may use equations (5-24) and (5-25) to infer the shadow price of physician time (P_H) implicit in any particular input combination (H_o, L_o, K_o) the physician is observed to employ in his practice. This shadow price is given by the expression

$$\hat{P}_H = (W_o^* + E_o^*) \cdot \frac{f_H(H_o, L_o, K_o)}{f_L(H_o, L_o, K_o)} \tag{5-28}$$

The estimated value of P_H is of some interest, for it may be compared to the value of physician time implicit in the physician's fee schedule.[f]

   Finally, one can turn the previous problem around and posit some value of P_H—perhaps that implicit in the physician's fee schedule. Using once again equations (5-24) and (5-25), one can then infer the psychic costs or benefits (P_L) implicit in the physician's actual input combination (H_o, L_o, K_o) and in the shadow price P_{H_o} he seems to incorporate into his fee schedule. The estimated value of $\hat{P}_L$ is given by the equation

$$\hat{P}_L = P_{H_o} \cdot \left[\frac{f_L(H_o, L_o, K_o)}{f_H(H_o, L_o, K_o)} \right] - (W^* + E^*) \tag{5-29}$$

P_L, incidentally, is reminiscent of the "discrimination coefficient" occasionally estimated in analyses of racial or sex discrimination in the labor market. P_L has several alternative interpretations. On the one hand, it may be taken as a measure of the physician's "marginal distaste of" or "marginal delight in" employing aides. On this interpretation one would assume his actual input combination (H_o, L_o, K_o) to be a rational and economically efficient choice. An alternative interpretation is that the physician is inherently neutral in his attitude toward the size of his staff (that is, that P_L is truly zero) and that the estimated value $\hat{P}_L$ is simply a measure of his economic inefficiency. In empirical research there is, of course, always the further possibility that the underlying estimates are somehow biased. For example, it might be that one's production-function estimate overstates the marginal productivity of auxiliary personnel (perhaps as a

[e]If one applies equation (5-27) to solo practitioners or physicians in small partnerships, the solution values $\hat{L}$ should be constrained to multiples of the minimum basic units in which aides can be hired (e.g., half-days).

[f]As a rough approximation, one may obtain an estimate of P_H by comparing the fees for individual services with the time physicians normally devote to these services. For estimates of this sort, see Tables 6-4 and 6-5.

result of the management factor M_i discussed in the previous section) so that equation (5-29) suggests a higher value of P_L than would be obtained from the production function on which the individual physician in question actually operates. This possibility must constantly be kept in mind in the evaluation of empirical production functions.

In Chapter Six we will apply the analyses described above to the production-function estimates presented in that chapter. Thus we estimate optimal levels of aide input $(\hat{L})$ for alternative values of the arguments in equation (5-27) above. However, since neither Q nor $f_L(H, L, K)$ are found to be very sensitive to changes in the value of K (as we are forced to measure it in this analysis), we do not solve for an optimal value of K for an assumed price R_o^*, but instead hold K constant at the observed sample average. R_o^* is therefore eliminated from equation (5-27), and some value K_o is added to its arguments. Estimates of P_H and P_L implicit in the sample averages of the arguments in equations (5-28) and (5-29) are presented in Chapter Six as well.

Production Functions in Health Manpower Forecasting

In Chapter Two it was noted that the number of physicians required at some future time t may be calculated from the expression

$$M_t = \frac{D_t N_t}{Q_t} \tag{5-30}$$

where D_t denotes the per capita demand for physician services at time t; N_t is the size of the population to be served; and Q_t is the average output of physician services per active physician at time t. If one could assume that all physicians at time t used the same combination of practice inputs, equation (5-30) could be restated as

$$M_t = \frac{D_t N_t}{f(H_t, L_t, K_t)} \tag{5-31}$$

where (H_t, L_t, K_t) is the common input combination used by physicians. Using this expression, one could then examine the effect of health manpower substitution (changes in the ratio L_t/H_t) on future physician requirements (M_t). Alternatively, one could use equation (5-31) to develop trade-off functions (isoquants) indicating alternative combinations of L_t and M_t capable of meeting an assumed aggregate demand for physician services $(D_t N_t)$ for given values of H_t and K_t. Finally, one could posit growth paths for $M_t N_t$, and the input rates H_t, L_t and K_t and project the consumption stream D_t made possible by these growth paths. The easiest way to accomplish this would be to restate equation (5-31) as

$$m_t = d_t + n_t - e_{Ht} h_t - e_{Lt} l_t - e_{Kt} k_t \tag{5-32}$$

where lower-case letters denote the growth rates, at time t, in the variable defined by the corresponding upper-case letters—thus $m_t = [\partial M_t/\partial_t]/M_t$, and so on—and e_{Xt} is the elasticity of output with respect to the input denoted by X (either H, L or K). For example,

$$e_{Ht} = \left[\frac{\partial f(H_t, L_t, K_t)}{\partial H_t}\right] \cdot \left[\frac{H_t}{f(H_t, L_t, K_t)}\right]$$

and similarly for e_{Lt} and e_{Kt}. Given the very general form of the production function used in this analysis, these elasticities obviously vary as a function of the inputs and may well be zero or negative at some points on the production surface. Depending upon the particular form of the production function, equation (5-32) may be easier to work with than equation (5-31).

In using equations (5-31) or (5-32) in this way one must remain conscious of two stringent assumptions underlying the analysis. First, it is assumed explicitly that all physicians use an identical combination of inputs. Second, one may be assuming implicitly that all input rates are continuously variable. If the future supply of physicians includes a substantial number of physicians in solo practices or small partnerships, neither assumption may be warranted. The second assumption in particular is vulnerable because auxiliary personnel cannot normally be hired by the hour.

It may be tempting in this case to view the input rates inserted into the production function $f(H_t, L_t, K_t)$ as averages over the physician population. On that interpretation, continuous variation in all input rates would certainly be meaningful. Although that approach is not uncommon in applied economic research, it would be strictly valid only if the production function itself were linear in the input rates. In the absence of linearity,

$$f(\bar{H}_t, \bar{L}_t, \bar{K}_t) \neq \sum_{i=1}^{M_t} [f(H_{it}, L_{it}, K_{it})/M_t] \tag{5-33}$$

(where $\bar{H}_t$, $\bar{L}_t$, and $\bar{K}_t$ are averages over M_t physicians). It is, however, the right-hand side of this nonequality that is properly inserted into equation (5-30).

A number of ways to cope with this problem suggest themselves. First, it is clear that the degree of inaccuracy generated by the use of $f(\bar{H}_t, \bar{L}_t, \bar{K}_t)$ in conjunction with equation (5-30) depends, on the one hand, on the degree of nonlinearity in the production function and, on the other, on the empirically relevant range of variation in the input rates. One may get a feel for the probable degree of distortion through sensitivity analysis. Alternatively, one may posit a number of distinct input combinations (H, L, K) that span the relevant range of input rates and simulate the future by positing some change in the distribution of physicians over this set of distinct input combinations. If one is concerned with solo practitioners, for example, one might assume that all of them will use roughly the same amount of H and K,[g] but that they will employ either no aide, or one, or two or three aides, and so on. If r_z denotes the proportion of physicians employing Z aides per physician, then variable Q_t in equation (5–30) would be defined as

$$Q_t = \sum_{z=0}^{A} [r_{zt} f(H_t, Z_t, K_t)] \tag{5-34}$$

where H_t and K_t are assumed to be common to all physicians. The time path of Q_t would be generated by the assumed time paths of variables $r_{zt}(z = 0, 1, \ldots, 4)$.

In Chapter Seven we use the production-function estimates from Chapter Six in two distinct forecasting exercises. First, we estimate the number of office-based physicians that would be required 10, 20, or 30 years hence if all office-based physicians used 1, 2, 3 or 4 aides per physician.[h] In that exercise we proceed directly with equation (5–31). As a variant of the approach suggested with equation (5–34), we combine our manpower forecasting model described in Appendix A (and used for Figures 1–2 and 2–2) with the assumption that medical students in the future will be trained specifically to work with auxiliary personnel and that all future graduates will employ two aides per physician during the first Y years after establishing their office-based practice, three aides per physician during the next Y years, and four aides thereafter. Underlying this simulation is the assumption that all physicians are capable and willing to work with a large auxiliary staff, but that it may take some time to build up their practice loads to levels requiring a staff of four aides. The simulation will generate a time path of the supply of physician services $(Q_t M_t)$ that can then be compared to the time path $(Q_0 M_t)$ one would observe if the average productivity of physicians in the future remained at its base-year value of Q_0. The results from the exercise are shown in Figure 7–2.

NOTES

1. This and the next chapter draw heavily on Reinhardt [1972] and Reinhardt [1973b].
2. If inputs can be hired only in lumpy units (e.g., 40 hours per week), then the activity-analysis model can be solved for the cost-minimizing set of proportions p_i^r subject to the constraint that certain inputs can be

[g]It must be remembered that K is thought to be floor space and equipment over and above the strictly complementary capital required by health manpower. It is therefore legitimate to hold K constant while letting L vary.

[h]A maximum of four aides is used because the optima derived via equation (5–27) are generally found to lie between 3.5 and 4.5.

hired only in discrete amounts. The solution in this case would be obtained via integer programming. If the problem is posed in this way, one may solve it for various levels of output (perhaps by multiplying the output vector Q by scalars) and thus examine the effect of scale on production costs.

For a fairly detailed description of activity-analysis models in this context and a discussion of the problems of estimating such models, see Reinhardt [1973b]. For empirical applications of these models to health-care productions, see Dowling [1972], Smith et al. [1972]; Golladay et al. [1974]; and Uyeno [1971].

3. In his study of ambulatory care production in group medical practices, for example, Kovner [1968] used a quadratic function whose first-order terms were dropped (presumably because their inclusion among the regressors resulted in severe multicollinearity). His estimates suggested that the marginal product of any input *increases* throughout the domain of the function, a result that was dictated strictly by his *a priori* specification of the function, and one that is certainly inconsistent with reality.

4. One of the earlier descriptions of pure transcendental functions is given in Halter et al.[1957].

5. If one is interested in estimating a production function indicating the maximum rate of output technically attainable for given combinations of inputs, then other estimation techniques must be used. For a description of such a technique, see Farrell [1957].

6. See, for example, Marschack and Andrews [1944], Hoch [1958], Walters [1963], and Nerlove [1965]. The discussion in this chapter draws considerably on these publications.

7. See Hoch [1958].

8. Figure 5–1 is an adaptation from Konijn [1959].

9. An unsuccessful attempt to use the indirect approach in an analysis of medical practices is described in Kimbell et al. [1973].

10. For such applications of production functions see Feldstein [1967], and Epple and Reinhardt [1972].

11. For an example of derived cost functions, see Reinhardt and Yett [1972], pp. 77–92.

Chapter Six

Empirical Estimates of Physician-Care Production Functions

In the previous chapter the nature and uses of physician-care production functions were examined at the conceptual level. In this chapter we present empirical estimates of such functions, and explore their statistical and economic properties. Section I contains a brief description of the cross-section sample underlying these estimates. The estimates themselves are presented in section II.

Throughout section I it is tacitly assumed that the production function to be estimated is a specific version of equation (5–8) in Chapter Five, converted into some linear form

$$Q_i = a + \sum_{j=1}^{n} [b_j f_j(X_i)] + e_i \qquad (6\text{-}1)$$

where i denotes the individual physician; Q_i is an index of his output; vector X_i denotes his inputs (including his own time); e_i is a stochastic error term; f_j depicts the jth regressor as some function of the inputs; and b_j along with a are the parameters to be estimated. Based on the arguments presented in section I of Chapter Five, we proceed as if e_i were distributed independently of the elements of X_i, with zero mean and a constant variance for all i, so that the parameters of the function can be estimated by single-equation least-squares regression.

I. THE EMPIRICAL BASIS OF THE ESTIMATES

The empirical information used in this chapter has been taken from the 1965 and 1967 *Medical Economics* Continuing Surveys of self-employed physicians in the United States. These surveys are two of a series of annual surveys undertaken by Medical Economics, Inc., publisher of the fortnightly *Medical Economics*. The surveys retrieve information by way of questionnaires mailed to a fairly large, nationwide sample of physicians who are selected at random on an nth name basis. For each respondent the surveys—hereafter referred to simply as MEDEC surveys—provide data on annual gross and net income, the physician's typical number of weekly office, hospital, and home visits with patients, the number of hours per week the physician typically spends in various types of activities, the number of various types of aides employed by the physician and the salaries he pays them, the physician's fees for a number of standard procedures, and his professional expenses broken down by categories. A more detailed description of these surveys can be found in Appendix D.

The MEDEC surveys cover physicians in all medical specialties and all modes of medical practice. Since the technology of health-care production must be assumed to vary by specialty, a separate production function has been estimated for each of the following major specialties: general practitioners, pediatricians, obstetricians-gynecologists, and internists. With respect to the mode of practice, it was decided to include in our sample only solo practitioners or physicians in *single-specialty* groupings of two or more physicians (hereafter referred to as groups). Of the physicians thus retained, between 65 and 80 percent were solo practitioners in the survey years, the exact percentage depending upon the medical specialty. The great bulk of the remainder worked in single-specialty groups with a total of between two and four physicians.

Physicians in multispecialty group practices were excluded from our sample for the following reason. In general, the participants in single-specialty groups share the use of certain equipment and personnel, but otherwise conduct their practices more or less as would an independent solo practitioner. It may therefore be legitimate to compare such physicians with solo practitioners on the basis of weekly patient visits or patient billings, and to ascribe any difference in visits or billings for given combinations of inputs solely to the mode of practice. The category of multispecialty groups, on the other hand, is rather heterogenous. It represents an entire spectrum of professional and economic arrangements, ranging from almost complete independence of individual practitioners to highly integrated teamwork. As has already been noted in Chapter Four, one can never be certain just what is being measured when physicians in such practices are compared to solo practitioners. To eliminate the danger of unfounded or misleading interpretation, it was therefore considered safer to exclude altogether physicians in multispecialty groups from our analysis. In this connection it may be noted, however, that the type of physicians retained in the sample do represent between 80 and 90 percent of all office-based physicians rendering patient care in this country [American Medical Association 1972, pp. 4 and 32].

Measurement of the Physician's Output

Given the information contained in the MEDEC surveys, the physician's output may be measured either by his *weekly patient visits* or by his *annual gross billings to patients*. Problems in the use of either index as a measure of output have already been touched upon in Chapters Three and Four. A few additional comments, more narrowly focused on the problem of production function estimation, may nevertheless be in order.

Patient Visits: It is clear that for a given number of total practice hours, the physician's weekly rates of office, hospital, and home visits with patients are related to one another through a common input constraint. If the output index Q_i is to reflect all three types of visits, they must somehow be aggregated. One way to deal with this problem is to let Q_i be the sum of the three types of visits and to include the proportions of the physician's hospital and home visits in total visits among the regressors of the production function specification. On this method the technical rates of substitution among types of visits are not assumed *a priori*. The method does, however, require one to assume that the visit mix itself is exogenous from the physician's viewpoint. [1]

A reasonable alternative would be to focus the analysis solely on the office-based part of the physician's practice. It is reasonable to assume that any interdependence between the physician's office, home, and hospital visits arises solely from the fact that each type of visit requires the input of physician time; there is no reason to assume that the physician's office staff or equipment alters his productivity on housecalls or in the hospital. It would therefore be legitimate to measure the output from the physician's office-based practice solely by his rate of weekly office visits, and to relate that output index to the number of hours the physician actually spends in his office (and to the other inputs into his office-based practice).

Production functions using either specification of Q_i are presented in this chapter. Implicit in the use of either approach, however, is the assumption that the mix of services provided per patient visit does not vary intolerably over the physician population being sampled. This assumption is not as unfounded as it may appear at first glance, because the overall MEDEC samples have been stratified into the much more homogeneous medical specialties, and include only physicians in solo practices or single-specialty groups. Even so, we cannot rule out the possibility that some interphysician variation in the mix of services per average visit remains even within each sample stratum. Quite aside from the problem of potential differences in the *quality* of services provided, such variation in the *mix* of services per visit obviously introduces a measurement error into our output index.

From the point of view of regression analysis, such errors of observation in the dependent variable can be treated as part of the ordinary, stochastic disturbance term e_i of the postulated regression equation. If these measurement errors can be taken as independent of the explanatory variables X_i (inputs), then they will increase the standard error of estimate, but they will not by themselves introduce any systematic bias into the least squares estimators $\hat{b}_j$. On the other hand, an estimation bias will occur if the mix of services produced by the physician's practice is somehow systematically related to one or more of the inputs. The question therefore arises whether the employment of auxiliary personnel generally tends to alter the mix of services prescribed and produced per average patient visit and, if so, how damaging the resulting estimation bias is likely to be to productivity estimates based on the output measure "patient visits."

In approaching this question it is useful to recall our discussion in Chapter Four in which the services produced by a physician's practice were broken down into services of types I, II, and III. By definition, any interphysician and input-related variance in the mix of services per visit must be confined to services of type I and type II. In the case of type I services, such variances reflect merely a shift in the locus of production from outside facilities to the physician's practice. If one's interest centers on the effect of auxiliary personnel on the availability of medical services to society at large, then the failure of patient visits to take account of any interphysician variance in type I services is actually desirable, because the mere internalization of the production of these services by some physicians does not result in additional social output at all.

An estimation bias may arise, however, in connection with type II services. These services, it will be recalled, are prescribed by the physician only if he employs the appropriate staff to produce them. Failure of the visit measure to reflect any interphysician differences in the production of such services per patient visit therefore leads one to underestimate the true social productivity of auxiliary personnel—provided of course that the prescription of such services is medically necessary and not simply motivated by the profit margins physicians can earn on the delivery of such services. Should the latter be the case, then the type II services may not really have any social value in the first place and their omission from one's output measure is, once again, desirable.

Finally, there remains the possibility that observed interphysician differences in the number of patient visits per hour are more or less offset by differences in the *quality* of the physicians' services. If so, one's estimates will overstate the true productivity of auxiliary personnel in medical practice. As already mentioned, we shall address this point at length in the concluding chapter of the book. Briefly, it will be acknowledged there that increases in the physician's hourly patient load without some compensating change in the organization of his practice may very well come at the expense of quality. It will also be asserted that, if the increased patient load was achieved through the delegation of tasks to properly trained auxiliary personnel, then there is no reason to suspect a deterioration in the quality of the physician's services. The implication of this assertion for the estimation of physician-care production functions is illustrated in Figure 6-1.

In Figure 6-1 the curves $A, B, \ldots, F$ depict the assumed relationship between the effective (quality-adjusted) hourly output of the physician's practice (Y) and the physician's hourly rate of patient visits (Q) for various levels of aide input (L). By quality in this context is meant some objective standard of

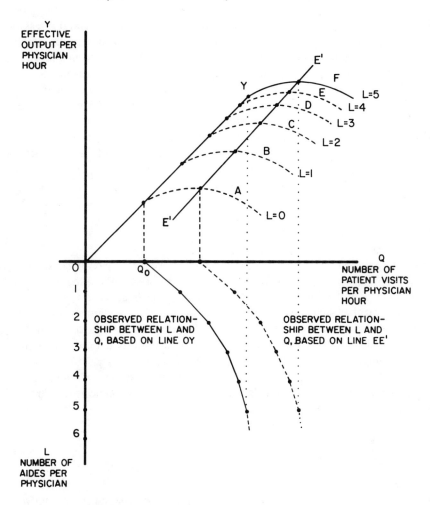

Figure 6-1. Hypothetical Relationship between Patient Visits per Hour and Effective (Quality-Adjusted) Physician Output per Hour

medical soundness. Thus it is assumed that a physician without assistants can increase his effective output and his rate of patient visits *proportionately* only up to a certain point, for example, Q_o. Beyond that point, the positive effects of increases in Q are dampened and eventually swamped by negative changes in the quality of the medical treatment dispensed, so that changes in Q are accompanied by less than proportionate changes in Y. But it is also assumed that the larger the physician's staff is, the later he will reach the point at which diminishing quality sets in, an assumption that is implicit in the relative positions of curves $A, B, \ldots, F$.

If one is willing to accept the notion that the hypothetical curves A,

$B, C, \ldots, F$ share a common, linear segment (the solid line OY),[a] and if one is mainly interested in the *marginal* contribution of aides to physician output, then it is of little consequence whether the physicians in one's cross-section sample are positioned exactly along the solid line OY, or somewhere on the broken lines $A, B, C, \ldots, F$. Nor is it crucial that all physicians in one's sample adhere precisely to a common standard of quality (for example, are all positioned on some line such as EE'). It need merely be assumed that the objective quality of the physicians' services is not systematically related to the number of aides they employ (that is, that the physicians in one's sample are more or less symmetrically distributed about a line such as EE'). For as long as the latter assumption is valid, Y could still be taken as roughly proportionate to Q, and an estimated production function in terms of patient visits would be meaningful. Since there is no *a priori* reason or empirical evidence to suggest otherwise, we proceed on that assumption here.

Patient Billings: It has been argued above that whatever variation there may be in the mix of services provided by the respondents to the MEDEC surveys, it will probably not result in any undesirable estimation *bias*. Nevertheless, it is clear that such variation will tend to increase the standard error of the estimate. It is therefore desirable to experiment with a measure of output that can be thought to reflect the responding physician's product mix: his annual patient billings.

On the assumption that the individual physician generally applies a single fee schedule to all of his patients, one may define his annual gross billings as

$$B_i = F_{1i} \sum_{j=1}^{z} (S_{ji} f_{ji}) = \frac{Y_i}{C_i} \qquad (6\text{-}2)$$

In this expression, vector $\mathbf{f}_i = (1, f_{2i}, f_{3i}, \ldots, f_{zi})$ may be regarded as the relative value scale (or its average) underlying the physician's fee schedule, and F_{1i} as the absolute fee of some basic service (usually a routine initial or follow-up visit) determining the physician's overall fee level. Finally, element S_{ji} of vector $\mathbf{S}_i$ denotes the number of services of type j the physician produces. From the MEDEC surveys, B_i can be obtained by dividing the physician's annual gross income from his practice (Y_i) by his collection ratio (C_i).[b]

B_i is obviously sensitive to the mix of services $(\mathbf{S}_i)$ produced by the physician. Unfortunately, vector $\mathbf{S}_i$ includes also the so-called type I services

---

[a]Since the employment of auxiliary personnel tends to act as a mild form of "peer review," line OY may, in fact, have a positive second derivative, at least up to a point.
[b]The collection ratio is defined as the average proportion of annual patient billings actually collected. For the MEDEC samples as a whole, this ratio had an average of 0.90 with a standard deviation of 0.07.

discussed earlier so that an approximation of the physician's output by B_i may lead one to overestimate the true social productivity of auxiliary personnel in medical practice. Furthermore, in the context of production-function estimation, B_i is a meaningful measure of output only to the extent that the relative aggregation weights (the elements of vector $\mathbf{f}_j$) it assigns to individual services are the same for all physicians in one's cross-section sample and, furthermore, are proportional to the relative resource inputs embodied in these services.

If American physicians operated in perfectly competitive nationwide product markets, and if the medical services supplied by physicians were well-defined standard products, then one would not expect to find much interphysician variation in either absolute or relative fees. It would also be reasonable to assume that the relative fees for the various services provided vary strictly as a function of factor costs. Under these conditions the use of fees as aggregation weights would be an acceptable procedure.

In fact, however, it is almost impossible to establish a clearcut definition of even as simple a procedure as an annual checkup, a tonsillectomy or an obstetrical delivery. Furthermore, American physicians typically work in local, semi-isolated product markets. Even if physicians acted on balance as price takers in their locality (for whatever reason), the absolute level of fees would nevertheless vary from locality to locality.

Table 5-1 presented the sample averages of the absolute fees typically charged by general practitioners in the 1965 MEDEC sample for a number of standard medical procedures. As is evident from the standard deviations associated with these averages, there is a considerable degree of interphysician variation in absolute fees in that year. Much of this variation does of course reflect regional differences, primarily in patients' ability to pay. Table 6-1, for example, presents the estimated coefficients of a linear regression of the absolute fee for a routine follow-up visit on certain locational variables. As can be seen from the coefficients of determination (R^2), the equations explain roughly one-third of the observed interphysician variation in fees. Had these regressions been based on county rather than the cruder state data, they would probably have explained an even greater proportion of the sample variance in absolute fee levels.

As a minimum, then, a production function specification with output measured by patient billings must include some control for interphysician variation in absolute fees. One way to accomplish this would be to deflate the billings reported by the physician by some appropriate fee index. For example, in terms of equation (6-2) one might divide B_i by F_{1i}, where the latter might be measured by the physician's fee for a routine office follow-up visit. An alternative to outright deflation would be to include F_{1i} among the regressors of the production function. Finally, if one is uncertain that there is a single fee that can adequately reflect the physician's overall level of fees, one might use the per capita income in the physician's locality as a reasonable proxy for the overall level.

Table 6-1. Variation of Absolute Fee Levels with Certain Locational Variables, General Practitioners and Pediatricians, 1967

Variable		General Practitioners		Pediatricians	
		Coefficient	t-Ratio	Coefficient	t-Ratio
Sample mean and (standard deviation) of dependent variable:					
Fee for routine follow-up visit		5.08 (1.15)		6.02 (1.20)	
Intercept (Urban-Western Region-Solo)		1.91	2.92	2.71	2.72
Per capita income of state	I	1.11	6.04	1.35	4.38
Physician's collection ratio	C	1.94	3.35	0.90	1.20
Group practice dummy variable	G	0.01	0.10	0.26	1.75
Rural practice dummy variable	R	-0.53	-5.26	-0.62	-1.51
Suburban practice dummy variable	SU	-0.11	-1.06	0.09	0.64
Regional dummy variables:					
Southern States	S	-0.77	-4.19	-0.47	-1.46
Eastern States	E	-0.81	-5.81	-0.49	-2.08
Midwestern States	MW	-1.02	-7.79	-0.86	-3.60
Mountain States	M	-0.62	-2.95	-1.50	-3.42
Coefficient of Determination R^2		0.37		0.32	

Source: Based on cross-section data from *Medical Economics*, Continuing Survey, 1967. Unfortunately, the 1967 surveys did not include information on the time devoted to particular medical procedures. The 1965 survey, on the other hand, did not include information on rural or suburban location.

Even after adjustment for interphysician differences in absolute fee levels, patient billings will not measure physician output well if *relative* fees (vector f_i) vary greatly over one's sample. If American physicians still followed the traditional sliding scale of fees (under which each patient is charged in accordance with his ability to pay), then relative fees would vary almost capriciously among physicians. Gross billings should then not be used at all as a measure of physician output. But there is growing evidence that during the postwar years the sliding scale of fees has gradually been replaced by more rigid fee schedules uniformly applied to all of a physician's patients.[2] Indeed, many state medical societies have followed California's lead and issued relative value scales that individual members may take as a guide. A comparison of the relative value scales used in the various states has indicated a fair degree of uniformity among them [Brewster and Seldowitz, 1965]. As is shown in Table 6-2, the American scales also seem to be quite similar to the relative value scales implicit in the fee schedules used in the Canadian provinces during the mid-1960s. Although some differences still persist in the value points assigned to individual procedures, the overall uniformity in the relative value scales shown in Table 6-2 is remarkable. Unfortunately, individual physicians do seem to deviate from their state's relative value scales, as may be inferred from the rather wide variation in the coefficients of variation in Table 5-1 and from the matrix of first-order correlations among medical fees charged by individual physicians in Table 6-3. The elements of vector f_i can therefore not be assumed to be constant over the MEDEC sample.

One explanation for the often rather low first-order correlation among medical fees may be that the services listed in Tables 5-1 and 6-3, although fairly common, are nevertheless not completely standard. There may be substantial interphysician differences in the resource intensity of ostensibly standard services, and medical fees may reflect these differences. The linear regression estimates shown in Table 6-4 support that hypothesis. These estimates are based on the responses of individual physicians to the 1965 MEDEC survey. As is evident from the standard deviation of the time physicians normally devote to a comprehensive check-up (variable M) the nature of that service seems to vary substantially among physicians. And the estimated coefficients and t-ratios of variable M suggest that physicians who devote an above average amount of time to a comprehensive check-up also tend to charge a correspondingly higher fee for that service, *ceteris paribus*.[c]

That relative medical fees are strongly influenced by relative factor costs also emerges from the fee data contained in Table 6-5, which shows the relationship between the sample averages of fees for a variety of distinct medical

[c]In interpreting Table 6-4 one should be mindful of the possibility that the relatively higher resource input per procedure observed for some physicians may simply reflect the operation of Parkinson's Law and not necessarily superior quality. In this connection, the reader is reminded of the discussion in Chapter One.

Table 6-2.　Relative Value Scales[a] of Certain Medical Procedures—United States and Canada, 1965

State or Province	Tonsillectomy	Hysterectomy	Repair of Hernia	D&C	Obstetrical Delivery	Caesarian Section
United States						
Calif.	0.4	1.5	0.9	0.4	0.8	1.3
D.C.	0.5	2.0	1.2	0.5	0.7	1.7
Haw.	0.4	1.5	0.9	0.4	0.8	1.4
Ill.	0.5	2.0	1.0	0.5	1.0	1.7
Iowa	0.5	1.7	1.0	0.3	1.0	1.3
Mont.	0.4	1.8	1.0	0.5	1.0	1.7
Nebr.	0.4	1.7	1.0	0.4	0.8	1.2
Pa.	0.5	1.7	1.0	0.5	0.8	1.7
S. Dak.	0.4	1.8	1.0	0.3	1.0	1.5
Utah	0.5	1.7	1.2	0.5	0.8	1.7
Mean	0.4	1.7	1.0	0.4	0.9	1.5
Standard Deviation	0.1	0.2	0.1	0.1	0.1	0.2
Canadian Plains[b]						
B.C.M.S.I.	0.4	1.7	1.2	0.4	0.9	2.0
M.S.A.	0.4	1.8	1.1	0.3	0.9	1.9
M.S.(A.)I.	0.4	1.7	1.1	0.3	1.1	1.5
M.M.S.	0.4	1.7	0.9	0.3	0.7	1.3
P.S.I.	0.4	2.0	1.3	0.4	1.3	1.7
W.M.S.	0.2	1.7	1.1	0.3	1.0	1.5
M.H.S.A.	0.3	1.5	1.1	0.3	1.0	1.3
M.M.C.	0.3	1.3	0.9	0.3	0.6	1.1
Mean	0.3	1.7	1.1	0.3	0.9	1.5
Standard Deviation	0.1	0.2	0.1	0.0	0.2	0.3

[a] All fees have been normalized on the fee for an appendectomy.

[b] The Canadian Prepayment Plans are, in the order listed: (1) B.C. Government Employees Medical Services (British Columbia); (2) Medical Services Association (British Columbia); (3) Medical Services (Alberta) Inc.; (4) Manitoba Medical Service; (5) Physicians' Services Incorporated (Ontario); (6) Windsor Medical Services, Inc. (Ontario); (7) Maritime Hospital Services Association (New Brunswick); (8) Maritime Medical Care Inc. (Nova Scotia).

Source: A.W. Brewster, and E. Seldowitz, "Medical Society Relative Value Scales and the Medical Care Market," *Public Health Report* 80 (June 1965): 501–509, and data supplied by Trans-Canada Medical Plans, Inc, Toronto.

Table 6-3.   Correlations among Selected Medical Fees Charged by General Practitioners, 1965

Medical Services	1	2	3	4	5	6	7	8	9	10
1. Comprehensive diagnostic history and physical examination	1.00									
2. Initial visit (noncomprehensive)	0.38	1.00								
3. Follow-up visit, routine or usual	0.28	0.63	1.00							
4. House call—one person	0.64	0.51	0.69	1.00						
5. Follow-up examination and evaluation per day	0.28	0.38	0.55	0.57	1.00					
6. Appendectomy	0.21	0.30	0.57	0.60	0.60	1.00				
7. D&C diagnostic	0.21	0.33	0.54	0.56	0.51	0.69	1.00			
8. Complete obstetrical care	0.33	0.52	0.69	0.72	0.65	0.69	0.59	1.00		
9. T&A child	0.22	0.37	0.62	0.64	0.55	0.65	0.65	0.66	1.00	
10. Urinalysis	0.08	0.21	0.54	0.40	0.32	0.36	0.36	0.42	0.40	1.00

Source: Data from *Medical Economics*, Continuing Survey, 1965.

Table 6-4. Estimated Linear Relationship Between Medical Fees, Medical Inputs, and Patients' Ability to Pay, General Practitioners, 1965

Variable		Sample		Equation 1		Equation 2	
		Mean	Standard Deviation	Coefficient Estimate	t-Ratio	Coefficient Estimate	t-Ratio
Fee for comprehensive physical check-up	F	15.44	10.53	—	—	—	—
Intercept	—	—	—	-5.62	-1.93	-3.54	-1.02
Number of minutes devoted to procedure	M	45.84	20.66	0.29	13.13	0.29	13.09
Total professional expenses per visit	E	2.15	0.96	0.92	1.91	—	—
Nonsalary expenses per visit	NSE	0.73	0.60	—	—	1.21	1.58
Number of RN's per physician	RN	0.42	0.52	—	—	-3.91	-2.58
Number of Technicians per physician	TE	0.26	0.42	—	—	-1.93	-1.17
Number of Office Aides per physician	OA	1.22	0.79	—	—	-2.53	-1.92
$(RN + TE + OA)^2$	LSQ	4.38	4.41	—	—	0.94	3.33
Per capita income of state in which physician practices ($1,000s)	I	2.08	0.37	2.09	1.63	2.45	1.12
Percent of work week devoted to insurance claims	HI	2.87	2.69	0.29	1.68	0.18	1.12
Group Dummy Variable	G	0.33	—	1.51	1.54	1.43	1.48
Coefficient of Determination	R^2			0.37		0.40	
Number of observations		477		—		—	

Source: Based on data from Medical Economics, Continuing Survey, 1965.

Table 6-5. Comparison of Average Time Required and Fees Charged for Common Medical Procedures, General Practitioners, 1965[a]

Type of Service	Average Fee for Procedure	Average Physician Time (minutes) per procedure	Equivalent Hourly Fee for Procedure
Comprehensive examination and patient history	$15.00	45.9	$19.60
Initial office visit	5.20	17.8	17.60
Follow-up office visit	4.30	11.2	23.00
House call, one person	7.50	27.7	16.30
House call, two persons	10.10	35.0	17.30
Comprehensive examination of patient in hospital	14.10	50.1	17.00
Follow-up visit of patient in hospital	5.50	13.4	24.60

[a]The estimated relationship between average fee per procedure (F) and the average number of physician minutes required per procedure (M) is

$$\hat{F} = 0.9 + 0.28M; R^2 = 0.95$$

Source: Data from *Medical Economics,* Continuing Survey, 1965. The averages are based on 477 observations.

procedures and the corresponding sample averages of physician time devoted to these procedures. When these statistics are converted to equivalent hourly fees, it becomes apparent that there does exist a fairly close relationship between time input and fee levels. The same conclusion emerges from Table 6-6, which presents similar data from an independent Canadian study undertaken in 1964, and which implies a comparable hourly rate of remuneration.

It may be noted that the estimated marginal remuneration of physician time (in 1965) implied by Table 6-5 is quite close to that implied by Table 6-4. Furthermore, the estimated coefficient of the cost variable E in Table 6-4 also suggests that professional costs other than time costs (such as the cost of supplies, equipment, and auxiliary personnel) tend to reflect themselves in medical fees. This observation is consistent with Martin Feldstein's time-series analysis of medical fees, in the course of which he found that "greater use of paramedical personnel and supplies has increased the cost and [hence] price of physicians' services" [1970, p. 132]. However, according to equation (2) in Table 6-4, the increase of fees with aide input appears to set in only after a certain point (between one to two aides per physician), prior to which fees appear to fall with aide input.[d]

[d]Variables I and HI are included in the equations in order to account for the influence of ability to pay on fees. Unfortunately, the 1965 data did not include information on whether the physician practices in a rural or urban area. Ideally, of course, one would like to represent ability to pay by the average income and insurance coverage of *each* responding physician's clientele. Even so, our rather unsatisfactory proxies do have coefficients with the expected positive signs. It should be noted, incidentally, that identical regressions for the other medical specialties reflected broadly similar patterns.

Table 6-6.   Comparison of Average Time Required and Fees
Charged for Office Visits of Varying Duration, General Practitioners[a]

Average Length of Visits, in Minutes	*Average Fee of Visits*
Average length of office visit: 15.5 minutes	
Average gross fee for office visits	$ 4.65
under 10 minutes	3.55
11–20 minutes	4.25
21–31 minutes	7.57
31–45 minutes	9.41
over 46 minutes	9.47
Equivalent hourly gross fee for office visits	$17.75

[a]The above data are based on the activity of a multispecialty group practice in Saskatchewan, Canada. As part of that study, each physician in the group kept detailed statistics on every face-to-face contact with patients during the calendar year 1964. The data so collected included information on the duration of face-to-face contact with patients and on the corresponding fee payable by the government-operated Medical Care Insurance Commission in Saskatchewan.
Source: S. Wolfe, et al. [1968], p. 114.

One concludes from this brief examination of fee-setting in American medical practices that fees are perhaps not as capriciously set as would be the case under a full-fledged sliding-scale-of-fees system. There does appear to be a functional relationship between relative fees and relative factor costs for individual services, so that patient billings, adjusted for interphysician differences in the absolute overall fee level, can probably be used as a rough-and-ready proxy for the output produced by a physician's practice. It has to be conceded, however, that the relationship between relative factor costs and fees is not as close as one would like it to be from the view of econometric theory. The regression equations in Table 6-4, for example, explain at most 40 percent of the observed sample variance in fees.

There is also the possibility that above-average time input per procedure—and the correspondingly higher fee associated with that procedure— reflects the working of Parkinson's Law more so than socially useful output. (In this connection, see footnote c above.) Even so, an estimated relationship between annual patient billings and medical inputs is surely not uninteresting. In addition to the production-function estimates based on total patient visits and office visits as output measures, we therefore also present in this chapter estimates in which output has been approximated by the physician's annual patient billings.

Measurement of the Inputs into the Physician's Practice
The information contained in the MEDEC surveys enables one to distinguish among the following types of practice inputs: the physician's own

time, his use of auxiliary personnel, his use of medical supplies, drugs and small instruments, and his use of floor space and equipment. None of these measures is completely free of inherent shortcomings.

The Input of Physician Time: In connection with the input of the physician's labor, the MEDEC data for 1965 and 1967 are unusually detailed. The physician's total practice hours per week are broken down into office hours, hours spent on staff meetings, and time devoted to research, writing, and teaching. It may be noted in passing that the average breakdown of total physician hours into these various professional activities appears to be fairly constant from survey to survey.

For our present purposes, the input of physician time has been defined as the total number of hours per week spent on strictly practice-related professional activities. For the estimates using annual patient billings or total (office, hospital, and home) visits as an output measure, the input of physician time excludes the time devoted to reading, research, writing, teaching, and staff meetings. Where output has been measured strictly in terms of office visits only, the time spent in the hospital or on house calls has been excluded from the physician's time input as well.

Although the extent of a physician's engagement in reading, writing, research, or teaching may be taken as an index of the physician's medical competence, they are not likely to contribute to output as it is measured in this study. Its inclusion in physician input would therefore detract from the statistical fit of the production function. As it happens, the physicians in the MEDEC samples do not differ markedly with respect to the time devoted to strictly practice-connected activities. The mean percentage of time devoted to strictly practice-related activities was between 90 and 93 for all specialties; the standard deviation about this mean was only 7 percentage points.

Auxiliary Personnel: The MEDEC data include information on the number of paramedical and clerical aides employed by the physician (or by his group), differentiated in terms of medical technicians, registered nurses and clerical staff, on the one hand, and in terms of part-time and full-time status on the other. In the absence of better information, two part-time employees were considered the equivalent of one full-time employee. Conspicuously absent from this list of personnel are the newly emerging physician extenders (physician assistants, MEDEX, pediatric nurse practitioners, and so on) which were not in widespread use at the time the MEDEC surveys were taken. The health manpower with which we are concerned here thus includes only the traditional types of paramedical aides.

In principle, the occupational lines between registered nurses, medical technicians and clerical personnel are clearly drawn. In the hospital sector, the division of tasks among types of health manpower is severely constrained by these formal lines. Within the confines of their own practice, however, physicians tend to be rather flexible with respect to the use of their aides. For example, both the nurse and the technician will normally be involved also in the clerical side of the physician's practice, unless he also employs a full-time office aide. And if a physician does not employ either a nurse or a technician, he will generally train his office aides to perform a variety of medical tasks under his personal supervision, although the range of tasks he can delegate in this way is likely to be narrower than that delegatable to either nurses or technicians. Within the context of private medical practice the three ostensibly distinct types of aides can therefore be regarded as fairly close substitutes for each other, and our separation of aides into nurses, technicians, and clerical personnel is designed mainly to account for differences in the quality of aide input.

It would be tempting to measure any remaining differences in the quality of aides in terms of their salaries. But over a nationwide cross-section of physicians the salaries individual practitioners pay their aides are likely to reflect the market power of local hospital associations [3] more so than the quality of the physician's aides. Thus the use of salaries as proxies for labor quality would quite probably distort our measure of labor input even more seriously.

Medical Supplies: It is not clear what role the category of drugs and medical supplies (including nondepreciable, small instruments) play in the production of medical output, as it is measured in this study. On the one hand it may be argued that a physician's expenditures on these items are strictly a consequence, rather than a determinant, of the volume of medical services produced. If so, the treatment of medical supplies as a separate input will necessarily result in an estimated output elasticity close to 1. But to the extent that those supplies include a significant number of disposable items (syringes, sheets, towels, gloves), they will act as a substitute for the input of paramedical aides [Frederick 1968, p. 70].

At the present time, little is known about the extent to which the productivity of health personnel can be raised through the use of disposables. Although this area is one worthy of more research at the microeconomic level, it is doubtful that much can be learned from the MEDEC data in this respect. These data include information only on the physician's total annual expenditures on medical supplies. However, in many instances the use of disposables involves not only a time saving, but also a dollar saving in outlays for the particular items [Frederick, 1968, p. 70]. It is therefore impossible to measure a physician's use of disposables by the level of his medical-supplies expenditures. Since these expenditure data are likely to reflect for the most part supplies and drugs in their role as complementary inputs, the category of "supplies, drugs and small instruments" has been omitted altogether from the production function estimates presented here.

Capital: For the most part, a physician's capital stock consists of ordinary furniture, office, laboratory and x-ray equipment, and floor space, or, more specifically, the number of examination rooms at his disposition.

Given the size of a physician's staff, a physician may increase the productivity of *all* manpower inputs, including his own, by acquiring capital equipment that is more elaborate and expensive than is minimally necessary. For example, the acquisition of dictaphones and photocopying machines can yield a substantial savings in clerical time; a large and rather expensive autoclave reduces the aide-time which must be devoted to the sterilizing of instruments; in comparison with ordinary examination tables, a more expensive hydraulic table with flexible surface appears to reduce significantly the time in which a physician can examine his patients. It is clear, then, that the physician's capital stock is not purely a complement of health manpower; in some instances it acts as a substitute for the latter.

Ideally, one would like to dichotomize the physician's capital stock into that part which is purely complementary to health-manpower and that part which is in the nature of a substitute. Furthermore one would like to measure the input of the latter as a physical flow of services. Unfortunately, the MEDEC surveys were not sufficiently informative on this point. The best available proxy was the sum of the physician's annual depreciation expenses for medical and office equipment and his annual expense (depreciation or rent) for floor space. This figure was estimated by subtracting the physician's annual outlays on drugs, medical supplies and instruments, the annual cost of operating and amortizing his automobile, and his annual payroll expenses from his total professional expenses.

It is quite obvious that this estimate of capital is at best a rough approximation to the true flow of services from the physician's capital stock. [4] Furthermore, it lumps together the services from all types of capital, including floor space and equipment that is purely complementary to health manpower. It can therefore be expected that a production function estimate including that measure of capital will yield a biased estimate of the capital-elasticity of output, especially if output is measured by patient visits. This potential bias notwithstanding, it is surely better to include at least some measure of capital in the production function specification than to omit the item from the analysis altogether. (In general, the omission of a relevant variable X_k from an estimate of the linear function

$$Y = \sum_{i=1}^{k} (b_i X_i) + e \qquad (6\text{-}3)$$

will bias the estimators $\hat{b}$ of the parameters b_i, $i = 1, 2, \ldots, k - 1$ by the corresponding factors $P_{ik} \cdot b_k$, where P_{ik} is the ith coefficient in the regression of X_k on the remaining X_i, $i = 1, 2, \ldots, k-1$, that is, in the equation

$$X_k = \sum_{i=1}^{k-1} (P_{ik}X_i) + v \qquad (6\text{-}3a)$$

If X_k is correlated with X_i, then $P_{ik} \neq 0$, and hence $E(\hat{b}_i) = b_i + (P_{ik}b_k)$. In this connection, see Griliches [1957].)

II. ESTIMATES OF PHYSICIAN-CARE PRODUCTION FUNCTIONS

Tables 6–7 to 6–10 present production-function estimates for general practitioners (GP), pediatricians (PD), obstetricians-gynecologists (OBG) and internists (IM) in solo practice or single-specialty groups. In these estimates the physician's output has been alternatively measured (1) by the sum of the physician's weekly office, home, and hospital visits (hereafter referred to as "total patient visits"); (2) by his weekly office visits; and (3) by his annual gross billings to patients.

The coefficients of multiple determination (R^2) of these regression equations range from a low of 0.42 to a high of 0.69. Depending on the specialty being considered and the output measure used, our estimates thus explain between 42 percent and 69 percent of the observed variation in the dependent variables about their sample mean. Given the fact that the estimates are based on cross-section survey data, these R^2 are not unexpectedly low.

With respect to the overall statistical significance of the estimated equations, it may be noted that the smallest observed F-ratio (27.0) in any of the equations is more than ten times the appropriate value of the F-distribution at the 99 percentage point. In other words, all of the equations can be taken to be statistically significant at better than a 1 percent level.

The fact that the estimates still leave a considerable residual of unexplained variance in the dependent variable does not destroy their usefulness. It has not been the main purpose of our empirical investigation to predict accurately the rate of visits of each individual physician in the MEDEC sample. Rather, the objective has been to obtain information on the probable influence of certain major inputs, particularly of auxiliary personnel, on a physician's rate of patient visits (billings). Since the estimated coefficients of these inputs are highly significant statistically, and barring any severe estimation biases, they can surely be taken as at least broadly indicative of that influence.[e]

[e]It is quite obvious that, given our present knowledge about medical care production and the paucity of available data, an analysis of this sort necessarily omits a great many minor factors that also influence a physician's rate of output. But in the absence of strong evidence to the contrary, it may be hoped that the omitted variables are essentially independent of the variables included in the regression.

Table 6-7.   Estimated Production Functions for General Practitioners in Private Practice

Variable	Sample Mean	Standard Deviation	Equation 1 Output Measured by Total Patient Visits		Equation 2 Output Measured by Office Visits		Equation 3 Output Measured by Patient Billings	
			Estimated Coefficient	Standard Error	Estimated Coefficient	Standard Error	Estimated Coefficient	Standard Error
$\text{Log } H^a$	4.06	0.24	1.671	0.234	—	—	1.038	0.182
H	60.98	14.29	-.015	0.004	—	—	-.0086	0.003
$\text{Log } OH^b$	3.53	0.28	—	—	0.671	0.039	—	—
$\text{Log } K$	4.06	0.96	0.044	0.011	0.040	0.012	0.084	0.009
$L_1(RN)$	0.46	0.63	0.274	0.029	0.364	0.032	0.282	0.026
$L_2(TE)$	0.26	0.49	0.245	0.032	0.312	0.035	0.277	0.028
$L_3(OA)$	1.24	0.88	0.240	0.024	0.306	0.028	0.264	0.022
$(\sum L)^2$	5.13	5.62	-.024	0.004	-.035	0.005	-.026	0.004
G	0.21	—	0.045	0.023	0.051	0.025	0.055	0.018
PPR	1.31	0.36	-.058*	0.033	-.102	0.031	-.044*	0.024
PHV	0.15	0.12	0.217	0.092	—	—	0.222	0.075
PHC	0.04	0.05	-.457	0.234	—	—	-.514	0.186
$\text{Log } F$	1.82	0.36	—	—	—	—	0.494	0.126
$YEAR$	0.52	—	—	—	—	—	0.051	0.017
$CONSTANT$	—	—	-1.174	—	2.084	—	-1.403	—
$\text{Log } Q^c$	—	—	5.14	0.44	4.94	0.44	3.94	0.42
R^2	—	—	0.52		0.50		0.67	
δ_u	—	—	0.29		0.31		0.21	
N	862		—		—		—	

[a]H denotes total weekly practice hours, including time spent on hospital visits and housecalls, but excluding time spent on teaching and research.
[b]OH denotes only hours spent in the office, excluding time spent on teaching and research.
[c]Q denotes either total weekly patient visits, total weekly office visits, or annual gross billings in thousands of dollars.
*Significant at a 10 percent level only.

Table 6–8.   Estimated Production Functions for Pediatricians in Private Practice

Variable	Sample Mean	Standard Deviation	Equation 1 Output Measured by Total Patient Visits		Equation 2 Output Measured by Office Visits		Equation 3 Output Measured by Patient Billings	
			Estimated Coefficient	Standard Error	Estimated Coefficient	Standard Error	Estimated Coefficient	Standard Error
Log H^a	3.92	0.21	0.809	0.092	—	—	0.482	0.074
H	52.00	10.86	—	—	0.570	0.080	—	—
Log OH^b	3.52	0.25	—	—	0.061	0.026	—	—
Log K	4.18	0.83	0.059	0.025	0.383	0.048	0.107	0.020
L_1(RN)	0.43	0.58	0.355	0.045	0.324	0.058	0.372	0.036
L_2(TE)	0.18	0.41	0.234	0.058	0.378	0.058	0.331	0.044
L_3(OA)	1.07	0.80	0.298	0.042	−.041	0.047	0.309	0.036
$(\Sigma L)^2$	4.32	8.70	−.027	0.004	−.041	0.006	−.034	0.005
G	0.35	—	0.060**	0.042	0.079	0.040	0.100	0.031
PPR	1.40	0.36	0.126**	0.206	−0.36*	0.055	—	—
PHV	0.13	0.10	−.782	0.399	—	—	—	—
PHC	0.03	0.36	—	—	—	—	—	—
Log F	1.91	0.39	—	—	—	—	.457	0.142
YEAR	0.70	—	—	—	—	—	0.017**	0.033
CONSTANT	—	—	1.171	—	2.129	—	0.185	—
Log Q^c	—	—	4.97	0.42	4.82	0.43	3.85	0.38
R^2	—		0.46		0.43		0.60	
$\hat{\sigma}_u$	—		0.31		0.32		0.24	
N^d	270		—		—		—	

*Significant at a 10 percent level only.
**Not significant at a 10 percent level.
For other notes, see Table 6–7.

Table 6-9.   Estimated Production Functions for Obstetricians/Gynecologists in Private Practice

Variable	Sample Mean	Standard Deviation	Equation 1 — Output Measured by Total Patient Visits		Equation 2 — Output Measured by Office Visits		Equation 3 — Output Measured by Patient Billings	
			Estimated Coefficient	Standard Error	Estimated Coefficient	Standard Error	Estimated Coefficient	Standard Error
Log H[a]	3.99	0.28	2.041	0.326	—	—	0.525	0.059
H	57.00	16.34	-.024	0.005	—	—	—	—
Log OH[b]	—	—	—	—	0.560	0.067	—	—
Log K	4.31	0.78	0.077	0.029	0.074	0.031	0.135	0.021
L_1(RN)	0.49	0.54	0.337	0.063	0.384	0.071	0.432	0.049
L_2(TE)	0.16	0.43	0.269	0.080	0.265	0.086	0.368	0.058
L_3(OA)	0.89	0.78	0.243	0.062	0.268	0.071	0.337	0.050
$(\Sigma L)^2$	3.25	4.61	-.024	0.012	-.028	0.014	-.043	0.009
G	0.38	—	0.130	0.047	0.129	0.045	0.117	0.033
PPR	1.42	0.45	-.134	0.051	-.093*	0.053	—	—
PHV	0.24	0.13	0.575	0.173	—	—	—	—
PHC	0.003	0.01	—	—	—	—	—	—
LT2	0.06	—	-.155*	0.091	—	—	—	—
MT25	0.13	—	-.102*	0.067	—	—	—	—
Log F	2.29	0.42	—	—	—	—	0.350	0.140
YEAR	0.60	—	—	—	—	—	0.104	0.034
CONSTANT	—	—	-2.576	—	2.004	—	-.047	—
Log Q	—	—	4.71	0.51	4.41	0.50	3.97	0.41
$\bar{R}^2$	—	—	0.56		0.42		0.63	
$\hat{\sigma}_u$	—	—	0.34		0.38		0.25	
N	271		—		—		—	

*Significant at a 10 percent level only.
For other notes, see Table 6-7.

Table 6-10. Estimated Production Functions for Internists in Private Practice

Variable	Sample Mean	Standard Deviation	Equation 1 Output Measured by Total Patient Visits — Estimated Coefficient	Standard Error	Equation 2 Output Measured by Office Visits — Estimated Coefficient	Standard Error	Equation 3 Output Measured by Patient Billings — Estimated Coefficient	Standard Error
$\text{Log } H^a$	3.99	0.26	0.709	0.075	—	—	0.423	0.053
H	56.00	13.35	—	—	—	—	—	—
$\text{Log } OH^b$	3.36	0.37	—	—	—	—	—	—
$\text{Log } K$	4.15	0.84	0.039	0.004	0.695	0.053	0.098	0.017
$L_1(RN)$	0.29	0.46	0.346	0.071	0.045	0.025	0.391	0.049
$L_2(TE)$	0.30	0.44	0.277	0.077	0.377	0.076	0.402	0.053
$L_3(OA)$	1.00	0.65	0.365	0.066	0.280	0.081	0.405	0.049
$(\Sigma L)^2$	3.21	3.48	-.026	0.015	0.392	0.075	-.043	0.011
G	0.29	—	0.039**	0.043	-.028	0.017	0.057	0.029
PPR	1.46	0.43	-.208	0.051	-.002**	0.045	-.069**	0.043
PHV	0.31	0.18	0.526	0.109	-.003**	0.047	0.186	0.076
PHC	0.04	0.04	-.909	0.452	—	—	-.827	0.303
$\text{Log } F$	2.14	0.37	—	—	—	—	0.267	0.139
$YEAR$	0.47	—	—	—	—	—	0.079	0.026
$CAP4$	2238.	357.	—	—	—	—	0.000119	0.00005
$CONSTANT$	—	—	1.216	—	1.306	—	0.453	—
$\text{Log } Q$	—	—	4.75	0.49	4.31	0.51	3.86	0.37
R^2	—	—	0.58		0.59		0.69	
$\hat{\sigma}_u$	—	—	0.31		0.33		0.21	
N	296	—	—		—		—	

**Not significant at a 10 percent level.

For other notes, see Table 6-7.

The regression equations shown in Tables 6-7 to 6-10 are minor variants of the production-function specification

$$\log(Q_i) = a_0 + a_1 \log(H_i) - b_1 H_i + a_2 \log(K_i) + \sum_{j=1}^{3}(c_j L_{ji}) - d\left[\sum_{j=1}^{3}(L_{ji})\right]^2$$

$$+ \sum_{s}(m_s D_{si}) + e_i \qquad i = 1, 2, 3, \ldots, N. \tag{6-4}$$

In this specification, i denotes the ith physician in a cross-section sample of size N, and e_i is a stochastic error term whose presumed properties have already been described in conjunction with equation (6-1) above. Variable Q_i represents the physician's rate of output (measured either by weekly patient visits or annual gross billings); H_i denotes the input of the physician's own time (total weekly practice hours if output is measured by total patient visits or gross patient billings, and weekly office hours if output is measured by weekly office visits only); K_i measures the services from the physician's capital stock (an annual-expense figure); L_{1i}, L_{2i} and L_{3i} denote the number of registered nurses (RN), technicians (TE) and office aides (OA), respectively; and the elements of vector D_i are quantitative indexes further characterizing the nature and location of the physician's practice. It is worth emphasizing that variables H, L and K are all expressed on a "per physician" basis. Since the *flow* of services rendered by auxiliary personnel is measured by *stock* variables, it is implicitly assumed that this flow of services is roughly proportional to the stock of aides.

Equation (6-4) will be recognized as a specific version of the fairly general production function (5-8) developed in the previous chapter. In equation (6-4), variables H and K play the role of "essential" inputs (denoted by X_j in equation (5-8)). Variables L_1, L_2 and L_3, on the other hand, are treated as analogues of the "nonessential" inputs (denoted by Y_j in equation (5-8)). The general function $g(X, Y; c)$ in equation (5-8) is thus given the specific algebraic form

$$g(H, K, L; c, d) = \sum_{j=1}^{3}(c_j L_{ji}) - d\left[\sum_{j=1}^{3}(L_{ji})\right]^2 \tag{6-5}$$

In principle it would have been desirable to disaggregate the squared term in equation (6-5). Since the majority of physicians in the MEDEC sample were solo practitioners, however, L_1, L_2 and L_3 were frequently either zero or unity. Disaggregation of the squared term would therefore have led to severe multicollinearity. The procedure reflected in equation (6-5) was adopted instead.[5]

Equation (6-5) has the admittedly undesirable property of reaching a maximum independently of the values of H and K. If the sample variances of H and K were large, this would be an intolerable drawback. Variables H and K in equation (6-4), however, are expressed on a per physician basis, a procedure that considerably reduces the sample variances of H and K. Since L_1, L_2 and L_3 are expressed as the number of full-time equivalent aides per physician, it does not seem unreasonable to postulate that the values of L_1, L_2 and L_3 at which equation (6-5) reaches a maximum are more or less independent of the precise number of hours the physician works per week, and similarly for K. A preferred method would, of course, have been to include cross-products among H, K and **L** among the arguments of equation (6-5). It became obvious during the pilot phase of the study, however, that this approach was vitiated by intolerable multicollinearity among the regressors.

The nature and measurement of H, **L** and K have already been discussed in section I of this chapter and hence require no further comment. The variables represented by vector **D**, on the other hand, require further explanation. Included in this vector are the physician-population ratio of the state in which the physician practices (identified in the tables by the mnemonic variable-name *PPR*), the percentage of hospital visits and house calls in total patient visits (*PHV* and *PHC*, respectively); a dummy variable (YEAR) set equal to zero if the *i*th observation was taken in 1965 and equal to one if it was taken in 1967; and a dummy variable (*G*) set equal to zero if the *i*th physician was a solo practitioner and equal to one if he belonged to a single-specialty group or partnership.

The inclusion of the physician-density index (*PPR*) among the regressors seems advisable because the *hourly* patient load of physicians in high-density areas (such as California or New York state) tends to be lower than that of physicians in low-density areas (such as the southern or midwestern states). (In this connection the reader may wish to refer back to Table 2-5.) Ideally one would like to have a variable characterizing relative physician density in the physician's immediate environment. Such information was unfortunately not contained in the MEDEC surveys; the best approximation to physician density was the statewide physician-population ratio. *A priori* one would expect the coefficient of *PPR* (where significant) to have a negative sign, as in fact it does.

As has been mentioned in section I, the mix of the physician's office, home, and hospital visits in total visits can be accounted for by including the percentage of hospital and home visits in total visits (*PHV* and *PHC*) among the explanatory variables. It was noted in Chapter Three that both home and hospital visits tend to be relatively more time-consuming than office visits (see Table 3-8). One would therefore expect both *PHV* and *PHC* to have negative coefficients. Where statistically significant at all, the coefficient of *PHC* did indeed have the expected negative sign. The coefficient of *PHV*, on the other hand, turned out to be positive where significant. *PHV* apparently acted as a proxy for other factors influencing the physician's hourly productivity and failed to play the role it was initially thought to play in the equation.

All estimates presented in Tables 6-7 to 6-10 are based on the combined 1965 and 1967 MEDEC surveys. The two annual surveys were pooled in order to include a sufficient number of nonsolo practitioners in the sample for each specialty. This pooling proceeded on the assumption that, over the short span of two years, the technology of private medical-care production has not changed significantly. On this assumption, the two independent surveys may be considered as one large sample.

On inspection of the Medical Economics data, the assumption of a more or less unchanged technology for 1965–67 does not appear to be unreasonable. For example, the inclusion of a year-of-survey dummy variable (*YEAR*) in the patient-visit equations—either in the form of an intercept adjustment or in the form of input-coefficient adjustments or both—failed to yield statistically significant coefficients for any of the four medical specialties and was therefore dropped from these equations; it was left in the patient-billings equations for reasons indicated further on.

The years-in-practice (*LT2, MT25*) dummy variables were included among the regressors on the notion that very young and very old physicians tend to spend relatively more time per visit with their patients. One would expect young and inexperienced physicians to move more cautiously on any procedure, while older physicians may have an outright preference for the traditional, more slowly paced medical practice. As it happens, however, the estimated coefficient of *LT2* and *MT25* were statistically significant only for the OBG specialists. They were therefore exluded from the estimates for the other medical specialties.

A word about the manner of incorporating the descriptive variables D_{si} in the production function may be in order. As these variables have been entered into equation (6-4), they are assumed to affect the productivity of all inputs in the same direction and to the same degree. In principle, of course, these variables can be assumed to affect both the intercept (or constant term) and the individual input elasticities. A perfectly flexible *a priori* specification should therefore include also the cross-products between each of the inputs and each of the descriptive variables in (6-4).

It must be recognized, however, that this increased flexibility in the *a priori* specification engenders certain statistical problems. For one, the inclusion of cross-product terms in equation (6-4) increases enormously the number of regressors. Worse still, the inclusion of numerous cross-products tends to result in serious intercorrelation among the regressors, and therefore detracts from the reliability of the individual coefficient estimates. In view of these difficulties, our approach has been to experiment with both intercept and input-coefficient adjustments during the pilot phase of the study. In the end only those estimates that resulted in the best fit, as indicated by the statistical significance and plausibility of the individual coefficient estimates, were retained. On these criteria, it was found that there was typically no compelling reason to prefer input-coefficient adjustment to intercept adjustment. On the contrary, the attempt to adjust input coefficients usually resulted in intolerable multicollinearity.[6]

In addition to the descriptive variables mentioned above, some or all of the patient-billings equations also include the per capita income of the state in which the physician practices (*CAPY*), the year-of-survey dummy variable already defined earlier, and a variable $\log F_i$, where F_i is the average of the physician's customary fees for a routine initial and a routine follow-up visit. These variables are intended to control jointly for any interphysician differences in the absolute level of fees.

The per capita income variable turns out to be statistically significant only in the equation for internists, and even there its absolute magnitude is very small. A statewide variable seemingly fails to portray adequately the physician's immediate environment. The year-of-survey variable, however, was invariably significant and positive. This variable was included primarily to capture changes in billing practices in response to the introduction of the Medicare/Medicaid programs in 1966. These programs provide insurance coverage for ambulatory care patients who would otherwise be unable to pay for such care and whom physicians may have treated at fees below their customary charges prior to the Medicare/Medicaid programs. The introduction of these programs may have had one or both of the following effects. First, physicians now were able to charge their (higher) customary fees for the treatment of these patients. Second, physicians may have increased the number of services rendered these patients per patient visit in the secure knowledge that these added services would not place an undue financial burden on their patients. Either effect would not be picked up by the fee variable *F*—hence the inclusion of the year-of-survey variable in the patient billings equations.

If physicians generally could change their rates of output without having to change the level of their fees, and the fee variable *F* acted solely as a proxy for the physician's absolute fee level, one would expect $\log F$ to have a coefficient close to unity. Actually that coefficient—the so-called fee-elasticity of patient billings—had a value below 0.50 in all four medical specialties. So large a deviation from unity can probably not be ascribed to the possibility that *F* is not a wholly reliable proxy for the absolute fee level; the explanation for the low fee-elasticity must be sought elsewhere.[7]

One possibility is that much of the fee effect was in fact picked up by the year-of-survey dummy variable (*YEAR*), for medical fees did rise almost everywhere during 1965–67. An alternative explanation is that the individual physician's pricing behavior is effectively market-constrained—specifically, that he prices his services on a less than perfectly elastic demand curve. Other things being equal, this pricing behavior implies a negative correlation between the physician's overall fee level (F) and his rate of output (Q). The latter, however, is partially a function of the error term in the production function (for example, variable e in equation 6-2). Given a negative correlation between F and Q, a negative correlation therefore exists also between $\log F$ and the error term e. Consequently the estimator of the fee-elasticity of gross patient billings will be subject to a downward estimation bias.[f]

III. THE APPARENT EFFECT OF MEDICAL INPUTS AND OF THE MODE OF PRACTICE ON PHYSICIAN PRODUCTIVITY

After this survey of the overall statistical properties of the production-function estimates and of the role played by the subordinate variables (vector $\mathbf{D}_i$) in these functions, we concentrate henceforth on the apparent effect of H, $\mathbf{L}$, K and G on the rate of physician output. Since the estimated functions for pediatricians, obstetricians-gynecologists, and internists are not strikingly different from those for general practitioners, our attention will for the most part be focussed on the latter.

As may be seen in Tables 6-7 to 6-10, in all equations the estimated coefficients of physician time ($\log H$, H and OH), of capital ($\log K$), and of auxiliary personnel (L_1, L_2, L_3 and $[\Sigma L]^2$) are statistically significant at at least a 5 percent level, the majority of them being significant even at a 1 percent level. All of the coefficient estimates have the expected signs and, with the exception of the capital coefficient, have plausible magnitudes. The coefficient of the group-practice dummy variable (G) also is generally positive and statistically significant, the exception being the specialty of internists (see Table 6-10).

The Apparent Role of the Mode of Practice: On the basis of their overall 1966 sample including *all* medical specialties surveyed, the editors of *Medical Economics* computed the *median* weekly patient visits of solo practitioners to be 118, while that for partnerships or groups was 144 [Owens, 1967b]. The corresponding *averages*, for general practitioners only, in the 1965-67 samples, were 183 and 213, respectively. In either case, the weekly patient load

[f]This proposition can be demonstrated mathematically, or with a simple hypothetical example. Suppose all physicians in one's sample employed an identical mix of inputs, and faced an identical demand for their services. Under these circumstances, any observed interphysician variance in the rate of output reflects differences solely in the error term e, perhaps differences in technical efficiency. Relatively more efficient practices would then be observed to produce relative higher rates of output and to charge relatively lower fees. If one regressed the observed rates of gross patient billings on the observed level of fees (F) and on the (common) rates of medical inputs, the effect of the unobservable, interphysician differences in technical efficiency would be loaded onto the coefficient of F. A physician whose fee level was found to be 10 percent below the sample average would be found to report gross patient billings less than 10 percent below the sample average, because his rate of output would exceed the sample average, and so on. The estimated fee-elasticity of gross patient billings would then clearly be below unity.

of physicians in single-specialty groups would be predicted to be between 11 and 16 percent higher than that of solo practitioners.

A simple comparison of weekly patient visits in solo and multi-physician practice, however, can be quite misleading if the various practice modes being compared differ systematically with respect to the relative amounts of factor services they employ. In this connection it is illuminating to examine the statistics in Table 6-11, which indicate that, on average, solo practitioners tend to work slightly *fewer* hours and employ *fewer* aides than do their colleagues in single-specialty group practice. In a comparison of unadjusted (total) patient visits per week—the sort of comparison one usually finds in the literature—the positive effect of additional factor employment by groups is simply loaded onto the practice-mode effect and hence exaggerates the latter. A production-function approach, on the other hand, is more likely to disentangle the separate effects of practice mode and factor usage.

Once adjustment has been made for interpractice-mode differences in levels of factor usage, the positive effect of group practice on factor produc-tivity appears to be somewhat lower, as is evident from Table 6-12. Further-more, the rate of patient visits or patient billings in internal medicine does not appear to be at all affected by group practice membership. It may be recalled that Richard Bailey [1968] in his study of internists in San Francisco did not find

Table 6-11. Average Weekly Patient Loads, Practice Hours, and Aides per Physician in Solo- and Single-Specialty Group Practice, 1965-1967[a]

Medical Specialty	Average Patient Visits per Week	Average Practice Hours per Week	Average Number of Aides per Physician
General Practitioners			
Solo	183	60	1.81
Group (single-specialty)	213	64	2.12
Group as percent of solo	116	107	117
Pediatricians			
Solo	154	52	1.66
Group (single-specialty)	169	52	1.90
Group as percent of solo	110	100	115
OBG Specialists			
Solo	117	56	1.51
Group (single-specialty)	138	58	1.60
Group as percent of solo	118	104	106
Internists			
Solo	125	54	1.48
Group (single-specialty)	140	58	1.82
Group as percent of solo	112	108	123

[a]Includes single-specialty partnerships. Figures are sample averages.

Source: Based on data from *Medical Economics,* Continuing Survey, 1965 and 1967.

Table 6–12. Estimated Percentage[a] by which Weekly Patient Visits or Billings of Group Practitioners Exceed Those of Solo Practitioners at Given Levels of Inputs H, L and K

Medical Specialty	Total Patient Visits Function	Office Visits Function	Patient Billings Function
General Practitioners			
Point Estimate	4.5%	5.1%	5.6%
Confidence Interval	(0.7% to 8.5%)	(0.9% to 9.5%)	(2.5% to 8.5%)
Pediatricians			
Point Estimate	6.0%	8.0%	10.5%
Confidence Interval	(−0.9% to 13.7%)	(1.3% to 15.5%)	(4.9% to 16.2%)
Obstetrician/Gynecologists			
Point Estimate	13.8%	13.7%	12.2%
Confidence Interval	(5.2% to 23.1%)	(8.2% to 23.0%)	(6.5% to 18.5%)
Internists			
Point Estimate	3.9%	−0.2%	3.7%
Confidence Interval	(−3.2% to 11.6%)	(−8.0% to 7.8%)	(−1.1% to 9.0%)

[a]Percentages have been calculated as $100(e^x - 1)$, where x is either the estimated coefficient ($\hat{g}$) of the group-practice dummy variable G in Tables 6–7 to 6–10, or the upper limit ($\hat{g} + 1.65\hat{s}_g$) or lower limit ($\hat{g} - 1.65\hat{s}_g$) of the 90 percent confidence interval for coefficient $\hat{g}$. In these expressions, $\hat{s}_g$ is the standard error of the estimate $\hat{g}$.

internists in groups to process more visits per physician hour either, although the incomes in groups were, in fact, somewhat higher.

In general, a physician's membership in a partnership or group appears to increase his billings somewhat more than it does his rate of patient visits. This disparity cannot be explained in terms of higher fees; for the MEDEC sample, at least, fees in solo practice were not found to be consistently lower than those in single-specialty group practices. Instead, the somewhat larger effect on billings probably reflects the fact that group practitioners tend to internalize the production and sale of many procedures that solo practitioners refer to outside facilities. In Chapter Four, such procedures were referred to as type I services.

In evaluating the results shown in Table 6-12 a number of caveats should be kept in mind. First, the comparison shown in the table is strictly between solo practitioners and physicians in single-specialty partnerships or groups of rarely more than three to four physicians. The test is therefore hardly an evaluation of the group-practice concept as that term is used in the literature. Second, it will be noted from Tables 6-7 to 6-10 that the estimated coefficient of the group-practice dummy variable (G) typically has a rather large standard error, especially in the patient-visit equations. The confidence intervals implicit in the coefficient estimates—shown in parentheses in Table 6-12—are therefore rather wide. Finally, the estimates are once again subject to the caveat that variable G may reflect more than just the mode of practice. As was noted earlier, one cannot rule out the possibility that physicians who find it comfortable to work in a group setting differ also in other respects from their peers in solo practice. They may, for example, be inherently more or less efficient than solo practitioners.

The Apparent Role of Capital: The estimated capital-elasticity of output (coefficient a_2) turned out to be fairly low in all equations, clustering around 0.05 in the patient-visit equations and around 0.10 in the billings equations. The differential between the visit and the billings equations probably reflects the fact that physicians with more elaborate facilities tend to internalize the production of services that would otherwise be referred to outside facilities, so that patient billings per visit increase as a function of capital input.

It is, of course, the case that the production process in medical practice is highly labor-intensive and that capital in that context plays the role primarily of a complement to health-manpower. Although capital in this role is a crucial ingredient in the health care production process, one suspects that its effect is likely to be picked up by **L** in a production function estimate. Even so, the estimated coefficients of log K in Tables 6-7 to 6-10 are very small, indeed, and may reflect also the inadequacy of the measure of K available in the MEDEC surveys. As noted earlier, a superior measure of K would probably be the number of examination rooms in the physician's practice.

In their more recent study, "Physician Productivity and Returns to Scale," Kimbell and Lorant [1973] had information on the number of examination rooms in the physician's practice, and the estimated capital-elasticity of output based on that measure did, in fact, tend to be higher than the estimates presented here. Kimbell and Lorant's overall sample included roughly 2,500 physicians responding to the American Medical Association's Seventh Periodic Survey of Physicians and its Survey of Medical Groups, both conducted in 1971. For the subsample of solo general practitioners (a subsample coming closest to the sample of general practitioners underlying the estimates in Table 6-7), Kimbell and Lorant obtained an estimated capital-elasticity of output between 0.10 and 0.13 when output was measured by weekly patient visits, and between 0.26 and 0.28 when output was measured by gross revenue [see their Table 2, p. 10]. One suspects that these estimates are a relatively more accurate reflection of the true role of capital equipment and floor space than those shown in Tables 6-7 to 6-10.

The Apparent Role of Auxiliary Personnel: As was noted in Chapter Four, the various tasks performed in a medical practice can be divided into those that can be performed only by the physician, those that can be delegated only to registered nurses (RN), those that can be delegated only to technicians (TE), and those that can be delegated as far down the occupational hierarchy as an office aide (OA). Since registered nurses and technicians can perform tasks delegatable to office aides while the obverse is not always true, one would expect the regression coefficients of RN and TE in Tables 6-7 to 6-10 to exceed those for OA. With the exception of the estimates for internal medicine, this pattern appears to prevail in fact. The differences among the coefficients of RN, TE and OA, however, are actually not very large. This finding suggests that in practice the three types of aides function—or are made to function—as closer substitutes than one would expect them to be purely on the basis of their formal training.

One can test for the statistical significance of these observed differences in coefficient estimates by using the criterion

$$t(n - k; i, j) = \frac{c_i - c_j}{[S_{ii} + S_{jj} - 2S_{ij}]^{1/2}} \qquad (6\text{-}6)$$

where c_i and c_j are the estimated coefficients for aide types L_i and L_j respectively, S_{ii}, S_{jj} and S_{ij} are the appropriate elements from the variance-covariance matrix of the estimated coefficients, and ratio $t(n - k; i, j)$ has the t-distribution with $n - k$ degrees of freedom. Table 6-13 shows the numerical values of the t-ratios for the total-visit, office-visit, and billings equations.

The difference between c_i and c_j is deemed to be statistically significant at the 5 percent level if $t(n - k; i, j) \geqslant 1.96$. This criterion is met only for the difference between the registered-nurse coefficient and the office-aide

Table 6–13. **Numerical Values of $t(n - k; i, j)$ for General Practitioners**[a]

Equation based on	$i = 1, j = 2$	$i = 1, j = 3$	$i = 2, j = 3$
Total visits	1.01	1.18	0.22
Office visits	1.85	2.80	0.23
Patient billings	0.25	1.15	0.65

[a]For all three equations, $n - k > 120$.

coefficient in the office-visit equation (Table 6–13). With the exception of that ratio, Table 6–13 does convey the impression that the estimated coefficients of the three types of aides in general practice are essentially the same. In what follows, we therefore adopt the analytic expedient of treating the three types of aides as one category by letting L be the sum $L_1 + L_2 + L_3$ and by assigning to it the coefficient $c = (c_1 + c_2 + c_3)/3$.

Figure 6–2 depicts the relationship between total weekly patient visits or weekly office visits on the one hand and the number of aides per physician (L) on the other. In the calculations underlying this diagram, the values of all other variables in the production function have been held constant at their sample means. From the diagram it is seen that the marginal product of aides ($\partial Q/\partial L$) increases up to a point, whereafter it decreases continuously and eventually falls to zero and below. The marginal product of aides reaches its maximum at a value of $L_m = (c/2d) - (1/[2d]^{1/2})$ and zero at a value of $L_0 = c/2d$, where c, it must be remembered, is equal to $(c_1 + c_2 + c_3)/3$. For the total-patient-visit equation, L_0 is equal to 5.3 and L_m is equal to 0.7. The corresponding figures for the office-visit equation are 4.7 and 0.8, respectively. For the billings equation they are 5.3 and 0.9, respectively.

Finally, the expression for the aide-elasticity of physician output can be obtained from equation (6–4) above as $e_L = cL - 2dL^2$. At the observed sample average of 1.96 aides per general practitioner, e_L has an estimated value of 0.31 for the total-visit equation, 0.36 for the office-visit equation, and 0.34 for the patient-billings equation. Thus although the estimates of parameters c and d vary considerably from equation to equation, these estimates imply roughly the same aide-elasticity of output at the sample means of the inputs.

It is worth noting that these elasticity estimates are corroborated by the more recent estimates presented in Kimbell and Lorant [1973]. For solo general practitioners, for example, Kimbell and Lorant report an estimated aide-elasticity of output between 0.31 and 0.34 for production functions based on patient visits as an output measure, and between 0.38 and 0.39 for estimates with output measured by gross revenue [see their Table 2, p. 10.] The production-function specification underlying the Kimbell-Lorant estimates, incidentally, was a conventional Cobb-Douglas production function with aides being measured simply by the sum of all types of aides employed in the physician's practice.

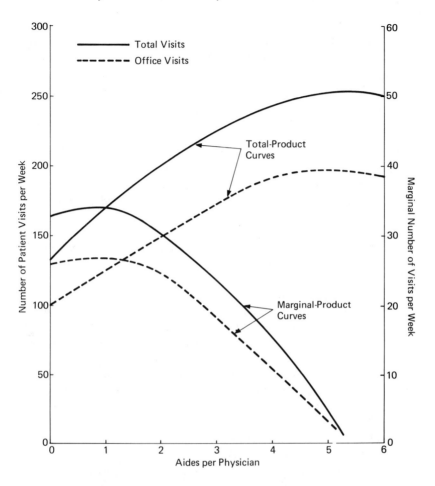

Figure 6-2.   Total-Product and Marginal-Product Curves—General Practitioners.

The Apparent Role of Physician Time: As is to be expected, the number of hours the physician works per week is the most important determinant of his weekly rate of output. From equation (6-4) above, the elasticity of output with respect to physician time is obtained as $e_H = a_1 - b_1 H$. At the observed sample averages of 60 total practice hours, e_H has a value of 0.77 for the total-visit equation and of 0.52 for the billings equation. In the office-visit equation, the inclusion of both log OH and OH (where OH denotes weekly office hours) introduced multicollinearity sufficiently strong to render the estimates of the coefficients of both variables seemingly insignificant statistically. For that reason, OH was dropped from the equation, so that the estimated elasticity of output with respect to physician time simply becomes a_1, or 0.67.

These output elasticities are, once again, corroborated by those recently presented in Kimbell and Lorant [1973]. In a production-function estimate obtained from a cross-section sample of roughly 2,500 physicians covering all specialties and modes of practice, the estimated physician-hours elasticity of weekly patient visits reported by these authors was 0.59 [see Kimbell and Lorant, Table 1, p. 9]. For general practitioners in solo practice (the subsample most closely resembling the sample used in this study) the estimates obtained by Kimbell and Lorant ranged from 0.80 to 0.85 for total patient visits, from 0.65 to 0.75 for office visits only, and from 0.61 to 0.62 for equations using gross revenue as an output measure [see their Table 2, p. 10]. The absolute and relative magnitudes of these estimates are very similar to those presented here.

The basic production-function specification underlying Tables 6-7 to 6-10 (equation (6-4) above) implies that the marginal product of physician time increases up to an inflection point $H_m = (a_1 - a_1^{1/2})/b_1$ whereafter it decreases and reaches zero at a rate $H_0 = a_1/b_1$. For the total-visit equation, H_m turns out to be 25 total practice hours per week and H_0 is a hypothetical rate of 111 hours. Since b_1 is equal to zero in the office-visit equation, H_m and H_0 are not defined. According to that equation, the marginal product of physician time decreases throughout the entire range of time input. Almost the same is true for the patient billings equation. Although in that equation $b_1 \neq 0$ and both the coefficient of log H and that of H are statistically significant, the relative magnitudes of a_1 and b_1 are such that H_m is reached at 2.2 practice hours per week, and H_0 at a hypothetical rate of 120 hours. Little information would therefore have been lost by altogether dropping variable H from the billings equation.

The Apparent Potential of Health Manpower Substitution in Medical Practice and the Optimal Number of Aides per Physician

Figure 6-3 illustrates the estimated joint and separate effects of physician time, of auxiliary personnel, and of the mode of practice on the number of total patient visits per week in general practice. In producing that diagram all variables other than the physician's weekly office hours (OH), his auxiliary staff (L) and his mode of practice (G), have been held constant at their respective sample averages. The diagram clearly suggests that a given number of weekly patient visits can be produced with a variety of alternative combinations of H and L (as can be seen by drawing a horizontal line through any particular rate of weekly office visits). These technically feasible trade-offs between physician time and auxiliary personnel are rendered even more visible in Figure 6-4, where the production function underlying Figure 6-3 is restated as a set of isoquants. A particular isoquant (trade-off curve) in that diagram indicates the various combinations of physician time and auxiliary personnel apparently capable of producing the rate of weekly office visits written next to that isoquant. In the real world all of the points on a given isoquant may, of course, not be economically feasible because solo practitioners cannot hire aides in small amounts. The set of input combinations viewed by producers as practical alternatives may therefore not form a truly continuous trade-off curve of the sort depicted in Figure 6-4.[8]

The general practitioners (GP's) in the sample underlying the estimates in Figure 6-4 reported to spend an average of about 36 hours per week in their office (not necessarily in direct contact with patients), to employ an average of about 1.96 aides per physician, and to handle an average of 152 office visits per week. This particular input combination is identified by a solid star in Figure 6-4. Since the isoquants plotted in the diagram and the average input combination have been estimated from the same data base, it is not surprising

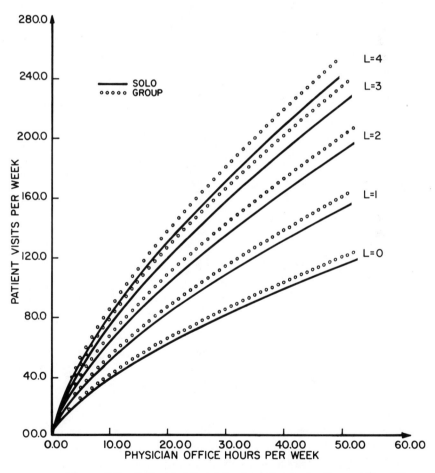

Figure 6-3. Estimated Total Product Curves for General Practitioners-Office Visits

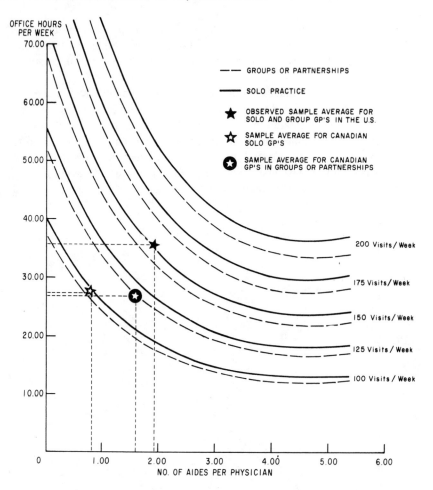

Figure 6–4.   Estimated Feasible Trade-Offs between Physician Time and Auxiliary Personnel, General Practitioners. Source: Reinhardt [1972b] , p. 172.

that the average input combination lies on the isoquant for an output rate very close to the observed sample average of 152 weekly office visits. It appears, however, that the estimated isoquants are compatible also with statistics from a quite independent sample of Canadian physicians.

The Canadian data were obtained from a survey of Canadian physicians conducted in 1962 under the auspices of the Royal Commission on Health Services in Canada. The relevant statistics to be used here are reported in Judek [1964]. At the time of the survey the delivery of ambulatory health care in Canada was not yet covered by universal, national health insurance. One may therefore assume that Canadian and American medical practices were then fairly similar. According to the statistics cited in Judek [1964], during the survey year Canadian GP's in solo- and group-practices employed an average of 0.8 and 1.6 aides per physician, respectively [Table 6-19, p. 243]. They were reported to have worked an average of 51 hours per week, of which roughly 55 percent, or 28 hours, were spent in the office, the remainder being spent in the hospital or on house calls. Finally, GP's in partnerships or groups apparently spent an average of 27 hours in the office [Appendix 5-2, p. 344]. These input combinations are plotted and appropriately labeled in Figure 6-4.

Judek reports that at the time of the survey, general practitioners in solo practice reported handling an average of 148 total patient visits per week. The comparable figure for GP's in partnerships or groups was 176 [p. 344]. Although these figures are not broken down by type of visit, Judek reports elsewhere that "on the average, a GP saw 16-20 patients (a day) in his office, 6-8 patients in [the] hospital and 1-4 patients at home" [p. 175]. In other words, office visits alone amounted to roughly 67 percent of total patient visits. If one applies this percentage of the total visit figures cited above, it seems that GP's in solo practice handled about 99 office visits per week during the year of the survey, while those in partnerships or groups handled about 118. In Figure 6-4, it is seen that the estimated isoquants presented there would lead one to predict roughly similar rates of output. The input combination OH = 28 hours and L = 0.8 (for Canadian solo GP's) lies very close to the solo practitioners' isoquant for 100 weekly office visits; the combination OH = 27 and L = 1.6 (for Canadian GP's in group practices) falls onto the isoquant for 125 visits, which is only slightly higher than the estimated average of 118 office visits for the Canadian physicians. In other words, the estimates presented in Figure 6-4 seem to have external validity.

As is illustrated in Figure 6-4, our production-function estimates capture the fact that there is a technical limit to health manpower substitution. This limit is reached when the marginal product of auxiliary personnel ($\partial Q/\partial L$) has descended to zero. In principle, health manpower substitution could be pushed to this limit, and prior to reaching it physician productivity would thereby be automatically increased. As was noted earlier, however, even prior to reaching the technically feasible limit a point is likely to be reached beyond which further gains in the productivity of medical manpower cease to justify the cost of additional auxiliary personnel. From the perspective of the individual physician—a perspective that is highly relevant in a society in which health manpower policy must operate through the decisions of individual physicians—the optimal size of the auxiliary staff is one that maximizes his net income per hour he works. Using the production-function specification (equation 6-4) underlying the estimates in Tables 6-7 to 6-10, this optimum implies a value $\hat{L}$ that satisfies the input-decision equation

$$(P^* - S^*)(c - 2d\hat{L})AH^{a_1}K^{a_2}e^{(-b_1 H + c\hat{L} - d\hat{L}^2 + \sum_s(m_s D_s))} = W^* + E^* \qquad (6\text{-}7)$$

This equation will be recognized as a specific version of the first-order condition (5-25) in Chapter Five. P^*, S^*, W^*, and E^* denote, respectively, the revenue earned from the sale of the marginal unit of output (for example, patient visits), the outlay on drugs and supplies for the marginal unit of output, the outlay on salaries and fringe benefits occasioned by the employment of the marginal aide, and the outlay on complementary floor space and equipment necessitated by the employment of the marginal aide. $(P^* - S^*)$ will henceforth be referred to as the "net proceeds per unit of output," and $(W^* + E^*)$ as the "marginal cost of employing aides." For given values of these input and output "prices" and for H and K, the optimum $\hat{L}$ can be obtained from equation (6-7) via iterative procedures.[g] Figure 6-5 depicts this solution graphically. In that diagram, $\hat{L}_{ij}$ denotes the optimal number of aides per physician corresponding to the set of "prices" $(P_i^* - S_i^*)$ and $(W_j^* + E_j^*)$.

To make any headway in solving equation (6-7) for $\hat{L}$, it is best to assume that P^* is constant at all empirically relevant rates of output. This assumption is useful in virtually all contexts other than one in which physicians act as market-constrained monopolists. Similarly it is useful and realistic to assume that the individual physician is a price-taker in the market for auxiliary personnel, so that W^* can be taken to be constant at all empirically relevant values of L.

It is difficult to obtain reliable estimates of the incremental costs S^* and E^*. The latter, in particular, is apt to vary with the physician's location, because E^* includes the cost of the incremental floorspace required for additional aides. In obtaining optimal values of L from the patient-visit equations, these difficulties can be met simply by solving equation (6-7) for sufficiently broad ranges of $(P^* - S^*)$ and $(W^* + E^*)$ to include the empirically relevant values of these variables. Tables 6-14 and 6-15 present such solutions for general practitioners and pediatricians; similar tables for obstetricians-gynecologists and internists are included in Appendix C (Tables C-2 and C-3). As would be expected, L is fairly sensitive to the relative magnitude of the input and output "prices."

Table 5-2 of the previous chapter indicates that in 1965 the GP's in the MEDEC sample paid registered nurses an average of $4,200 per year, technicians an average of $4,000, and office aides an average of $3,300. Even with an allowance for fringe benefits, this annual salary figure is the equivalent of at most $100 per week. Average gross billings per patient visit during the period were about $6.60 (calculated on a total-visit basis). As was shown in Table 4-9, the *average cost* of medical supplies and drugs per office visit was between $0.50 and $0.60. Since this figure includes the cost of small medical instruments, one

---

[g]As was noted in Chapter Five, in principle one should solve simultaneously for the optimum $\hat{L}$ and $\hat{K}$ corresponding to a given number of hours H_O. It turns out, however, that the coefficient a_2 of K is so low as to render the solution value $\hat{L}$ virtually insensitive to changes in K. Little information is therefore lost by setting K_O equal to the observed sample mean for all values of L, a procedure adopted here.

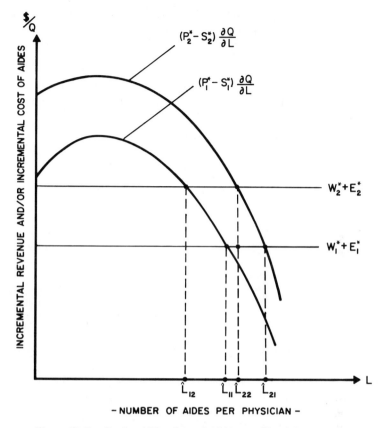

Figure 6–5. Optimal Number of Aides per Physician

suspects that the *marginal cost* of these items (S^*) was typically lower than average costs. In fact, in order to obtain at least a rough indication of the value of S^* in the 1965 MEDEC sample, the physicians' annual expenditure on drugs, medical supplies and small instruments was regressed on their weekly office visits. The resulting estimates suggested a value of S^* between $0.27 and $0.29.[9]

Given these cost and revenue data and our production-function estimates in Table 6–7, it would seem that the average general practitioner in the MEDEC sample could have profitably employed close to four aides per physician, or roughly twice the observed sample average of 1.96. Much the same conclusion is reached if one estimates the optimal value of L from the patient-billings equation. For that production function, the relevant first-order condition becomes

$$\frac{\partial Y}{\partial L} - S^* \frac{\partial Q}{\partial L} = W^* + E^* \qquad (6\text{–}8)$$

Table 6-14. Estimated Optimal Aide Employment at Alternative Input and Output Prices, General Practitioners[a]

Net Proceeds per Visit	Weekly Cost per Aide[b]			
	$70	$100	$130	$160
	Based on the Office-Visit Function			
$5.00	3.7	3.2	2.6	1.6
7.00	4.0	3.7	3.3	2.9
10.00	4.2	4.0	3.7	3.5
15.00	4.4	4.2	4.1	3.9
	Based on the Total-Visit Function			
$5.00	4.3	3.7	3.1	2.3
7.00	4.6	4.3	3.9	3.5
10.00	4.9	4.6	4.4	4.1
15.00	5.0	4.9	4.7	4.6
	Based on the Patient-Billings Function			
—	4.5	4.1	3.6	3.1

[a]Based on the production function estimates in Table 6-7 with G set equal to unity, $H = 60$, $OH = 35$ and all other variables, except L, set equal to their respective sample means. The 1965 sample average of gross billings per total patient visit was $6.70; the sample average number of aides per physician was 1.96. Estimates of $\hat{L}$ for solo practitioners are only slightly below those presented here.

[b]Defined to include fringe benefits and the cost of incremental floor space.

Here Y denotes gross patient billings (expressed not on an annual, but on a weekly basis) and Q is the number of weekly office visits. The derivative $\partial Y/\partial L$ can be obtained from the patient-billings function (equation 3 in Table 6-7) and $\partial Q/\partial L$ from the office-visit function (equation 2). In solving equation (6-8) for $\hat{L}$ it is, of course, necessary to make an explicit assumption about the value of S^*; for that purpose, a value of $0.28 was taken as a reasonable estimate. Upon insertion of this value into equation (6-8), solution of that equation for $\hat{L}$ yielded the estimates shown in the bottom row of Table 6-14. These estimates seem consistent with those derived from the patient-visit equations.

An evaluation of the production functions for the other medical specialties reinforces the conclusion that the typical American physician has not pushed the delegation of tasks to the point that seems technically feasible and economically sensible. Table 6-15, for example, presents the estimated values of $\hat{L}$ for pediatricians. The 1965 sample average of gross billings per pediatric patient visit was about $7 and pediatricians must have faced roughly the same labor costs as did general practitioners. These figures suggest that the average pediatrician in the 1965 MEDEC sample could have profitably employed about four aides per physician. The sample average number of aides per pediatrician, however, was only 1.68. Expansion of the auxiliary staff from that level to about four aides per pediatrician would yield an estimated increase between 30 percent and 40 percent over the observed rate of patient visits and patient billings. As is apparent from Tables C-2 and C-3 (Appendix C), a broadly similar pattern is observable among obstetricians-gynecologists and internists.

One can never escape the feeling in analyses of this sort that one's conclusions may simply be a statistical artifact possibly at variance with the underlying reality. It is therefore reassuring to note that the optima calculated here are not far off the norms suggested by management consultants in the health field.[10] As one of these consultants has been quoted by the editors of *Medical Economics*,

> Even now patients are knocking down doctors' doors . . . and in the next five years we'll see more changes and more pressures than we've seen in the past 20. Our clients [that is, medical practitioners] average two and a half aides apiece [per physician] now, *and that figure should go to four or more in the foreseeable future.*[11] [Emphasis added.]

This assertion, coming as it does from a practitioner in the field, gives aid and comfort to an ivory-tower economist.

Table 6-15. Estimated Optimal Aide Employment at Alternative Input and Output Prices, Pediatricians[a]

Net Proceeds per Visit	Weekly Cost per Aide[b]			
	$70	$100	$130	$160
	Based on the Office-Visit Function			
$5.00	3.5	3.1	2.5	1.7
7.00	3.8	3.5	3.2	2.8
10.00	4.0	3.8	3.6	3.7
15.00	4.1	4.0	3.9	3.7
	Based on the Total-Visit Function			
$5.00	4.4	3.8	3.1	1.9
7.00	4.7	4.4	4.0	3.5
10.00	4.9	4.7	4.5	4.2
15.00	5.1	4.9	4.8	4.6
	Based on the Patient-Billings Function			
	4.4	4.1	3.8	3.4

[a]Based on the production function estimates in Table 6-8 with G set equal to unity, $H = 50$, $OH = 35$ and all other variables, except L, set equal to their respective sample means. The 1965 sample average of gross billings per total patient visit was about $7; the sample average number of aides per physician was 1.66. Estimates of $\hat{L}$ for solo practitioners are only slightly below those presented here.

[b]Defined to include fringe benefits and the cost of incremental floor space.

The Apparent Shadow Price of Physician Time: As noted in Chapter Five, if one assumes that the individual physician does not associate any psychic benefits or costs with the employment of aides as such, then one may use the production-function estimates to infer the so-called shadow price of physician time implicit in the input combination (H, L, K) actually used by the physician, and in the wages he faced in the labor market at the time of the MEDEC survey. Applying production function (6-4) above to equation (5-28) of the previous chapter, this shadow price can be written as

$$\hat{P}_H = \frac{(W^* + E^*)\,(a_1/H - b_1)}{c - 2dL} \tag{6-9}$$

where $\hat{P}_H$ is understood to be the pretax shadow price of physician time.

If the sample averages of $H = 60$, $OH = 36$ and $L \simeq 2.0$, and a value of $(W^* + E^*) = \$100 + \$20$ are inserted into this equation, [12] $\hat{P}_H$ is found to be \$9.8 for the coefficient estimates in the total-visit equation and \$11.9 for those in the office-visit equation. In other words, our production-function estimate suggests that a general practitioner working, say, 36 hours per week in his office and employing roughly two aides whom he pays \$100 a week each (and for whom he incurs incremental overhead costs of about \$20 per week each) would seem to be assigning a value of about \$10 to \$12 to his marginal hour of leisure. From the fee data presented in Tables 6-4 and 6-5 above, however, one infers that general practitioners in 1965 seemed to price their own time out at an average rate of about \$17.50 (60 times the coefficient of M in Table 6-4). It would appear, then, that in selecting his aide-hour combination the average general practitioner in the MEDEC sample tended to treat his own time as a resource far cheaper than he thought it to be when setting his fees, and, thus, far below the price patients were obviously willing to pay for his time.

An alternative to the preceding interpretation of the MEDEC data might be that the monetary costs $(W^* + E^*)$ of aides do not actually reflect the *total costs* physicians tend to associate with the employment of aides. As noted earlier, physicians may view the administration of an auxiliary staff as a burden of sorts. If so, an equivalent weekly "psychic cost" (denoted by P_L in Chapter Five) must be added to the monetary cost of employing aides. Using equations (5-29) of the previous chapter and (6-4) of this chapter, these equivalent weekly psychic costs may be estimated as

$$\hat{P}_L = P_H \left[\frac{c - 2dL}{a_1/H - b_1} \right] - (W^* + E^*) \tag{6-10}$$

For $L = 2$, $P_H = \$17.50$, $W^* = \$100$ and $E^* = \$20$, $\hat{P}_L$ is equal to about \$94 for the parameter estimates of the total-visit equation, and to about \$56 for those of the office-visit equation. If the production-function estimates underlying these calculations are at all reliable indicators of the relative marginal productivities of aides and of physician time, and if the average general practitioner in the MEDEC sample considered his auxiliary staff optimal (taking into account the psychic costs of employing aides), then these psychic costs must have been very high indeed. Because any policy to increase physician productivity ultimately stands or falls on the physician's attitude toward task delegation, the determinants of these psychic costs, if any, merit careful investigation in future research.

  It behooves a careful researcher to offer yet another explanation for the observed gap between the actual and the estimated optional employment of paramedical aides—or between the actual and the estimated shadow price of physician time—namely, that the production-function estimates presented in this chapter may be subject to an estimation bias. The nature of this potential bias has been explored at length in Chapter Five. Its source, it will be recalled, lies in the fact that all physicians may not be equally adept, technically, in using auxiliary personnel, a phenomenon we had described as interphysician variance in technical efficiency. If this variance were large relative to the variance in observed input combinations, then the marginal productivity of aides ($\partial Q/\partial L$) one infers from the production function estimates in Tables 6-7 to 6-10 would be larger than that faced by the typical physician. More concretely, a physician observed to employ only two aides would not in fact increase his output by 30 percent were he to employ four aides instead. Equation (6-7) shows that such a phenomenon would lead one to overestimate the number of aides the physician could profitably employ. Similarly, it is clear from equations (6-9) and (6-10) that such a bias would lead one to underestimate P_H, the implicit shadow-price of physician time, and to overestimate P_L, the implicit psychic cost of employing aides.

  Unfortunately, it was impossible with the data available to this study to test for the presence or absence of this estimation bias. As was argued in Chapter Five, however, the very nature of medical training and practice in this country leads one to expect the bias to be relatively small. Furthermore, it is the case that the potential for productivity gains estimated here lies in the lower end of the range of productivity gains elsewhere attributed to task delegation (see Chapter Four).

  The need for objectivity in research of this nature dictates that the potential for estimation bias be candidly acknowledged. On the other hand, this author is persuaded that the potential marginal product attributed to aides in this chapter is, if anything, too low, primarily because certain legal constraints (real or imagined) may actually deter physicians from using their aides as efficiently, technically, as they would otherwise deem it safe and desirable to do. In the concluding chapter of this book we proceed on the implicit assumption that the production-function estimates presented here are in fact a reasonably reliable reflection of the productivity gains potentially available to the typical American physician. In that chapter, we explore some of the policy issues emerging from our analysis.

NOTES

1. This approach was followed by Griliches [1963] in his study of agricultural production functions, and by M.S. Feldstein [1967] in his study of British hospitals.
2. See, for example, Brewster and Seldowitz [1965], p. 501, and Anne Scitovsky [1967]. In the 1965 Medical Economics *Continuing Survey*, general surgeons in the sample were asked to respond to the question: "What is your usual basis for setting fees?" About 43 percent of the respondents reported to adhere to their own fee schedule, 17 percent used the Blue Shield fee schedule, and only 17 percent reported to take patients' ability to pay into account.
3. In this connection, see Greenfield [1969], p. 95.
4. The difficulty of measuring the physical *flow* of services per period rendered by a given capital *stock* is a problem that has plagued virtually all empirical production analyses. Depreciation expense is one of the most commonly used indexes of this flow of services; its inadequacies are too obvious to require elaboration. In this connection, see especially Walters [1963].
5. Subsequent to the completion of this study, there has emerged in the literature a fair amount of discussion concerning production-function specifications. See Christensen, Jorgenson and Lau [1971], Berndt and Christensen [1973], and Diewert [1973]. Of particular interest in these discussions has been the so-called "translog" production function, which is essentially a higher order Taylor-Series approximation in the logarithms of the arguments of some general function about some point on the production surface. Although the translog function has great appeal at the theoretical level, it is difficult to estimate its parameters statistically because the regressors include numerous cross-products among inputs, a circumstance that easily leads to multicollinearity among the regressors. Quite aside from these problems, the author no longer has access to the data base underlying this study and hence could not experiment with the translog function.
6. In this connection, see Table 5–1 in Reinhardt [1970], pp. 95–6.
7. In their paper, "Physician Productivity and Returns to Scale," Kimbell and Lorant [1973] also report a fee-elasticity of patient billings generally below 0.50 and below 0.10 for some specialties. The estimated fee-elasticity of patient visits, on the other hand, is found to be negative. The authors conclude from this result that the fee index captures not only a pure price effect, but also a complexity and quality effect. In other words, it is assumed that fees are high where the average time input per patient visit is high, and that the latter

reflects correspondingly high complexity and/or quality. While this
may be a reasonable interpretation, it is also possible that the
relatively higher input of physician time per patient reflects the working of Parkinson's Law in areas with high physician population
ratios (and high fees), a phenomenon already commented on in
Chapter One.

8. It is customary in economic theory to characterize the nature of isoquants by
the elasticity-of-substitution implicit in them. For the production
function underlying our estimates, this elasticity varies over the
production surface and reaches zero at some points. With the aid of
a computer it is a relatively easy matter to calculate the elasticity-of-
substitution (at alternative input combinations) for the production-
function estimates in Tables 6–7 to 6–10. These elasticity coefficients
are not presented in this volume, because it is felt that they are not
likely to be illuminating in the context of our discussion. The estimates may be obtained from the author upon request.

9. Two distinct estimates of S^* were obtained. In the first of these, the physicians' total professional expenses per week, exclusive of payroll
expense and depreciation and up-keep of their automobile, (C) was
regressed on the number of aides per physician (L) and the number
of office visits per week (Q). The resulting estimate was

$$C = 52.07 + 0.276Q + [19.32 + 5.06G] \cdot L \qquad R^2 = 0.24$$
$$(5.54) \qquad (6.94)\ (1.92)$$

where G is the familiar group-practice dummy variable and the
figures in parentheses are t-ratios. In an alternative estimate, the
annual expenditure on medical supplies only was regressed on weekly office visits. The resulting estimate was

$$MS = 1386.2 + 14.149Q \qquad R^2 = 0.11$$
$$(9.76)$$

If one converts this estimate to a weekly basis by dividing both sides
by 48 workweeks, the coefficient of Q is seen to be equal to 0.294.

10. Verbal communication from Systemedics, Inc., a Princeton-based management consulting firm specializing in the operation of private medical
practices.

11. See "Step Up Your Productivity?" *Medical Economics* (September 1968),
p. 67.

12. The $20 are an estimate of E^*. In this connection, see note 9 above.

Part Three

Public Policy and the Economics of Health Manpower Substitution

Chapter Seven

Health Manpower Substitution and Policy

The estimates presented in Chapter Six indicate the effect the employment of registered nurses, medical technicians, and office aides by medical practices appears to have on the physician's rate of output, with the latter measured alternatively by his rate of total patient visits (office, hospital, and home visits), by his rate of office visits only, or by his annual gross billings to patients. The types of support personnel considered in the study may be thought of as "traditional allied health manpower." The study excludes the various types of manpower commonly lumped together under the titles physician extender or physician assistant, a concept that was only just emerging when the sample surveys used in the study were taken.[1] There are currently well in excess of a hundred ostensibly distinct training programs for such personnel, ranging, in terms of length of training, from as short a period as four months to as long as five years.[2] Although graduates from some of these programs are unlikely to bring greater skill and competence to their job than do the traditional types of allied health manpower,[3] the premise underlying the whole concept of the physician assistant is that ultimately such personnel will be able to perform medical tasks now beyond the competence of even an experienced nurse. In view of this potential development, one is justified in regarding the productivity estimates presented in the previous chapter as lower limits.[4]

While failure of the present study to evaluate the potential role of physician assistants represents a weakness in one sense, it strengthens the analysis in another. First, the objective of the entire discussion has been to demonstrate that, because of a sizeable and as yet unexploited potential for raising physician productivity, the present and future need for medical manpower in this country is not likely to be nearly as acute as some authors believe. In offering that proposition, it is proper to be conservative in one's estimate of the alleged productivity potential. Furthermore, the concept of the physician assistant is still sufficiently controversial to cast some uncertainty on the rate at which such manpower will come forth in the future, and on the reception it is likely to find among both patients and physicians. The present study suggests what can be accomplished with the traditional types of allied health workers to which both patients and physicians have long been accustomed—and therein lies a certain virtue.

In this chapter the empirical results developed in Part II of the book are recapitulated in summary fashion and for a less technical readership. Section I is devoted to the technically feasible productivity gains potentially attainable through health manpower substitution. An attempt is made to apply our estimates to some basic forecasting exercises. The discussion in section II focuses on the economics of health manpower substitution, in particular on its potential impact on the cost of physician services. Finally, section III examines some of the policies the public sector might pursue to encourage the realization of productivity gains that seem both technically feasible and economically justifiable.

I. HEALTH MANPOWER SUBSTITUTION AND PHYSICIAN PRODUCTIVITY

Table 7-1 summarizes in index form the estimates developed in Part II of the book. The first column of the table shows the absolute number of weekly total patient visits, of weekly office visits, and of annual patient billings (in 1965–67 prices) that would be expected, on average, from a physician employing two aides of the traditional type. These estimates have been obtained from the production-function estimates in Tables 6-7 to 6-10 of the previous chapter. The next five columns contain indexes of weekly total- or office-visits, or annual patient billings, at alternative assumed numbers of aides per physician. The indexes are set equal to unity at a level of two aides per physician. The predicted absolute rate of visits or billings for any particular size of auxiliary staff (L) can be obtained from Table 7-1 by multiplying the appropriate figure in the first column by the index corresponding to that staff size. Thus, our estimates suggest that a general practitioner employing three aides should, on average, be able to handle $1.16 \times 156 = 181$ office visits per week, or that a pediatrician employing only one aide would, on average, handle $0.80 \times 165 = 132$ total patient visits per week, and so on. Finally, the last two columns in the table present the observed sample averages of the number of aides per physician and of the rates of patient visits and patient billings. Appendix Table C-4 is virtually identical to Table 7-1, except that the productivity index is set to unity at the observed sample-average aide input per physician rather than at two aides per physician.

It can be inferred from Table 7-1 that if the average American physician currently employed as many as two aides per physician and expanded

Table 7-1. Estimated Effect of Auxiliary Personnel on Physician Productivity[a]

Output Measured by:	Predicted Rate of Visits or Billings at 2 Aides per Physician	Estimated Index of Productivity at Alternative Assumed Numbers of Aides per Physician (L)					Sample Averages	
		$L=0$	$L=1$	$L=2$	$L=3$	$L=4$	No. of Aides per Physician	Rate of Patient Visits or Billings
		INDICES FOR:						
		General Practitioners						
Total Patient Visits/Week[b]	200	0.66	0.83	1.00	1.15	1.26	—	189
Office Visits/Week	156	0.60	0.80	1.00	1.16	1.26	1.96	152
Annual Patient Billings (1965–67)[c]	$60,000	0.63	0.81	1.00	1.17	1.29	—	$55,000
		Pediatricians						
Total Patient Visits/Week	165	0.60	0.80	1.00	1.18	1.33	—	159
Office Visits/Week	139	0.57	0.79	1.00	1.17	1.26	1.68	133
Annual Patient Billings (1965–67)	$57,000	0.56	0.78	1.00	1.20	1.35	—	$52,200
		Obstetricians/Gynecologists						
Total Patient Visits/Week	149	0.60	0.80	1.00	1.19	1.35	1.54	125
Office Visits/Week	94	0.61	0.80	1.00	1.18	1.32	—	92
Annual Patient Billings (1965–67)	$64,000	0.52	0.75	1.00	1.22	1.37	—	$57,200
		Internists						
Total Patient Visits/Week	137	0.57	0.77	1.00	1.23	1.42	—	129
Office Visits/Week	89	0.56	0.77	1.00	1.23	1.43	1.59	81
Annual Patient Billings (1965–67)	$57,000	0.52	0.76	1.00	1.21	1.35	—	$51,000

[a]Calculated from the production-function estimates in Tables 6–7 to 6–10, with all inputs other than aides held constant at their sample averages, and G set equal to zero. Setting G equal to unity will not materially affect these productivity ratios.

[b]The sum of weekly office, hospital, and home visits.

[c]Annual patient billings observed for a sample of physicians surveyed in 1965 and 1967.

his auxiliary staff to double that number, physician productivity as measured in the table would be expected to increase by about 26 percent to 40 percent, depending on the specialty being considered. Actually, with the exception of general practitioners, the physicians in the underlying sample typically employed fewer than two aides per physician (see column7 of Table 7-1). More recent surveys undertaken by the American Medical Association and by Medical Economics, Inc. indicate that there has been little change in this staffing pattern since 1965-67, as can be inferred from Tables 7-2 and 7-3.

If the number of aides per physician were to increase from the actually observed *averages* to about four, the productivity gains so generated would exceed those suggested in Table 7-1. Appendix Table C-4 conveys a rough idea about the magnitude of these gains. It is seen that with the exception of general practice, a move from the observed sample average number of aides per physician to a level of four would tend to increase physician productivity by roughly 40 percent to 55 percent over current levels, depending once again on the physician's specialty.

Toward the end of Chapter Five, alternative methods were suggested by which productivity estimates of the sort presented here could be incorporated into health manpower forecasting models. Figures 7-1 and 7-2 are illustrations of such forecasting exercises. The focus in Figure 7-1 is on the absolute number of medical doctors (that is, physicians excluding osteopaths) in office-based practice, a category for which our production-function estimates were developed; Figure 7-2 presents the corresponding number of office-based M.D.'s per 100,000 resident population—a number that can be read off the scale on the left-hand side—and the equivalent number of office visits per capita—a figure given on the scale on the right-hand side. The projections in these diagrams are based on the forecasting model described in Appendix A. As in

Table 7-2. Average Full-Time Equivalent Allied Health Personnel per Physician, United States, 1970

Type of Health Personnel	General Practice	Pediatrics	Obstetrics/ Gynecology	Internal Medicine	All Physicians
RN's	0.357	0.330	0.416	0.242	0.257
LPN's	0.185	0.138	0.167	0.095	0.100
Medical Assistants	0.411	0.272	0.448	0.338	0.304
Laboratory Technicians	0.127	0.066	0.065	0.188	0.186
Medical Secretaries	0.174	0.144	0.218	0.281	0.225
Secretary/ Receptionists	0.646	0.500	0.422	0.377	0.461
Other	0.184	0.125	0.144	0.124	0.195
Total	2.084	1.573	1.880	1.644	1.729

Source: American Medical Association [1972], Table 60, p. 129.

Table 7-3. Number of Aides per Physician, United States, 1973

Number of Aides[a] per Physician	*Percentage of Physicians Employing Aides*					
	General Practice		*Internists*		*Pediatrics*	
	Solo	*Partnership/ Group*	*Solo*	*Partnership/ Group*	*Solo*	*Partnership/ Group*
None	17%	1%	11%	4%	11%	3%
One	32	15	41	21	34	24
Two	28	36	33	39	37	43
Three	13	26	10	21	14	16
Four or More	10	22	5	15	4	14
Total	100%	100%	100%	100%	100%	100%

[a]Full-time equivalent employees other than physicians or physicians' assistants.
Source: *Medical Economics,* Continuing Survey, 1973, presented in Owens [1974].

earlier chapters, the projections are based on a number of assumptions that require explicit statement and some explanation.

The lowest of the curves in Figures 7-1 and 7-2 represent the projected number of office-based M.D.'s likely to be generated by the number of graduations from American medical schools currently forecast under existing health manpower legislation. This series of graduations has been developed by the Division of Manpower Intelligence of the Department of Health, Education and Welfare and probably is the best such estimate available at this time.[5] The forecasting model in Appendix A projects the *total* number of professionally active physicians as a function of this time series of graduations. For purposes of Figures 7-1 and 7-2, the number of M.D.'s in internship and residency was subtracted from this total. Next, it was assumed that roughly 75 percent of physicians who have completed their graduate training will choose to go into office-based practice, with the remainder joining a hospital staff or engaging in medical research.[6] The diagrams project only the office-based portion of these graduates. As in earlier chapters, any immigration of foreign-trained physicians after 1970 has been excluded. The projections are therefore to be viewed as lower limits that have already been exceeded during the period 1970-73.

The upper curves in the two diagrams represent the effect of productivity gains on the "effective supply" of office-based physicians. The premise underlying this concept is that a physician who is twice as productive as another physician is the effective equivalent of two physicians of the latter kind. In making these projections, it was assumed that physicians already in practice in 1970 employed two aides per physician and would continue to do so throughout their professionally active life.[a] (As shown in Table 7-2, the actual average

[a]Strictly speaking, it is assumed that every physician in 1970 was supported by two aides per physician, rather than that the average number of aides per physician was two. As was noted in Chapter Five, in conjunction with a production function that is nonlinear in the number of aides per physician, these two assumptions are not equivalent, at

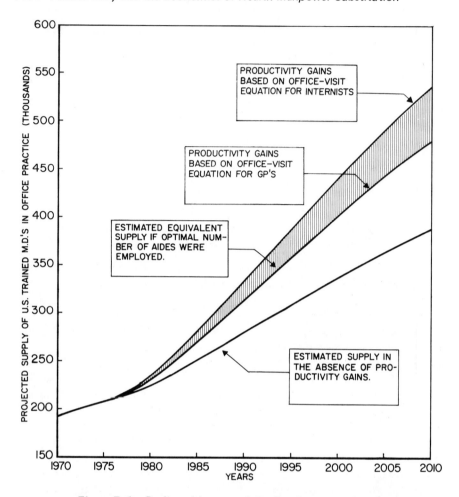

Figure 7-1. Projected Impact of the Employment of an Optimum
Auxiliary Staff on the Effective Supply of U.S.-Trained, Office-Based
Medical Doctors, 1970–2010

number of aides per physician in 1970 is estimated to be somewhere around
1.7.) It was further assumed that physicians graduating from medical school
after 1970 have been or will be specifically trained to function as part of
a wider health team, and therefore are or will be capable and willing to work
with as many as four aides per physician, provided they have a sufficiently
heavy practice load. Because it generally takes some time to build up a private
practice, it was assumed that the newly established physician will build up his
support staff in step with his practice load. Thus it was assumed that during

----

least not in theory. Depending upon the distribution of the number of aides per physician
over the universe of physicians, one may observe different average rates of patient visits for
the same average number of aides per physician.

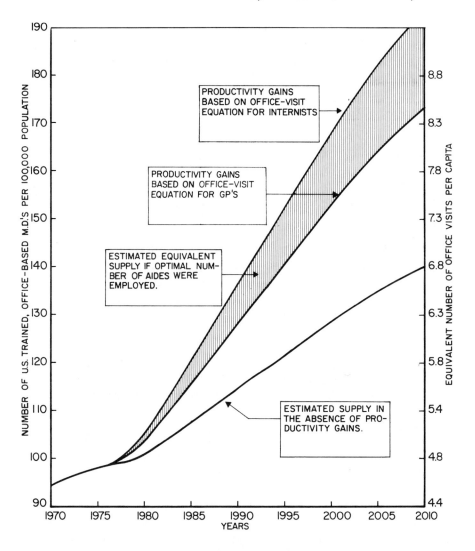

Figure 7-2. Projected Impact of the Employment of an Optimum
Auxiliary Staff on the Number of U.S.-Trained Office-Based M.D.'s
per 100,000 Population and on the Supply of Office Visits per Capita,
1970–2010

the first two years of his practice the physician will employ only the traditional
two aides per physician, that he will employ three aides during the following
two years, and finally hire the fourth aide in his fifth year in practice.

Given these assumptions, the baseline forecasts in Figures 7-1 and
7-2 (represented by the lowest of the three curves in each diagram) can be

converted into the *effective equivalent* supply of physicians (the top two curves) by incorporating the productivity indexes in Table 7-1 into the forecasting model set forth in Appendix A. As noted, these projections exclude from the total physician supply all M.D.'s in internship or residency training, all physicians on hospital staffs or engaged in research, and all foreign-trained M.D.'s entering the United States after 1970. Of the remainder, those M.D.'s who had graduated from medical school prior to 1971 are assumed to practice throughout their working life with a staff of two aides per physician. In the supply simulations, the total of these physicians is given a weight of (is multipled by) 1.00. Office-based M.D.'s graduated after 1970 are given a weight of 1.00 during the first two years of their practice, and weights equal to the appropriate productivity indexes in subsequent years. For example, in the simulation using the productivity indexes implicit in the production function for internists—a simulation represented by the upper of the top two curves in the diagrams— the total number of M.D.'s graduated after 1970 and in their third or fourth year of practice is multiplied by the index 1.23. Similarly, the total number of M.D.'s graduated after 1970 and in office-based practice for more than four years is multiplied by 1.43. The corresponding weights for the simulation using the productivity indexes of general practitioners are 1.16 and 1.26, respectively. This simulation is represented by the lower of the two top curves in Figures 7-1 and 7-2.

The productivity indexes for general practitioners and those for internists span the range of estimates presented in Table 7-1. Since these indexes are predicated on the assumption that physicians in 1970 employed an average of two aides per physician—rather than the actual average of about 1.7—the overall productivity gains projected by the top two curves in Figures 7-1 and 7-2 are clearly conservative. Had the diagrams been drawn for the productivity indexes in Appendix Table C-4 (indexes based on an expansion of the physician's auxiliary staff from 1.7 to 4 aides), the top two curves would naturally be steeper.

The concept of the effective equivalent physician supply is perhaps more readily understood if one thinks in terms of office visits rather than numbers of physicians. According to estimates published by the American Medical Association, in 1970 there were 192,436 office-based M.D.'s in this country, producing an average of 101.5 office visits per week and practicing an average of 47.5 weeks per year.[7] For a population of roughly 204 million, these figures suggest an average annual consumption of about 4.55 office visits per capita, almost precisely the number reported by the U.S. Public Health Service.[8] If one assumes that the annual average of 4,821 office visits per office-based M.D. is a constant, then the number of office visits per capita (the right-hand scale in Figure 7-2) can be obtained from the projected physician-population ratio on the left-hand scale by multiplying that ratio by 4,821/100,000.

Consider now the number of office-based M.D.'s in 1995 per 100,000 population as projected under the baseline forecast. According to Figure 7-2, this number is estimated to be about 122. On the assumption that these physicians will produce an annual average of 4,821 visits, the projected average annual number of office visits available per capita is roughly 5.9. With the productivity gains implicit in the lower of the top two curves, however, the average annual rate of office visits produced per M.D. would be close to 5,600, a rate that corresponds to an annual average of about 6.8 office visits per capita. To produce this higher per-capita rate in the absence of any productivity gains would have required not 122 but 141 office-based M.D.'s per 100,000 population. In other words, 122 M.D.'s per 100,000 with the productivity gains contemplated by the lower of the top two curves is the *effective equivalent* of about 141 M.D.'s per 100,000 population in the absence of productivity gains. If the assumed productivity gains generated the upper of the two curves, the effective equivalent number of M.D.'s corresponding to the actual forecast of 122 per 100,000 population would be as high as 153. This relationship between actual and effective equivalent manpower projections is more clearly brought out in Figure 7-3, which is an exact replica of Figure 7-2 without the internal labeling.

Projections such as those presented in Figures 7-1 and 7-2 have important implications for the role of health manpower forecasting in the formulation of the nation's health manpower policy. The typical problem in that context is to estimate, say, the number of M.D.'s or registered nurses required to meet some projected future demand for health services. As was indicated in Chapter Two, the analytic approach to this problem has traditionally been to posit a rigid proportionality between the projected utilization of health services and the numbers of various types of health manpower needed to meet that demand. Once this crucial assumption is made, it is an easy matter to translate the projected utilization into so-called point estimates of future health manpower requirements—one number for each type of health manpower. Policymakers find it easy to react to such firm numbers.

It is never quite clear from the literature on what particular factors the assumed proportionality between health services and health personnel rests. One assumption may be that, regardless of the technical potential for health manpower substitution, the health-care sector simply will not deviate from fixed manpower proportions, and that public policy cannot influence that behavior. An alternative assumption may be that the technology of health-care-production itself is of a kind that dictates more or less fixed proportions between health services and each type of health manpower, and hence also among various types of health manpower. Figures 7-2 and 7-3 suggest that this assumption is clearly not warranted. The health-care production process appears to offer those organizing it and those planning for it considerably more flexibility in staffing patterns.

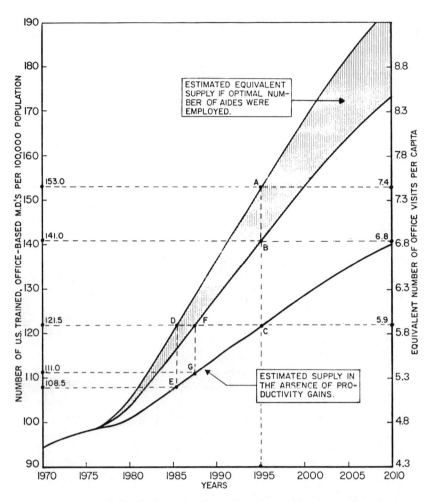

Figure 7–3. Estimation of the Number of Physicians Required to Meet a Projected Demand for Office Visits

Suppose, for example, that one's model of the demand for physician care predicted an average annual demand of 5.9 M.D. office-visits per capita by, say, 1995. In the absence of productivity growth after 1970, this demand would imply a requirement of close to 122 per 100,000, as may be seen by drawing a horizontal line from the level 5.9 on the right-hand scale of Figure 7–3 to the left-hand scale. If the productivity gains contemplated in the lower of the top two curves were realized, on the other hand, only about 111 office-based M.D.'s per 100,000 population would be required to meet the projected demand. This may be seen by dropping a vertical line from point F in Figure 7–3 to the baseline forecast and reading the number corresponding to the intersection (point G) off the left-hand scale. Similarly it is found that only about 108 M.D.'s per 100,000 population would be required if the productivity gains implicit in the uppermost curve were realized by 1995.

The productivity gains postulated in Figures 7-1 and 7-2, of course, imply a correspondingly larger pool of support personnel, for these gains were assumed to result from health manpower substitution. The nature of these trade-offs is brought out in Table 7-4. That table may be viewed as a menu of alternative manpower configurations capable of meeting a given present and future demand for patient visits at physicians' offices. The productivity indexes underlying this table are calculated from the office-visits equation for internists (equation 2 of Table 6-10). It is assumed that the actual number of office visits delivered in 1970 was produced by roughly 192,400 office-based M.D.'s employing the full-time equivalent of 1.75 aides per physician, a figure close to the average observed for all physicians in that year (see Table 7-2). It follows that Table 7-4 does not exactly mirror the uppermost curves in Figures 7-1 to 7-3. The latter, it will be recalled, are based on the assumption that 2 aides per physician, rather than 1.75, were employed in 1970; they are therefore relatively more conservative. To provide the reader with an exact mirror image of these more conservative projections, Table 7-4 has been replicated on the assumption that the actual number of office visits in 1970 was produced with 2 aides per physician. The resulting manpower estimates are shown in Table C-5 of Appendix C.

The productivity indexes underlying Table 7-4 and the annual rates of office visits to which they correspond are shown in the top two rows of the table. In assessing the realism of these indexes it is well to recall that they reflect only the use of "traditional allied health workers." It seems reasonable to assume that the postulated productivity gains would be anything but over-optimistic if the physicians' support staff in future years included substantial numbers of "physician extenders" who have more advanced training in patient care, and hence are capable of performing tasks not delegatable to traditional aides.

The remaining rows in Table 7-4 indicate alternative estimated combinations of medical and traditional auxiliary personnel capable of producing given rates of aggregate demand for office visits. The first pair of rows shows estimated manpower requirements for the base-year, 1970. The next pair indicates alternative manpower mixes capable of meeting the demand for office visits in 1990 if the per capita demand for visits remained constant over the period 1970-90. Finally, the third pair of rows suggests manpower requirements in 1990 if between 1970 and then the per capita demand for visits were to grow at an average annual rate of 3 percent. The population projections underlying these estimates are those used in Appendix A and published by the U.S. Bureau of the Census [1972a, Series E].

One of the more valuable contributions health manpower forecasters

Table 7-4. Estimated Technically Feasible Trade-Offs between Office-Based M.D.'s and Support Personnel, United States, 1970 and 1990[a]

	Number of M.D.'s and Support Personnel Required if the Number of Aides per M.D. (L) is equal to					
	0	1	1.75	2.0	3.0	4.0
Estimated Annual Rate of Office Visits per M.D.[b]	2,850	3,391	4,821	5,124	6,311	7,345
Index Set Equal to 1.00 for L = 1.75	0.59	0.82	1.00	1.06	1.31	1.52
1970						
Size of Resident Population: 204 million						
Average Annual Visits per Capita: 4.6[c]						
No. of M.D.'s required ('000s)[d]	326	236	192	181	147	126
No. of Aides required ('000s)	0	236	337	362	441	505
1990						
Size of Resident Population: 245 million[e]						
a) Zero Growth in per Capita Demand:						
Av. Annual Visits per Capita: 4.6						
No. of M.D.'s required ('000s)	391	283	231	217	176	152
No. of Aides required ('000s)	0	283	404	434	529	606
b) Annual Growth in per Capita Demand: 3%						
Av. Annual Visits per Capita: 8.3						
No. of M.D.'s required ('000s)	712	516	421	396	321	276
No. of Aides required ('000s)	0	516	736	792	964	1,104

[a]Based on the assumption that physicians in 1970 employed the equivalent of the time of 1.75 aides each. For an analogous table based on the assumption that physicians in 1970 employed 2.00 aides each, see Table C-5 of Appendix C.

[b]Based on the productivity index for the office-visit equation estimated from the sample of internists.

[c]Office visits only.

[d]Office-based M.D.'s rendering patient care.

[e]U.S. Bureau of the Census [1972a], Series E.

could make to the process of policy formulation would be to provide policymakers not with a single set of point estimates of a prospective manpower
situation, but instead with the entire technically feasible trade-off frontier faced
by the health-care sector now and in the future. Figures 7-1 and 7-3 and Table
7-4 are modest examples of this type of information. Although these displays
are intended to be merely illustrative, an effort has been made to tailor the
assumptions underlying them as closely as possible to reality. The estimates presented in the displays can therefore be taken as rough-and-ready guides to technically feasible health manpower trade-offs in the production of ambulatory
care. It may be noted that for a given aggregate demand of office visits, the
physician requirements shown in Table 7-4 are functions solely of the postulated
productivity gains, regardless of how these gains are achieved. The estimated
requirements of physician-support personnel, on the other hand, reflect the
assumption that the postulated productivity gains (or losses) are brought about
by changing the number of full-time equivalent aides per physician from a base
value of 1.75 to whatever number is indicated at the top of the table. As noted,
the category of aides considered in this analysis includes only the so-called traditional allied health workers. If the physicians' support personnel actually
included a substantial number of "physician extenders," the required number
of support personnel would probably be somewhat smaller than those indicated
in the table. For example, a 50 percent increase in physician productivity over
current levels might readily be achievable with merely two traditional aides and
one physician extender. Whether or not that manpower configuration would be
less costly than one involving four traditional aides would, of course, depend on
the relative remuneration received by physician extenders.

II. THE ECONOMICS OF HEALTH
MANPOWER SUBSTITUTION

The preceding estimates indicate the range of gains in physician productivity
that seem technically attainable. Such information is clearly fundamental in the
development of a health manpower strategy. There remains the question
whether the indicated productivity gains are worth their price. Table 7-4, for
example, shows that a per capita demand of 8.3 visits per year in 1990 could
be met by 396,000 M.D.'s supported by two aides each, or by only 276,000
M.D.'s supported by four aides each. The question policymakers must ask is
whether it makes economic sense to train and employ an additional 312,000
allied health workers merely to reduce physician requirements by 120,000.
Put another way, the task faced by health manpower planners is to steer the
health-care sector toward the most *economic* of all *technically* feasible alternative manpower mixes.

   Precisely what is meant by "the most economic health manpower
combination" probably requires some elaboration. It can readily be agreed that

the least-cost alternative of reaching a stated goal is the economically optimal one. The problem lies in the definition of costs. Before turning our attention to the economics of health manpower substitution, we must digress to develop an operationally meaningful concept of costs.

Real Resource Costs vs. Transfer Costs

In evaluating alternative public policies, economists invariably think of the so-called *real social resource cost* associated with each alternative. By real resource costs in this context is meant the so-called opportunity cost of a course of action, that is, the goods and services collectively forgone by following that particular course of action rather than the next best alternative. Thus the real resource costs of deploying a particular manpower combination in office-based medical practice is said to be the goods and services society forgoes by training that manpower for and retaining it in medical practice rather than training it for and employing it in the next best alternative activity, not necessarily within the health-care sector.

This approach to the costing of public policies emerges from the premise that, for analytical purposes, the human and physical resources owned by the members of a given body politic can be viewed as the collective property of society as a whole, and that any public policy affecting the use of these resources should seek, first of all, to encourage their deployment in a way that maximizes the collective returns from them, whereafter thought can be given to the problem of distributing these collective returns equitably among individual members of society. It can be shown that minimizing the real social resource costs of reaching given goals—for example the delivery of a certain set of health services—generally contributes to the maximization of this proverbial collective "pie," otherwise known as the national product.

Unfortunately it is not easy to work with this cost concept in the area of health manpower policy. First, it is extremely difficult to estimate empirically the real social resource costs of alternative manpower mixes. In a perfectly competitive market environment one can take the remuneration earned by various types of manpower as an index of their social opportunity costs.[b] As we have noted repeatedly, however, the market for health services seems a far cry from the competitive norm. The market for physician services, in particular, is widely held to contain monopolistic elements that enable physicians to earn incomes probably in excess of the true social opportunity costs of that type of manpower. Under these circumstances, it is inappropriate to view the relative remuneration of different types of health manpower as indexes of their relative real resource (opportunity) costs.

It is difficult also to identify the long-run direct resource costs of training various types of health manpower. The problem is probably not insur-

---

[b]This is strictly true only if the manpower being considered is marginal relative to society's overall labor pool.

mountable in the case of paramedical assistants. Estimation of the long-run direct cost of a medical education, on the other hand, is a more intractable problem because it is difficult to ascertain how much of the cost of medical schools should be allocated to patient care, how much to medical research, and how much to medical education proper. In short, then, the estimation of the real resource costs of alternative health manpower combinations is a major research project in itself.

Quite aside from these purely methodological difficulties of estimating real resource costs, the general public and their legislative representatives are not always receptive to the normative implications of that cost concept. Consumers, legislators, and the media—in fact, virtually all noneconomists—react primarily to the so-called *transfer costs* of alternative courses of action. The transfer cost of deploying a given health manpower combination in medical practice, for example, can be defined as the total purchasing power consumers and taxpayers individually or collectively must transfer to physicians and their aides as a group in order to train that manpower for medical practice, and in return for the delivery of physician services. They are, so to speak, an index of the slice of the collective "pie" that the nonphysician sector must carve out and hand over to physicians and their aides. Concerned legislators usually think of these costs when they deplore the "high cost of medical services" or the proportion of the gross national product devoted to health care.

(It may be noted in passing that some legislators take the more parochial posture of reacting primarily to the so-called *budget-costs* of alternative health policies, namely, that portion of the implied transfer costs which is channeled to the health sector through the particular budgets over which these legislators preside. In debating the relative merits of alternative health insurance proposals, for example, some politicians in this country have shown a manifest tendency to rank these proposals in terms of estimated budget costs. On this cost concept, a health insurance scheme is considered "cheap" when the bulk of its transfer costs are channeled to health care providers through the private sector (for example, through private insurance companies), and similarly for health manpower policies. It is self-evident that to evaluate public policies strictly on their budget cost is defective policymaking. We shall not consider that cost concept further here.)

Although it is obvious that the budget and transfer costs of alternative policy measures need not coincide, it may be less obvious why these transfer costs may deviate also from the real resource costs implicit in the policies. A theorist can certainly envision market environments in which the two cost concepts do coincide. As already noted, however, the earnings transferred by consumers to particular types of health manpower may not reflect the true opportunity costs of that manpower, so that the two cost concepts and the optima they imply may deviate from each other. A simple and purely hypothetical example may help to clarify this point.

Suppose a given commodity can be produced by alternative combinations of type X and type Y manpower. Next suppose that the real social opportunity costs of X is $10,000 per year and per person of that type of manpower, and that the analogous figure for Y is $30,000. Suppose further, however, that while manpower of type X is indeed paid $10,000 per year, a degree of monopoly power enables manpower of type Y to extract from consumers an annual amount of purchasing power equal to $60,000 per person of type Y manpower employed. If one defines the least-cost combination of manpower capable of producing a given rate of that commodity as the optimal combination, then the optimal ratio of Y to X defined on the basis of real resource costs will clearly exceed that defined on the basis of transfer costs. It is clear that adherence to the first of these optima reduces the sacrifice (in terms of foregone goods and services) *society as a whole* must bear to obtain the stipulated output of the commodity. It is not at all clear, however, whether the consumers of that commodity reap any of these efficiency gains. In fact, it is not difficult to construct hypothetical examples in which the extra transfer consumers must make to manpower of type Y as a group actually exceeds the total savings from greater real resource efficiency.[c] Under these circumstances, an economist's assurance that the move to greater efficiency has somehow served to increase the collective "pie" available to society as a whole may be small comfort to the impoverished consumer of the commodity.

The preceding discourse may strike the reader as an excruciating piece of pedantry. In fact, it strikes at the very heart of the apparent communications gap between economists and policymakers. The truth is that the economist's rules for efficient social choice are invariably developed in abstraction from the distributional impact of alternative policy options. It is a bit of handwaving that occasionally flabbergasts policymakers who tend to be highly sensitive to the distributional consequences of their decisions. One hastens to add that the economist's motivation in offering his rules is anything but sinister; these rules are based on the quite sensible notion that once the returns from society's

[c]Consider the hypothetical case in which it is technically feasible to produce the assumed rate of output only with two alternative combinations of *Y* and *X*: combination A, calling for 3 units of *Y* and 5 units of *X,* and combination B calling for only 2 units of *Y* but 9 units of *X.* Given the cost data assumed in the text above, combination A has a real resource cost of $140,000 and a transfer cost of $230,000. Combination B, on the other hand, has a real resource cost of $150,000 and a transfer cost of $210,000. Suppose initially combination B were chosen because of the relatively lower transfer costs associated with it. An economist might point out that a move to combination A would lower real resource costs by $10,000. As a result of the move, however, one extra person would enter the pool of type *Y* manpower and receive $60,000, of which $30,000 are monopoly gains. In other words, although consumers of the commodity would be saved $10,000 in real resource costs, they would pay a "price" (in the form of monopoly gains) of $30,000 for these gains, and would hence be poorer by a net amount of $20,000 in the end. Although our example is obviously designed to generate this result, it does illustrate the general nature of the problem alluded to above and, as this author suspects, the nature of the dilemma faced by health manpower planners in this country.

resources are maximized, it should always be possible to compensate the losers from moves toward greater overall efficiency out of the enhanced collective sweepstakes. The nagging fear laymen and their legislative representatives seem to have is that the potentially feasible compensation may never actually be paid—hence their preoccupation with the transfer costs of alternative public policies. In the context of health manpower policy these transfer costs do, after all, determine *inter alia* the average price consumers must pay directly or indirectly for the receipt of health services, and therefore the proportion of the consumers' incomes that must be set aside for that purpose. To the consumer it matters not one whit whether the average physician income implicit in the physician's fees is smaller or larger than the true social opportunity costs of physician manpower. The consumer is interested solely in seeing the transfer cost of adequate health maintenance minimized. Given the overall orientation of this book, our discussion on the economics of health manpower substitution emphasizes this cost concept as well, as is apparent in Table 7-5.

Health Manpower Substitution and the Cost of Physician Services

Table 7-5 indicates the estimated total and average *direct* transfer costs of alternative health manpower combinations capable of meeting an assumed demand for office visits in medical practices. By direct costs in this context is meant the sum of the physician's net income, his payroll costs, and his nonlabor overhead costs. On this definition, the direct cost per patient visit is, of course, identical to the average price per visit charged by the physician—a variable of great interest to consumers and policymakers alike. It will be noted that these direct costs are not exactly the same as the true net total transfer costs associated with a given manpower combination, because the latter include also the subsidies consumers indirectly pay for the training of health manpower and exclude the sum returned by physicians and their aides to the nonphysician sector in the form of income taxes. For suitable assumptions about these subsidies and taxes, Table 7-5 could easily be converted to reflect total net transfer costs.

The estimated manpower requirements underlying Table 7-5 are those presented in the last two rows of Table 7-4. It will be recalled that these requirements have been estimated from the productivity indexes implicit in the production function for internists. Analogous cost estimates based on the productivity indexes for general practitioners are presented in Appendix Table C-6. The estimated manpower requirements underlying Table C-6 can be found at the bottom of that table.

Tables 7 and C-6 are based on the implicit assumption that physicians price their services so as to reach a desired target income on the office-based part of their practice. In the first row of the table, for example, it is assumed that whatever number of aides the physician employs he prices his services so as

Table 7-5.   Illustration of the Effect of Health Manpower Substitution on the Direct Costs of Furnishing an Assumed Aggregate Demand for Office Visits in 1990[a]

Assumed average annual salary per aide, and assumed contribution to non-labor overhead and net profit per hour the physician spends in his office	Total cost and cost per office visit if the number of aides per physician is equal to:					
	0	1	1.75	2	3	4
Salary per aide: $7,500	*Total costs (billions of dollars)[b]*					
Contribution margin per hour:						
$20	$23.91	$21.20	$19.65	$19.23	$18.03	$17.56
30	35.87	29.87	26.72	25.88	23.43	22.20
40	47.82	38.54	33.79	32.53	28.82	26.84
	Average cost per office visit[c]					
$20	$11.79	$10.45	$ 9.69	$ 9.48	$ 8.89	$ 8.66
30	17.69	14.73	13.18	12.76	11.55	10.95
40	23.58	19.00	16.66	16.04	14.21	13.23
Salary per aide: $10,000	*Total costs (billions of dollars)*					
Contribution margin per hour:						
$20	$23.91	$22.49	$21.50	$21.21	$20.44	$20.32
30	35.87	31.16	28.56	27.86	25.84	24.96
40	47.82	39.83	35.63	34.51	31.23	29.60
	Average cost per office visit					
$20	$11.79	$11.09	$10.60	$10.46	$10.08	$10.02
30	17.69	15.36	14.08	13.74	12.74	12.31
40	23.58	19.64	17.57	17.02	15.40	14.60
Salary per aide: $15,000	*Total costs (billions of dollars)*					
Contribution margin per hour:						
$20	$23.91	$25.07	$25.17	$25.18	$25.26	$25.85
30	35.87	33.74	32.24	31.82	30.66	30.48
40	47.82	42.41	39.31	38.47	36.05	35.12

	Average cost per office visit					
$20	$11.79	$12.36	$12.40	$12.41	$12.45	$12.74
30	17.69	16.64	15.90	15.69	15.12	15.03
40.	23.58	20.91	19.38	18.97	17.78	17.32

[a]Calculated from the manpower requirements presented in Table 7–5 on the assumption that the per capita demand for office visits will grow at a steady annual rate of 3 percent. The costs shown in the table include only the office-based part of the physician's income; income earned in the hospital is thought to be excluded. It is assumed that the physician will spend an average of 35 hours per week in his office (not necessarily in direct contact with patients) and work an average of 48 weeks a year.

[b]Calculated as $X = CHM + SML$, where X is total cost, C is the assumed contribution margin per hour, S is the assumed annual salary per aide, L is the number of aides per office-based physician, M is the required number of office-based physicians, and H is the total number of office hours per year.

[c]Calculated as $P = X/(ND)$, where P is average cost per visit, X is total cost (as defined in note b), N is the size of the population to be served, and D is the per capita demand for office visits.

to cover his annual payroll costs and to leave himself with a so-called contribution to overhead and profits (gross revenues minus payroll) equal to $20 per hour he works in his office. For an assumed fixed number of office hours per year, this full-cost pricing formula automatically yields him a fixed annual income.[d] (In Table B-1 of Appendix B, incidentally, this pricing theory is identified by the label II-B.) It should be obvious that under this formula, any net economic benefits from task delegation are passed on to consumers in the form of lower prices. Conversely, any additional labor costs that cannot be met out of added revenues at given prices are passed on to consumers through price increases.

Table 7-5 indicates that under the preceding pricing formula, health manpower substitution tends to lower the direct cost per office visit for reasonable assumptions about desired contribution margins and the salaries paid to aides. This is true even for the more pessimistic productivity estimates incorporated into Table C-6. As is to be expected, the reductions in average direct costs diminish as the number of aides per physician increases. It is a manifestation of the law of diminishing marginal returns. For realistic combinations of contribution margins and aide salaries, direct costs per visit tend to bottom out and then begin to rise again somewhere between 4 and 5 aides per physician if one's estimates are based on the productivity indexes implicit in the production function for internists (that is, the figures in Table 7-5), and somewhere between 3.5 and 4.5 if one bases one's estimates on the productivity indexes for general practitioners (Table C-6).

One could envisage certain combinations of contribution margins and aide salaries at which health manpower substitution would increase the direct cost (price) per office visit, even at fairly low numbers of aides per physician. In such cases the price per visit would be so low that the gross revenues generated by more extensive task delegation would be insufficient to cover the associated payroll costs unless that price were raised from its previous level. The third and sixth rows from the bottom of Table 7-5 are illustrations of that possibility. One wonders, of course, whether the particular combination of salaries and contribution margins postulated there occurs frequently in the real world.

As noted, the pricing behavior postulated for Table 7-5 implies that the economic benefits from increased task delegation are fully passed on to consumers. This assumption was made to illustrate what seems possible if physicians could be constrained to a fixed annual income (perhaps by paying them a salary). In the absence of strong outside inducements, the typical self-employed practitioner in this country would probably not wish to follow so selfless a

[d]Actually his true net income may fall slightly with the level of aides (for any given contribution margin and aide-salary) because additional aides may generate some additions to the physician's overhead. In Chapters Five and Six we had overcome that problem simply by thinking of these incremental overhead costs as part of the salary figure ($W^* + E^*$).

pricing policy. A plausible alternative hypothesis would be that physicians generally seek to appropriate the economic gains from task delegation for themselves by selling the added patient visits so generated at a *constant* price. Under these circumstances the optimal number of aides per physician may be defined as one that maximizes the physician's average income per hour he works in his office.

Using this standard of optimality, it was found in Chapter Six that under the level of physician fees and aide salaries prevailing in 1965-67—and under those currently prevailing—the estimated optimal number of traditional allied health workers per physician tends to cluster closely around a value of 4 (see Tables 6-14 and 6-15, and Tables C-2 and C-3). Tables 7-6 and 7-7 illustrate this calculus in a somewhat different fashion. The figures in the body of these tables are the estimated hourly "contribution margins to the physician's nonpayroll overhead and net income" at alternative numbers of aides employed per physician. This contribution margin is defined as the sum of money left over from gross revenues after the physician has met his payroll expenses. For each level of aide input, the contribution margins in Tables 7-6 and 7-7 are calculated at alternative assumed prices and aide salaries. The hourly contribu-

Table 7-6. Estimated Effect of Health Manpower Substitution in Medical Practice on the Contribution to Nonlabor Overhead and Net Profits Earned per Hour the Physician Spends in His Office[a] (General Practice)

Assumed average revenue per office visit, and assumed weekly salary per aide	Contribution to nonlabor overhead and net profit if the number of aides per physician is equal to:[b]				
	0	1	2	3	4
Assumed average revenue per office visit: $7.50					
Average weekly salary per aide					
$100	$19.55	$23.09	$26.51	$28.79	$28.96
150	19.55	21.54	23.41	24.15	22.76
200	19.55	19.99	20.32	19.50	16.57
Assumed average revenue per office visit: $10.00					
Average weekly salary per aide					
$100	$26.06	$31.81	$37.41	$41.48	$42.73
150	26.06	30.27	34.31	36.84	36.54
200	26.06	28.72	31.22	32.19	30.35

[a]Calculated from the office-visit production function for general practitioners in Table 6-7. It is assumed that the GP spends an average of 35 hours per week in his office (not necessarily in direct contact with patients) and practices an average of 48 weeks a year.

[b]Calculated as $X = (PQ - SL)/H$, where X is the contribution margin, P is the average revenue per office visit, Q is the annual rate of office visits, S is the annual salary per aide (52 times the weekly rate), L is the number of aides per physician, and H is the annual number of office hours (weekly hours times 48).

Table 7-7. **Estimated Effect of Health Manpower Substitution in Medical Practice on the Contribution to Nonlabor Overhead and Net Profits Earned per Hour the Physician Spends in His Office**[a] **(Internal Medicine)**

Assumed average revenue per office visit, and assumed weekly salary per aide	Contribution to nonlabor overhead and net profit if the number of aides per physician is equal to [b]				
	0	1	2	3	4
Assumed average revenue per office visit: $12.50					
Average weekly salary per aide					
$100	$20.11	$24.13	$28.92	$33.67	$37.33
150	20.11	22.32	25.31	28.26	30.11
200	20.11	20.51	21.70	22.84	22.88
Assumed average revenue per office visit: $17.50					
Average weekly salary per aide					
$100	$28.15	$35.22	$43.38	$51.48	$58.04
150	28.15	33.41	39.77	46.06	50.82
200	28.15	31.61	36.16	40.64	43.59

[a]Calculated from the office-visit production function for internists in Table 6–10. It is assumed that the internist spends an average of 30 hours per week in his office (not necessarily in direct contact with patients) and practices an average of 48 weeks a year.
[b]See Table 7–6.

tion margins presented in Table 7–6 reflect the productivity indexes implicit in the office-visits equation for general practitioners; those in Table 7–7 are based on the office-visits equation for internists. The prices and salaries used in these tables are thought to bracket the range of relative prices and salaries faced by physicians in various parts of the country.

Tables 7–6 and 7–7 indicate that up to a point (generally somewhere between 3.5 and 4.5 aides per physician) the substitution of aides for physician time can have a highly salutary effect on the physician's income. Employment levels at which the contribution margin per hour reaches a maximum are the optima we seek to estimate. The fact that these optima are roughly the same as those suggested in conjunction with Table 7–5 should come as no surprise. These optima are mirror images of each other, because the average prices postulated in Tables 7–6 and 7–7 are mirror images of the "reasonable" contribution margins postulated in Table 7–5.[e] The essential difference between Table 7–5 on

[e]In more technical terms, this may be shown as follows. The average direct costs presented in Table 7–5 is defined as

$$C = \frac{(YM + SML)}{MQ}$$

where Y denotes the annual contribution to nonlabor overhead and profit the physician wishes to earn on the office-based part of his practice; M denotes the total number of the one hand and Tables 7-6 and 7-7 on the other is that the net economic benefits or costs from task delegation are assumed to accrue to different parties. Neither set of estimates, however, seems to be a mere statistical artifact. First, as was noted in Chapter Six, a level of four or more aides per physician also appears to be viewed as optimal by management consultants in the field of medical practice. Furthermore, the frequency distributions in Table 7-3 suggest that a good many American physicians already do employ in excess of four aides per physician. Table 7-8, taken from the same survey as that underlying Table 7-3, suggests that physicians can indeed benefit substantially from the employment of aides. The income figures in Table 7-8 may of course reflect still other factors that vary positively with the number of aides employed (for example, fees or hours worked per year). Such factors have been held constant in Tables 7-6 and 7-7. Even so, Tables 7-3 and 7-8 do encourage one to think that the optima suggested in the preceding discussion are both technically feasible and economically sensible in the real world.

In reaction to Tables 7-6 and 7-7 it may be felt by some that, even if the indicated profit margins are generated by physicians without raising the price of their services to consumers, there is something inherently inequitable in a situation in which an already well-paid professional can pocket benefits generated by other persons (auxiliary personnel) whom he obviously pays much less than their average economic contribution to his practice. Such critics should be aware that their argument is a perhaps unintended broadside against the capitalist system in general. If one accepts the ethical precepts underlying that system and, moreover, is willing to tolerate a situation in which even inefficient producers can earn a satisfactory profit—a situation that has long been tolerated in the area of medical practice—then the relatively high economic returns physicians can reap from the employment of three or four aides per physician must be viewed simply as rewards for relatively greater efficiency and compensation for the administrative chores created by a large auxiliary staff. They are rewards that cannot logically be viewed as ethically offensive by

---

physicians in office practice; L denotes the number of aides per physician; S is the average salary plus fringe benefits earned by an aide; and Q denotes the annual rate of office visits per physician. If one expresses Q by some production function $Q = f(H, L, K)$—where H denotes annual office hours and K is an index of capital—then the effect of changes in L on direct costs C can be inferred from the partial derivative

$\partial C/\partial L = [SQ - (Y + SL) \partial Q/\partial L]/Q^2$

This derivative will be negative as long as

$$S < \frac{(Y + SL)}{Q} \, \partial Q/\partial L$$

But $(Y + SL)/Q$ is also the definition of the price (P) per unit of output, and the physician finds it profitable to expand L as long as $(\partial Q/\partial L)P > S$. The two definitions of an optimum are thus mirror images of each other.

Table 7-8.   Relationship between Number of Aides per Physician and Gross Income per Solo M.D., United States, 1973

Number of Aides per Physician[a]	Median Gross Income per Self-Employed Solo M.D.	Increment in Gross Income per Solo M.D.	Income as a Percent of Income in the Absence of Aides
None	$ 40,900	–	100%
One	57,200	$16,300	140
Two	73,800	16,600	180
Three	87,200	13,400	213
Four or more	114,800	27,600	281

[a]Number of full-time equivalent aides other than physicians or physicians' assistants.
Source: *Medical Economics,* Continuing Survey 1973, presented in Owens [1974].

one who accepts the ethical precepts of capitalism and who tolerates inefficiency in medical practice elsewhere. By implication, those policymakers or
commentators who do find these rewards offensive ought to be prepared also
to recommend reimbursement schemes under which inefficient physicians
could not earn an adequate income. We shall return to this point later in this
chapter.

Health Manpower Substitution and the Supply of Physician Services

In the previous illustration it has been assumed that physicians
work the same number of hours per year regardless of the number of aides they
employ. This implies that they convert the economic benefits from task delegation wholly into added income. Formal economic theories of physician behavior—surveyed at length in Appendix B—suggest that at least part of these
benefits may be converted by physicians into added leisure time, not income.
If so, some of the added office visits postulated in the preceding exercises
would never materialize. Some students of the health-care sector consider this a
real possibility. They view any attempt to increase the supply of physician
services through enhanced physician productivity as potentially self-defeating.[9]

The empirical evidence on this issue is unfortunately inconclusive.
As was noted in Chapter Four (Table 4-9), over a cross-section of American
physicians one discerns a slight *positive* correlation between hours worked and
the number of aides employed per physician. This finding, however, provides
no clue on how average hours worked would respond to increases in the number
of aides employed by each in a given set of physicians. Some researchers—for
example, Feldstein [1970]—appear to have detected a *negative* relationship
between the number of physician services supplied and the price per unit of
service. This finding implies that when the physician's hourly remuneration
increases because the price per unit of his output increases, the physician tends
to convert some of this profit potential into added leisure. With constant
hourly productivity this necessarily means fewer units of output per physician.

The same result could obviously not obtain if the increase in the physician's hourly remuneration were due to more extensive task delegation and the average revenue per unit of output (patient visit) remained constant. Under these circumstances, there would have to be at least some additional output per physician as long as physicians do not accept an actual decrease in their net income. The reason, of course, is that the payroll cost of additional aides must be covered by gross revenues. At constant prices per unit of output, these additional revenues can obviously come only from the production and sale of additional output.

Recent empirical research, more directly focused on the relationship between average remuneration per physician-hour and hours worked, has indicated a remarkably low response of hours worked to hourly income, and only weak and statistically insignificant evidence for the hypothesized negative response.[10] Although the data base underlying this conclusion has some shortcomings, the finding nevertheless encourages optimism concerning policies to increase the availability of physician services through increases in physician productivity. In this connection it is well to remember also that public policy-makers need not stand by passively should physicians decide to trade produc-tivity gains for leisure, particularly not where physicians are reimbursed for their services under a national health insurance system. Under such a system the public sector could, if it chose to do so, constrain reimbursement rates so as to exert strong economic pressure on inefficient health-care providers, leaving, say, a physician bent on maintaining or improving his income no alternative but to enhance the productivity of his practice, presumably through more extensive task delegation or through whatever other means are feasible.

Health Manpower Substitution and the Service-Intensity of Physician Care

Some observers of the health system suspect that the employment of paramedical aides in a medical practice does not normally enhance the physician's hourly productivity at all, but merely serves to increase the service-intensity—and hence the cost—of medical treatment. The hypothesis is that the presence of auxiliary personnel in a physician's practice will not generally lead to bona fide task delegation as such, but instead induce the physician to have produced and to sell additional and often unnecessary ancillary services, pre-sumably at a net profit to him. Coupled with the potential problem of a nega-tive relationship between hourly physician income and hours worked per physician, this possibility would have ominous implications for the social usefulness of health manpower substitution. For, if the employment of aides served merely to increase the typical physician's hourly income without also increasing his true hourly productivity, and if he sought to convert even a mere fraction of this increased hourly income into added leisure, then the net effect of health manpower substitution in medical practice might well be to decrease the supply of physician services (such as office visits) supplied by a given stock of physicians, and in the process to drive up the cost of these services unnecessarily. This is clearly no trivial matter.

We have already touched upon this problem in Chapter Four where it was acknowledged that the employment of auxiliary personnel may induce the physician (a) to produce on his premises certain services that would otherwise be contracted to outside facilities (type I services) and (b) to prescribe and have produced on his premises certain services that would not be included in his prescribed treatment at all in the absence of appropriate auxiliary personnel (such as technicians). In Chapter Four the latter type of services were referred to as type II services. It is clear that the first type of reaction would not by itself increase the service intensity of medical treatments, but merely change these services' locus of production and the distribution of the profits they generate. Production of type II services, on the other hand, would ipso facto increase the service intensity of treatments and, to the extent that such services are not truly necessary from a medical viewpoint, needlessly increase the cost of medical care.

There is evidence that increases in type I and type II services per patient accounts for the major portion of any observed productivity differential between solo practices and small groups, on the one hand, and large-scale multispecialty groups on the other, if productivity is measured by gross billings [Bailey, 1970]. The relationship between service intensity and the number of aides *within* the category of solo practices and small groups, however, appears much less pronounced. Yankauer et al.'s analysis of pediatric practices (cited in Tables 4–6 and 4–7, Chapter Four) clearly indicates that the employment of aides in these practices does lead to substantial delegation of specific tasks from the physician to his aides, that there is only a mild tendency for greater service intensity per visit, and that physician productivity as measured by "patients seen" does respond strongly and positively to the number of aides employed. The production-function estimates presented in Chapter Six and summarized in Table 7–1 corroborate this conclusion. Although the annual rate of patient billings (adjusted for interphysician variation in the absolute fee level) generally does appear to rise somewhat more rapidly as a function of the number of aides than does either the rate of total patient visits or the rate of office visits (the exception being internal medicine), the observed difference is actually quite small, and the rate of patient visits is very responsive indeed to increases in staff size (L).

These empirical findings suggest that if the employment of aides really served no purpose other than to increase the service-intensity of the treatment given to an unchanged number of patients, then this increased service-intensity would have to take the form primarily of additional re-visits for given medical conditions. Although one cannot rule out this possibility *a priori*, it does not invalidate the argument advanced in this chapter (or in this book, for that matter). First, such additional re-visits might in fact be medically desirable and, in the absence of physician-support personnel, simply not feasible for want of physician time. But even if such visits were medically unnecessary—a case actually lacking plausibility at the theoretical level[f]—the present analysis has not really been concerned with the actual distribution of potentially available patient visits among individual consumers. The objective of the analysis has been to explore whether the hypothesized task delegation in medical practice does in fact tend to take place when physicians augment their auxiliary staff. The fact that the number of patient visits per physician hour increases substantially with the number of aides employed persuades one that the hypothesis can be maintained, and that the productivity gains commonly attributed to the employment of aides are potentially real and not just apparent. In the real world and under some circumstances this productivity potential may well be frittered away in added physician leisure or by the delivery of patient visits to patients not truly in need of them; it may even not be exploited at all. The point is that the potential seems available and that it could be tapped to meet a perceived shortage of medical manpower.

In reacting to this conclusion it is well to recall once more the overall focus of the book. The objective throughout our discussion has been to demonstrate empirically the inherent looseness of the link between *aggregate* demand for physician services and the *aggregate* number of physicians required to meet that demand, a looseness that is often not appreciated in discussions over health manpower policies. To that end we have attempted to estimate the aggregate supply of physician services (as measured by physician-patient contacts or patient billings) that could *potentially* be made available to society as a whole by alternative combinations of health manpower in medical practices. No attempt was made to predict the volume of physician services that will actually be made available by physicians in the future, nor even the volume that may probably be made available. The intent was merely to estimate the rate of production that seems technically attainable and economically sensible if physicians could somehow be induced to expand their support staff to the indicated optimum levels without reducing the length of their own workweek. Whether the estimated potential will ultimately be exploited will depend in

---

[f]It is entirely possible that where physicians are in relatively abundant supply, an attempt will be made to prescribe more re-visits for given medical conditions than would be prescribed in less well endowed areas or would be medically necessary. (The actual re-visit rate would depend in part also on the relative value patients assign to their own time.) There is no reason to suspect the number of visits per case to vary systematically and positively with the number of aides per physician, however. Where physicians are in relatively abundant supply, it is not necessary to hire support personnel to free physician time; if desired, added re-visits could presumably be delivered even in the absence of support personnel. If support staff *is* hired in such situations, it is likely to be employed either for noneconomic reasons or to enhance the physician's hourly income through the sale of ancillary services per patient visit. It is not obvious why the sale of these ancillary services should require additional re-visits.

part on the behavior of physicians themselves and on the influence policy-makers have over that behavior. It will, of course, depend also on whether policymakers choose to wield what influence they do have in this area. We now turn to a consideration of these policy options.

III. HEALTH MANPOWER POLICY AND RESEARCH

In exploring the policy implications of the preceding analysis, few insights are lost if one abstracts from the numerous distinctions that could be made among types of physician-support personnel and simply treats the latter as a homogenous category of manpower. This abstraction permits one to proceed as if there existed a single market for physician-support personnel. Public policies designed to encourage greater use of such personnel by physicians can then be viewed as public intervention into this otherwise private labor market, and the rationale underlying these policies, as well as their potential impact, can be explored within the framework of standard labor-market theory. Such an examination should, of course, always include the fundamental question of whether public intervention in this or related markets can reasonably be justified in the first place.

To structure the analysis of health manpower policies around the economic theory of labor markets is not an arbitrary choice made solely to serve an economist's convenience. The great majority of these policies operate directly or indirectly through the market system. They rely on market forces for their success. Failure to appreciate this fact, and failure to understand the particular markets through which proposed policies must work, can easily doom well-intentioned policy action from the outset. It can seduce policy-makers into the granting of subsidies where none are justifiable, or to tolerate market imperfections that reduce the potential power of public subsidies to naught. Although economic analyses of this sort rarely make easy reading—even if rendered in essentially nontechnical language—the clarity to be gained by working through the economics of health manpower policy will hopefully be worth the effort. We begin the analysis with a brief description of the conventional labor-market model.

Figure 7–4 is a diagrammatic characterization of the market for physician-support personnel in some hypothetical geographic area. The curves in that diagram may be thought of as compact summaries of the behavior of all of the region's potential employers of such personnel, and of all potential employees offering their services to these employers. Such curves are referred to as "market demand and supply schedules." They are not to be confused with the demand and supply schedules characterizing the individual medical practice. (Examples of the latter are presented in Figure 6–5.) Figure 7–4 is a standard labor-market model found in most textbooks on microeconomic

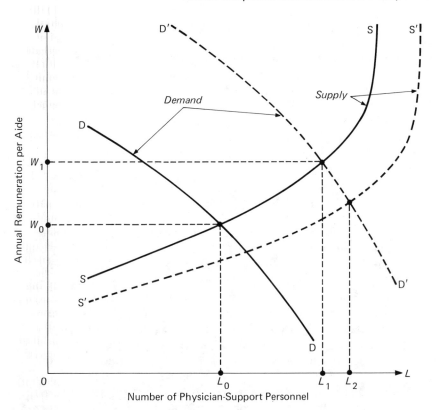

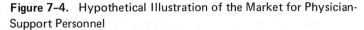

Figure 7–4. Hypothetical Illustration of the Market for Physician-Support Personnel

analysis. We shall find it convenient to develop much of the ensuing discussion in terms of this diagram.

The market demand schedules in Figure 7–4 (DD and D'D') indicate the total number of aides physicians as a group would hire at alternative levels of aide salaries. One reason these demand schedules slope downward to the right is that successive additions of support personnel to a given stock of physicians in an area tend to add successively smaller increments to the physicians' average productivity, and hence are increasingly more difficult to justify financially unless salaries are lowered in step. It is a reflection of the familiar law of diminishing marginal productivity. An alternative reason for the negative slope might be that successive additions to physician output generated by additional support personnel can be sold by physicians only if they lower the prices (fees) of their services. That circumstance—referred to as a monopolistic market structure—also would make it increasingly difficult for physicians to justify successive additions to their support staff unless the aides' salary were lowered in step.

The market-supply curves in Figure 7–4 (SS and S'S') indicate the total number of aides in the region that would be willing to work in physicians' offices at alternative salary levels. Underlying these schedules are (1) the characteristics of persons offering their labor services in the market for physician-support personnel (including these persons' attitudes toward the kind of work a physician's aide performs); (2) the features of competing labor markets in which these persons' services are in demand (primarily the hospital sector); and (3) the market for the kind of formal training physician-support personnel must have. The market-supply curves slope upward to the right because at successively higher salaries more and more potential physician-support personnel will be lured away from competing occupations (including the occupation of running a household), and more and more persons will find it advantageous to invest in paramedical training.

Any development that induces physicians as a group to hire more or fewer aides per physician *at a given salary level* is represented in Figure 7–4 by a corresponding shift of the entire demand schedule (for example, from DD to D'D'). Such shifts can occur either because, at given levels of aides per physician, the productivity of aides has somehow been enhanced, or because at given rates of physician output, the prices (fees) of physician services have changed. Similarly, any development as a result of which more or fewer persons offer their labor services in the market for physician-support personnel *at given salary levels*, is represented by a corresponding shift of the entire supply schedule (for example, from SS to S'S'). Such developments include changes in the salaries offered in competing labor markets, changes in attitudes toward working in medical practices, or increasing economic pressure (perhaps through unemployment of a spouse) forcing potential physician-support personnel out of a household occupation into the labor market. Changes in the cost of paramedical training would, of course, reflect themselves in shifts of the labor-supply curve as well.

In any regional market for physician-support personnel there currently prevails a level of aide salaries and a certain level of aides employed by medical practices. Level L_0 in Figure 7–4 may be thought of as such a prevailing level. Policies designed to increase the average number of aides employed per physician—say, from L_0 to L_1—must seek to induce a rightward shift in either the market supply curve or in the market demand curve, or in both. Some of the policy levers that may be employed for this purpose have been broadly hinted at above. In the following sections they are examined in finer detail.

Public Policy and the Supply of
Physician-Support Personnel

Critics of the notion that a perceived physician shortage might well be met through health manpower substitution sometimes accuse its proponents of a so-called fallacy of composition. It is conceded by these critics that an individual physician might be able to enlarge his support staff from, say, two to four aides, but that all American physicians could clearly not do so simultaneously. The reason given is that there is a shortage of physician-support personnel as well. As one of the more outspoken of these critics has put it:

> A practical problem arises [in implementing policies designed to enhance physician productivity] : Where are the paramedical personnel who will be trained to relieve physicians of some of their burden? . . . Allied health service personnel are in short supply, and training facilities for an appreciable improvement in the future are woefully inadequate. . . . The futility of depending upon "more efficient use of the physician's time by making him the leader of nonexistent people" has been previously called to the attention of the medical profession [Gerber 1967, p. 308].

This comment was made in 1967; its validity has in the meantime been eroded by events. Even so it is instructive to examine it within its own temporal context.

The proposition that there is an absolute shortage of physician-support personnel, in the short and perhaps even the long run, implies that the market-supply schedule for that type of personnel is very steep. In the economist's jargon, that supply curve would be described as *wage-inelastic* or *wage-insensitive*. It is assumed that any attempt by physicians to attract a large number of assistants must come at the expense of the hospital sector, and that this so-called zero-sum game would ultimately serve only to drive up the salaries of such personnel without increasing the total active labor pool from which both hospitals and physicians draw, at least in the short run. The validity of this proposition is clearly an empirical matter.

It can be readily conceded that all 180,000 or so office-based American physicians could not, in 1967, have doubled their support staff without drawing some of this personnel away from employment in other health-care facilities, chiefly hospitals. Yet it need not be assumed that *all* of the additional personnel would have had to be drawn from other parts of the health-care sector. In 1966, the average weekly salary of a registered nurse in the in the United States was roughly $100, and that of a practical nurse $72.50.[11] The salary paid registered nurses amounted to only about 69 percent of that paid public school teachers in that year, and was barely more than the average salary paid secretaries.[12] As was noted in earlier chapters (for example, see Table 5-2), the salaries physicians paid registered nurses during that period were roughly comparable, and perhaps somewhat lower. Under these circumstances it is hardly surprising that, at the wages they were ready to offer, physicians and hospital administrators perceived an aggregate shortage of nursing personnel. It is estimated, for example, that the roughly 650,000 registered nurses *professionally active* in 1966 constituted only about 55 to 60 percent of all reg-

istered nurses living in the United States at that time.[13] Although factors
other than salaries determine these so-called labor-force participation rates,
it can safely be assumed that many of the inactive nurses at that time could
have been drawn into the job market had physicians and hospitals been willing
to offer them a somewhat more adequate remuneration. In short, there is reason
to believe that even in the short run the supply of physician-support personnel
is rather more wage-elastic than is suggested by the above quotation.

      Failure to distinguish between a perceived shortage of manpower
at a given salary level, and shortages under which sufficient manpower does not
come forth at any salary level, is a common affliction among health care providers.[14] This distinction is not simply an academic nicety. It has important
implications for public policy. If the supply of physician-support personnel
were known to be wage-elastic, the focus of public policy should be primarily on
the demand side of that labor market. An attempt should be made, through
research, to identify the determinants of the demand for physician aides and to
discover among these determinants potential policy levers through which the
demand curve can be shifted to the right (for example, from DD to D'D' in
Figure 7-4). A number of policy options in this area will be examined shortly.
On the other hand, if one is convinced that the relevant labor supply curve is
wage-inelastic, the appropriate policy response would clearly be measures to
shift the supply curve to the right (and perhaps the demand curve as well).
Since most of the factors determining the position of the labor-supply curve lie
beyond the immediate reach of health manpower policy, the most practical
means of achieving a rightward shift in that curve is probably to intervene not
in the market for physician-support personnel, but instead in the market for
paramedical training.

      Public policy in the health manpower area has traditionally sought
to operate primarily through the supply side of the relevant labor market. In
Chapters One and Two this proposition was demonstrated in connection with
medical manpower. Recent legislation on allied health manpower exhibits a
similar pattern. By and large, public intervention in this labor market has had
the objective simply to increase the number of trained paramedical personnel
potentially available to the health-care sector, leaving decisions concerning
the use of that personnel to physicians and hospital administrators. The policy
instruments used to that end have been primarily general institutional support,
support for special training projects, and direct financial assistance to the
trainees. As a result of these measures, there have been substantial additions to
the capacity of nursing schools; the flow of graduates from these schools has
now reached proportions that have raised the prospect of a nursing surplus in the
near future. As noted earlier, there has also been much experimentation with
various types of specialized physician-support personnel, referred to under the
common label "physician extenders." Such experimentation has typically
taken the form of developing a new curriculum and of formally evaluating the

performance of graduates on the job, sometimes through costly time-and-motion studies.

Medical and nursing educators continue to design new training programs of this sort, and continue to press for increased federal support of both these and already-established programs. Social scientists stand ready to evaluate whatever new training programs emerge in this area, not, however, without generous federal research support. Since there is virtually no limit to the variety of new training programs that could be conceived, funded and evaluated in this manner, policymakers who control the flow of federal funds into this activity clearly face a dilemma. The educators and researchers who argue for federal support of their activities must be considered experts on health manpower issues. Their counsel can therefore not easily be brushed aside. Yet, these very same experts typically have a personal financial or professional stake in the survival of particular training programs, and may therefore argue from an unduly parochial perspective. Proposals for a termination of this experimental phase—or of subsidies to health professional schools in general—simply cannot be expected to come from these experts.

This circumstance forces on policymakers themselves resolution of t the following hard questions: (1) How much more information of the type now generated by these health manpower experiments is really needed before rational policy can be made in this area, and precisely what information is actually yielded by these experiments? (2) If, as it is claimed, there is a need for innovation in the training of health manpower, why can health-related professional schools not respond to this challenge without being explicitly rewarded for each new curricular development or, as is sometimes requested, merely for a willingness to make new curricula developed elsewhere part of their regular curriculum? Might not society expect its already well-supported training institutions to respond imaginatively to society's changing needs without additional financial inducements? And (3) precisely what is the economic and ethical foundation for the relatively large public subsidies that have traditionally been bestowed on health professionals of all types, and have come to be all but taken for granted by them? More specifically, how heavily should the training of physician-support personnel be subsidized on a long term basis? These are questions from which the guardians of the taxpayer's funds cannot, or at least should not, escape.

In principle it would seem reasonable to suppose that the desired attributes of new types of physician assistants for particular medical specialties could be identified by panels of competent and experienced practitioners in the field, that the appropriate training program for such personnel could be developed by educators in consultation with such panels, and that the competence of the trainees could be evaluated by the educators themselves as part of the training program in much the same way the competence of, say, a physicist is assessed at the end of his or her formal training. Why this evaluation needs to be buttressed with costly time-and-motion studies of on-the-job performance is not clear.

　　If the trainees are evaluated on the job, their observed performance will actually reveal much more about their employer—that is, about the manner in which the employer chooses to use the trainee—than about the inherent attributes of the trainee to be evaluated. Furthermore, the employer characteristics so revealed will be those of employers who have agreed to participate in the experiment. Precisely what such information reveals about the merits of the training program or about the impact of larger numbers of such trainees on the performance of the health-care sector as a whole is not immediately obvious. It depends to a large extent on the degree to which employers (physicians) *volunteering* for the experiment are representative of American physicians in general. Ultimately the success or failure of the entire physician extender concept stands or falls on the attitudes and behavior of this majority of physicians. In other words, if one is interested in the probable future potential of physician extenders, one had best concentrate one's research on the determinants of the market demand for physician-support personnel in general, and not on the performance of a select number of prototype graduates from particular programs, assigned to a nonrandom sample of medical practices (nonrandom in the sense that physicians who participate in experimental programs of this sort do so on a voluntary basis, presumably because they are well disposed toward using physician extenders in the first place).

　　Even if one deems the information yielded by continued experimentation with new forms of health manpower to be valuable and relevant for policy purposes, there is the question of how heavily the training of physician extenders should be subsidized in the long run. As was argued in Chapter One in connection with medical manpower, it is always useful to view training of any sort as a form of investment in the trainee. Economists refer to it as "human capital formation." On this perspective, publicly funded assistance to educational institutions or to their students is an investment subsidy in much the same way as would be public subsidies to private investments in the ownership of say, a service station, a restaurant, a barbershop or a trucking company. Such subsidies need to be defended explicitly; they should never be taken for granted. In the present case, for example, one should be able to explain to a taxpaying laborer who wants to own a business why his particular form of investing in his own future does not warrant a public subsidy while investments by health professionals in their own future merits substantial public assistance.

　　The traditional rationale for public subsidies to private investments in human capital—to education—has been that in the absence of public support, too few individuals would make that investment, and that higher levels of that kind of investment are in the public interest.[g] To make the latter case, however,

[g]Subsidies to professional schools are sometimes defended on the ground that they indirectly assist members from the lower income strata in gaining access to the occupa-

one must be able to argue that the investment in the trainees will ultimately generate benefits that accrue to society at large, but whose value will not be fully reflected in the income eventually earned by the trainees. The work of scientists, for example, is often thought to yield such unrequited "spillover benefits." These benefits go unrequited, first because scientific information once produced is essentially a free good, and second because the true value of a scientific discovery may come to be appreciated only decades or centuries later. One can think of public subsidies to investments in scientific training as a partial prepayment for unrewarded future spillover benefits.

It seems a natural tendency among educators in alsmost any discipline to attribute unrequited spillover benefits to the type of education they impart, and to argue for public support of that education, preferably in the form of untied institutional grants, which leaves the educator (who presumably knows what is best in this matter) free to allocate these funds as he sees fit. Only rarely is an attempt made to identify the nature of the alleged spillovers, perhaps because legislators have in the past responded to the educator's plea without asking for such an accounting. Since public subsidies of any kind imply a redistribution of wealth among members of society, policymakers granting such subsidies owe society that accounting.

Those who argue for federal assistance to the training of physician-support personnel appear to suggest, on the one hand, that such personnel can make a highly valuable contribution to society and, on the other, that society's representatives in the market for physician-support personnel—that is, physicians—are unlikely to pay such personnel a salary commensurate with their social contribution. In the economist's jargon, they suggest by implication that the prevailing demand schedule for physician-support personnel is lower than it would be if it reflected the true social value of such personnel. It may be noted that this implied allegation is certainly consistent with the empirical findings presented in Chapter Six and in earlier sections of the present chapter. Tables 7-6, and 7-7, for example, suggest that at observed levels of physician fees and aide salaries, the typical American physician could have gained financially from expanding the size of his auxiliary staff. If one takes the physician's fees as a measure of the value society attaches to physician services, then one is led to conclude that the value of the benefits added by the marginal aide to the typical physician's practice exceeds the salary he pays his aides by some margin.

If the alleged underpayment of physician-support personnel does

---

tion in question. The argument overlooks the fact that institutional grants typically are used to lower tuition fees across the board, so that they effectively constitute a transfer of wealth to students from the upper income classes as well. Tuition-free universities, for example, have traditionally had a regressive net financial impact on the community. If members from lower-income families are to be assisted in entering professional occupations, one had better grant them selective direct assistance in the form of scholarships or, preferably, in the form of low-interest loans.

indeed reflect imperfections in the relevant labor market, a sensible alternative to across-the-board training subsidies would be to eliminate these market imperfections. Upon elimination of these imperfections, the salary of aides would presumably rise, and it would then be quite reasonable to ask trainees for that occupation to absorb a greater proportion of the cost of their training. It goes almost without saying that such a policy would be feasible only if the trainees could borrow readily against future income. Although ready access to funds for investment in human capital is not now available in the private capital market—presumably because individual loans of this type seem risky— the public sector clearly has the wherewithal to create the requisite lending institution. Indeed, to make this type of financing more attractive to individual students, human-capital loans might be coupled with features of the so-called Yale tuition plan by limiting the maximum annual installment students would have to pay upon graduation to a fixed percentage of each year's income. That clause would eliminate the argument that human-capital loans impose undue economic hardship on those who do or must take advantage of them.

In the context of health manpower training, the policy proposed above involves more than an essentially neutral trade-off between subsidies now and income later. All too often public subsidies to the training of health manpower are predicated on the notion that once individuals have been trained for health professions, they will automatically be active in them. As the tra- ditionally low labor-force participation rates in nursing demonstrate, however, that assumption remains valid only so long as the trainees receive adequate remuneration upon completion of their training. If for one reason or another salaries in the health professions are below those in competing labor markets, many of the trainees may eventually desert the health professions for more lucrative employment elsewhere. They may even leave the labor force altogether. In the end, the public sector may thus find itself providing subsidies to two trainees for every one actually remaining active in health-care delivery. Efforts to assure adequate remuneration of paramedical personnel strikes one as a superior policy response.

To sum up at this point: federal efforts to encourage more extensive task delegation in medical practice have so far proceeded on the tacit assumption that the effective constraint on physicians has been an inadequate supply of paramedical personnel. To remove this presumed bottleneck, there has been substantial federal involvement in the financing of health-related professional training. The objective of this policy has been to increase the potential supply of physician-support personnel. Its underlying hope has been that the health- care sector will actually use the added health manpower, and use it judiciously

The proponents of this approach can certainly point to a need of physician-support personnel. It is now widely accepted that more extensive task delegation in medical practice would be in society's interest. The problem is that in the United States society's *needs* in this respect are communicated to the relevant labor market through the good offices of medical practitioners. The translation is communicated in the form of the physicians' *effective demand* for physician-support personnel. For reasons to be explored shortly, this translation of need into effective demand may be less than accurate. It is colored by the physicians' own perception of society's needs and, more importantly, by their personal preferences for particular practice styles. The preferred practice style may not call for extensive task delegation. As has been noted on several occasions in this book, the physician's market environment appears to be one that affords him wide discretion in catering to his personal preferences.

The recent development of the physician extender concept is a case in point. One remarkable aspect of this entire development is that it appears to have originated primarily in the minds of educators and health policy planners—who presumably perceived society's need for such personnel—and not actually from what may be called the representative medical practitioner in the field.[15] In fact, from the literature one infers that the concept is still being sold to the profession of medical practitioners, where it has not infrequently been met by a conspicuous lack of enthusiasm. How successful this sales pitch will ultimately be is still anybody's guess at this time. It will depend in large measure on how well the determinants of the physicians' demand for support personnel are understood by policymakers, and on how boldly the latter will manipulate these determinants. This aspect of health manpower policy has hitherto been neglected in both research and policy action.

Public Policy and the Demand for Physician-Support Personnel

The demand for any type of labor by a conventional profit-oriented business firm is fully determined by two factors: the *marginal physical productivity* of that type of labor, and the *marginal revenue* the firm can earn on the sale of additional units of output. At any given use-rate of the manpower in question, its "marginal physical product" is defined as the additional physical units of output generated by adding one more unit of that manpower to a given combination of all other inputs used by the firm. (In the case of medical practice, these other inputs would be the physician's own time, his office, and his equipment.) Unless the firm has to lower the price of the output to sell this marginal product, the so-called "marginal revenue product" associated with the additional unit of manpower is its marginal physical product times the prevailing price per unit of output. Unless the firm is willing to take a loss, the maximum wage it could afford to pay for the additional unit of manpower is precisely equal to its marginal revenue product.[h] Furthermore, since the

---

[h]Since in practice all labor of a given type within a business establishment must be paid the same wage, the marginal revenue product associated with the marginal addition to the work force actually determines the wage paid all workers of that type.

marginal product of any type of labor tends to diminish as more and more of
that labor is added to given amounts of other inputs, its marginal revenue
product—and hence the maximum wage the firm can offer for that type of
labor—tends to decrease in step. The entire schedule of such maxima at
alternative input rates is, of course, the demand curve for that type of manpower.

If the market for physician services were a perfectly and fiercely
competitive one in which only thoroughly efficient medical practices could
survive financially, and if the individual physician could hire any number of
aides at constant, market-determined salaries, then each physician in the market
could be assumed to employ an optimal number of aides, that is, one that
maximizes his hourly net income from the practice. This circumstance would
have two consequences of note. First, one could assume that the salary paid
aides reflects the social value of the contribution made by the marginal aide
to the physician's practice. Second, it would then be impossible to generate
further gains in physician productivity through health manpower substitution
without either (a) forcing the individual physician to suffer a financial loss; or
(b) lowering the salaries of aides through rightward shifts in the aide-supply
curve; or (c) inducing upward shifts in the demand for aides, either through
increases in physician fees or through increases in the productivity of the
physician's aides.

The conclusion emerging from Chapter Six is that American physicians typically do not find themselves in so constrained a financial position;
they seem to fall short of the optimum as defined above. In a way this finding
is paradoxical. The paradox lies in the fact that many areas in this country
are said to suffer from an acute shortage of primary-care physicians (the category of physicians on which our analysis has concentrated), that primary-care
physicians themselves commonly complain of excessive workloads, and that
there is in this country nothing ethically objectionable to increases in physician
incomes as long as the latter are brought about through enhanced productivity
gains rather than through price increases. Since lack of profitability does not
appear to have been an effective constraint on physicians' choices in this matter,
the explanation must be sought in more subtle factors. In keeping with the
analytic framework employed throughout this section, we focus our thoughts
on (1) the physician's perception of the marginal productivity of physician-
support personnel; and (2) the role physician fees play determining the demand
for physician-support personnel.

In exploring the determinants of the demand for physician-support
personnel it must be kept in mind that the position of that demand curve is
ultimately determined not by the true potential marginal productivity of such
personnel, but by the physician's perception of that potential. The perceived
productivity of aides may deviate substantially from reality. One cannot rule
out the possibility, for example, that many American physicians are simply
not aware of the economic potential of health manpower substitution. Information of this sort is routinely communicated to ordinary businessmen as

part of their training or through trade journals. It may not be sufficiently stressed in medical school curricula.

This constraint to task delegation in medical practice can obviously be overcome through dissemination of the requisite information. Probably the most fruitful way of accomplishing this would be to include training in teamwork in the clinical part of a medical education and, at the conceptual level, to expose prospective physicians to the basic economics of health-care delivery. A good many medical schools seem to be moving in this direction. An alternative is to disseminate the information through the professional literature. The fortnightly *Medical Economics*, for example, has for some years now been engaged in this educational effort (see, for example, "Step Up Your Productivity?" [1968] or Owens [1974]).

Appropriate changes in medical school curricula may help alert physicians to the potential of task delegation and teach them to use health manpower efficiently. In practice, however, the realized productivity of physician-support personnel might still fall short of its actual potential. Surveys of physician attitudes toward physician assistants, for example, have revealed a remarkable discrepancy between the range of tasks physicians feel *could* be delegated to physician assistants and the tasks they themselves actually *would* delegate to such personnel.[16] These surveys suggest that factors other than mere ignorance constrain the physicians' choice of a staffing pattern.

Constraints widely believed to inhibit more efficient use of health manpower are the various licensure laws governing the practice of medicine in this country. As Pauly has observed, the medical profession as a whole cannot view such laws as exogenously determined constraints, since physicians themselves determine the content and the very existence of such laws [Pauly, 1970, p. 115]. Individual physicians, on the other hand, may nevertheless feel severely constrained by them. First, they may disagree with the boundaries set in these laws. Second, they may interpret given laws with varying degrees of strictness, depending upon their own attitudes toward risk-taking. If their income is satisfactory even in the absence of task delegation, many physicians may prefer sacrificing additional income for the certainty of remaining within the law as they interpret it. Indeed, the more vague the laws and the more capricious their interpretation by the courts, the more likely will they deter physicians from pushing task delegation to the point that is actually permissible under these laws. Finally, it must be kept in mind that the various licensure laws now governing the conduct of health manpower have rarely been designed to keep up with the rapidly changing organizational and technical innovations that are potentially feasible in health-care delivery. Although, as noted, the medical profession as a whole must ultimately bear responsibility for the nature of these laws and their effect on resource allocation within the health-care sector, it is still possible that one generation of physicians feels effectively constrained by legal strictures conceived and formalized in prior decades.

Some students of licensure in the health field have advocated the abolition of these laws altogether. The reason given is that the advantages offered by such legislation—the protection of consumers—rarely match its social cost: that is, its deterrence to innovation in the delivery of health services and to efficient resource allocation in the health-care sector. Others have proposed sweeping changes in present licensing patterns, for example the licensing of entire health teams instead of the current rigid specification of the tasks individual members of a health team may or may not perform.[17] Changes of this sort are, of course, a prerogative of state legislatures. Federal health manpower policy can assist in this effort only indirectly, either by using fiscal levers in federal transactions with individual states or by providing individual states with technical assistance in the drafting of health manpower legislation. It may be noted in this connection that many states already have amended their medical practice acts to accommodate the newly emerging types of physician assistants and to permit more extensive task delegation even to traditional paramedical personnel. It can be hoped that ultimately such efforts will result in some upward shift in the demand for physician-support personnel, and an increase in the number of aides employed per physician.

Quite aside from the existence of legal constraints—whether real or imagined—many physicians may also fear patient resistance to more than the traditional degree of task delegation. There is some evidence that individuals in the very high and the very low income classes tend to shy away from group medical practice, presumably because it is viewed as "medicine for the poor." Similarly, it is to be expected that many patients would view more extensive task delegation in medical practice with suspicion, seeing it as an attempt to foist low-cost and hence low-quality care on the consumer. To the extent that physicians are sensitive to the consumers' sentiments in this regard, their demand for support personnel will thereby be depressed. Such a circumstance, for example, might explain why physicians frequently admit that they *could* use additional aides to advantage, but that they are actually not willing to hire them.[18]

It is not clear how effective public policymakers by themselves can be in altering patients' attitudes in this respect. Some progress in this direction can undoubtedly be made with a program of consumer education, perhaps at the high school or college level. But in this instance, once again, it is pertinent to ask whether patient resistance to organizational change in medical practice can truly be considered a constraint on physicians, or whether it is in fact a "constraint" of the physicians' own making. It is probably fair to suggest that the medical profession itself has contributed much to the mystique now surrounding the physician, and that mystique has undoubtedly contributed much to some of the misconceptions patients may have about the determinants of quality care. Studies have shown, for example, that patient acceptance of care from a physician assistant tends to be predicated on the personal endorsement of a family physician, but that such care *is* readily accepted once that endorsement is given.[19] Since the attitudes of patients mirror in so many ways those of their physicians, it is probably through the latter that any public policy in this area must seek to operate.

The preceding discussion has dealt with legal and social constraints that may introduce a gap between the perceived productivity of physician-support personnel—perceived, that is, by the pysician—and the true productivity potential of such personnel. Policies designed to reduce this gap are obviously a step in the right direction. In terms of Figure 7–4, they can be expected to shift the demand curve upward to the right. But there is also the possibility of raising the demand for physician-support personnel through changes in the level of physician fees. This possibility is almost always overlooked in discussions on task delegation.

One's natural inclination in this respect is probably to think here of increases in the level of physician fees. It is an inclination likely to be rooted in one's acquaintance with the theory or practice of conventional business firms. It may be thought that, other things being equal, an increase in physician fees will raise the so-called "marginal revenue product" of physician-support personnel and thus induce physicians to expand their support staff. Such a policy might work in the desired direction. A medical practice, however, differs in important respects from the textbook model of a profit-maximizing business firm. As a consequence, the most fruitful measure to induce upward shifts in the demand for physician-support personnel may turn out to be a decrease rather than an increase in the prices of physician services. This proposition may seem paradoxical and hence requires careful explanation.

Two factors in particular complicate the relationship between the price of physician services and the demand for physcain-support personnel: (a) the typical medical practice is an owner-operated enterprise; and (b) the practice setup *preferred* by the physician (including the extent of task delegation in the practice) may deviate substantially from what an objective efficiency expert would view as the most economically efficient practice setup. It can be hypothesized that the higher the physician's income is in the absence of economic efficiency, the less interested he will be in the profit potential of added task delegation.

Even if one abstracts entirely from the second of these factors, the theory of owner-operated enterprises suggests that the owner's work effort may either increase, remain unchanged, or decrease in response to a given change in the price of his output and hence in his hourly remuneration. In section II of this chapter we have already explored the implications of this theory for the number of hours worked by physicians. The theory also has implications for the economics of health manpower substitution in medical practice.

It is reasonable to suppose that at any level of aide input the marginal productivity of aides in medical practices rises or falls with increases or decreases in the number of hours the physician chooses to work himself. On this logic one would expect that, if an increase in the absolute level of the physician's fees leads him to work fewer hours per week and year, then such a price increase tends to shift his demand-for-aides curve downward to the left. It would be the natural consequence of a decline in labor productivity. The obverse would be the case if the physician chose to work longer hours in response to an increase in his fees. As noted in section II, the empirical evidence on this aspect of physician behavior is unfortunately inconclusive at this time. It is therefore not possible to predict with any degree of confidence how the typical American physician would actually respond to changes in the level of his fees. At this point it is sufficient to note that one's intuition in this matter may be a poor guide, for that intuition persuades one that a decrease in the price of physician services would unambiguously lead to a decrease in the number of hours worked by the physician, in the number of aides he employs, and in his rate of output. Economic theory suggests that the obverse may well obtain.

In assessing the probable effect of changes in physician fees on the extent of task delegation in medical practice, it is important to take account also of the second factor mentioned above, namely, the possibility that the typical medical practitioner in this country has an outright preference for a relatively simple practice setup, and deliberately forgoes the potential profits from more extensive task delegation for the sake of a more relaxed work setting. One way of incorporating this possibility formally into one's model of physician behavior is to assume that the physician associates certain "psychic costs" with the employment of support personnel. (In this connection, see also Chapters Five and Six, and Appendix B.) These psychic costs would reflect the physician's aversion to the administrative headaches of supervising a large auxiliary staff. Formally one envisages the physician as adding these nonmonetary psychic costs to the monetary costs (salaries) associated with the employment of aides. Other things being equal, the effect of these psychic costs is to shift the physician's demand for support personnel downward (or to the left). In Figure 7–4, for example, one might think of demand curve $D'D'$ as one obtaining in the absence of these psychic costs, and of curve DD as the demand emerging after these psychic costs have been taken into account.

If an outright aversion to task delegation were characteristic of the typical American physician, then the appropriate policy response would be to exert *downward* pressure on the absolute level of fees charged by physicians (if such a policy were administratively and politically feasible). It can be shown at the theoretical level that, other things being equal, the so-called psychic costs physicians are thought to associate with task delegation tend to decrease with decreases in income—that is, when the economic pressure on physicians mounts. The reason is straightforward. At relatively lower levels of income, the physician is likely to be more reluctant to sacrifice income for the sake of a congenial practice atmosphere; the latter is in a sense a "luxury commodity" of which less is "consumed" as income declines. If fees cannot be raised to augment income, the profit potential inherent in task delegation may become more alluring. In the vernacular, inefficiency in the conduct of his practice becomes a luxury the physician can no longer afford.

Health manpower policies designed to operate through economic pressure on medical practitioners may strike the reader as harsh, as they undoubtedly are. Such policies, however, would in effect be nothing more than an attempt to simulate precisely the kind of market pressure to which truly competitive enterprises are exposed as a matter of course, and which forces them to the high degree of efficiency commonly associated with competitive markets. The danger inherent in any attempt to constrain physician fees is that, in the absence of quality controls, the policy may backfire. As was acknowledged in Chapter Three, in the provision of physician care it is not always easy to distinguish genuine productivity gains from increases in, say, weekly patient visits purchased at the cost of lower quality. Suppose, for example, that a physician operating under a condition of excess demand for his services were constrained by an effective ceiling or downward pressure on his fees. His response to that constraint might be either to increase the efficiency with which his practice renders services of a given intrinsic quality (probably through more extensive task delegation), or simply to be less thorough and thus welch on the quality of his services. By diminution in the quality of care in this context is not meant simply a reduction in the amount of time the physician spends with his patients; such a reduction is implicit in the very notion of task delegation. The quality diminution referred to here is thought to be a quickening of the practice pace without benefit of additional support personnel. And even added task delegation can, of course, eventually be pushed beyond the medically safe.

Controls on physician fees under conditions of excess supply can also have undesirable consequences. It is conceivable that in such a market environment, downward pressure on physician fees would indeed induce physicians to employ more support personnel. That personnel, however, would be likely to be employed not to take over certain tasks from the physician, but instead produce added ancillary services that could be sold by the physician at a profit. Physicians could in this way partially or wholly offset the effect of fee controls on their hourly income. Even in the absence of additional auxiliary staff, physicians in this situation could, of course, restore their hourly income simply by increasing the service intensity of their treatments. In short, exertion of downward pressure on physician fees under conditions of excess supply is likely to trigger upward pressure on the per capita utilization of physician services, with potentially serious consequences.

The gist of the preceding remarks is that, even if control over physician fees were administratively feasible—as it might be under a regime of national health insurance—it should not be attempted unless that policy is accompanied by some form of quality control. Routine monitoring of statistical profiles on physician practices is one possible mechanism. Such monitoring now takes place under some of the provincial health insurance plans in Canada. The recently introduced Professional Standards Review Organizations (PSRO's) in the United States are intended to serve a similar function.

In concluding this section it is pertinent to comment briefly on one particular pricing scheme that unambiguously inhibits more extensive task delegation in medical practice. As noted earlier in this chapter, some observers find it objectionable on ethical grounds that physicians can charge patients or third-party payers their full regular fee for services partly or wholly performed by physician support personnel. The normative prescription implicit in this objection is that, if a physician's productivity is improved as a result of task delegation, then the economic benefits so generated should be passed on to consumers in the form of lower prices. Recent legislation on physician-support personnel had certainly envisaged that this would occur in practice. Indeed, under the Social Security Administration's current interpretation of Title XVIII, Part B, of the Medicare Act, a noninstitutional health-care provider cannot be reimbursed at all for services rendered solely by a physician extender in a physician's employ, unless these services are of a sort that have traditionally been performed by auxiliary staff incident to (and not in place of) services rendered by the physician himself. This is clearly an extreme variant of the pricing strategy under discussion here.

On the surface this pricing strategy may seem fair enough. It undoubtedly has political appeal among the constituents of budget-conscious legislators. Yet why would anyone wish to force efficient producers to lower their prices, all the while permitting inefficient producers to adhere to their customary (and higher) price schedules, as is apparently being proposed? In its application, this approach to the pricing of physician services leads to a two-tier price system under which identical medical services (for example, the suturing of a simple wound) fetch relatively high fees if the services are performed by a physician, and a relatively low fee if they are performed by a qualified physician assistant. In terms of Figure 7–4, and relative to a one-tier price system, such a policy would clearly induce a downward shift in the demand for physician-support personnel and thus impede the acceptance of such personnel among physicians. The pricing strategy therefore runs exactly counter to the government's effort elsewhere to encourage the employment of physician extenders by medical practitioners. Furthermore, since patients are accustomed to judging the quality of physician care partly by its price, such a pricing policy inevitably confirms the widely held suspicion among patients that task delegation reduces the quality of health services. Such a message is surely not intended by the proposed pricing scheme.

If one is really intent on reducing the cost of primary health care in this country, alternative approaches suggest themselves. One of these has already been alluded to earlier in this chapter. It is to constrain the fee schedules for medical services so as to preclude the existence of inefficiently organized medical practices. Concretely this means that the relative value scales for medical services would be patterned closely on the relative costs experienced in *efficiently* organized practices. Services judged to be safely delegatable to a physician assistant would be priced *as if* a physician assistant actually produced them in all cases. Physicians who actually had the service produced by an assistant would fare well under that pricing scheme.[i] On the other hand, physicians who failed to delegate tasks to the extent that is medically sound and economically efficient would obviously be penalized by the fee schedule. If such a physician produced a perfectly delegatable task himself, he would effectively price out his own time at the hourly rate of a physician assistant. The loss implicit in his behavior might soon become obvious to him. Quite obviously the strategy would fail if the absolute level of fees were so high that physicians could easily absorb the financial loss from inefficient task delegation. And, once again, the strategy would become administratively feasible only under a regime of national health insurance.[20]

If one is unwilling or if it is somehow not feasible to influence physicians through their fee schedules, one might consider another alternative, already discussed in Chapter One in connection with the maldistribution problem, namely, the establishment of independent paramedical practices offering patients with seemingly minor ailments access to relatively less expensive primary care. The merits and demerits of this approach have already been discussed in Chapter One. It may be added here that the strategy would make sense only in the absence of complete and comprehensive insurance coverage for primary health care. If patients do not share in the direct cost of the health care they receive—for example, through co-insurance—one would not expect them to shop around for cost-effective health services. Instead they would probably bypass paramedical practices even for minor complaints, resorting to them only to escape long queues occurring in full-fledged medical practices.

NOTES

1. Formal training programs for physician assistants appear to have emerged only in 1965, the best known among them being the Duke University Physician's Assistant Program (now Physician Associate) developed by Dr. Eugene Stead. In this connection, see Sadler et al. [1972], Chapter 2.
2. Ibid., p. 20.
3. In one of the training programs (Project Hope in Laredo, Texas) the requirement for entry is that the student be eighteen years of age. The training program itself covers four months. (Ibid., p. 21.)
4. Some authors, for example Pondy [1970] and Smith et al. [1972], have

[i]It would not be insurmountably difficult to develop a reasonably good approximation of such an ideal fee schedule. The empirical foundation for such an effort might be direct observation of medical practices, or task allocation patterns agreed upon by panels of experienced and imaginative medical practitioners in the various specialties.

attributed productivity gains up to about 75 percent to the employment of a physician assistant in medical practices.

5. Communicated to the author in private communication by the Division of Manpower Intelligence, Bureau of Health Resources Development, Department of Health, Education and Welfare.

6. This assumption reflects the distribution of physicians by activity in 1970. For details, see American Medical Association [1971], Table 10, p. 26.

7. See American Medical Association [1971], Table 1, p. 4; and American Medical Association [1973], Tables 22 and 28, pp. 56 and 62.

8. *United States Statistical Abstract, 1972*, Table 100, p. 69.

9. See, for example, Garbarino [1959].

10. Sloan [1973].

11. In this connection, see Altman [1971], Table 10, p. 29.

12. Ibid., Table 27, p. 80.

13. Ibid., Chapter 5.

14. In fairness to health-care providers, it must be mentioned that virtually all non-economists have difficulty with the concept of a shortage. The appearance of so-called shortages of meat, paper, disposable diapers and gasoline during 1973–74, for example, was not an indication that the country or the world was running out of these commodities, but simply a manifestation of the fact that prices were not permitted to equilibrate the relevant markets. An economist might be accused of hairsplitting, were it not for the fact that the popular misconception of the concept of a shortage frequently leads to highly questionable policies. The proposed rationing of gasoline in early 1974 was a case in point.

15. Todd [1972], p. 61.

16. Ibid.

17. For a perceptive analysis of the current status of licensure laws and the response of legislatures to newly emerging types of health manpower, see Boness [1973].

18. Todd et al. [1972], p. 1718.

19. Litman [1972], p. 346.

20. For a more extensive discussion of the policy potential of fee-for-service reimbursement under comprehensive national health insurance, see Reinhardt [1974].

Chapter Eight

Summary and Conclusions

Much diverse material has been covered in this book. Because of the often technical or controversial nature of the material it was occasionally necessary to stray somewhat from the main theme of the book. It will therefore be useful to pull together the various threads of the discussion into a more coherent and compact summary. This is done in section I. In section II we conclude the discussion with some comments on the relationship—real or imagined—between efficiency in the production of health services and the quality of health care.

I. SYNOPSIS

Our analysis began in Chapter One with an examination of the demand for and supply of medical manpower in the United States. Two schools of thought have emerged on this issue. One widely held view is that the nation currently faces a severe overall physician shortage, a shortage sufficiently serious to warrant continued expansion of the already substantial capacity of American medical schools. Evidence pointing to a physician shortage is seen in the lack of medical facilities in many localities and in the sustained influx of foreign-trained physicians into the United States. The fact that each year many more qualified Americans apply for admission to medical school than can be accepted is thought to make even more compelling the case for further expansion of medical school capacity. Continued or even enhanced federal support of medical education is expected to solve at once the perceived imbalances in both the market for physician services and the market for medical educations.

In contrast to this pessimistic view, a number of economists and some high public officials[1] are persuaded that concern over the *aggregate* supply of physicians in this country—as distinct from the geographic and specialty distribution of that supply—should by now have become a thing of

239

the past. Indeed, these observers feel that at the aggregate level this country may very well face the prospect of a physician surplus in the near future. This more sanguine view inevitably leads to the conclusion that the public sector should retreat somewhat from its heavy involvement in the financing of medical education. Alternatively, it is felt, if there must be federal support to medical education, then this support should be used (where possible) to influence the geographic and specialty distribution of medical school graduates rather than facilitating an expansion of medical school capacity beyond levels already contemplated under existing health manpower legislation.

The discussion in Chapter One favored the second view. It was shown, first of all, that the physician-population ratio in this country would increase for decades to come even if the capacity of American medical schools were constrained to its projected level for 1975, and even in the absence of any further immigration of foreign-trained physicians (see Figure 1–2). Thus, even if there currently were a shortage of physicians at the aggregate level—a conclusion not to be taken for granted, because the aggregate supply of physicians is a matter quite distinct from its geographic distribution—the phenomenon is likely to be a short-run problem calling for short-run solutions. A continued liberal policy toward the immigration of foreign-trained physicians strikes one as one such solution. An obvious alternative, though perhaps not as quick to provide relief, would be efforts to enhance the productivity of American physicians. Since that policy may turn out to be the most sensible response to the alleged physician shortage, the bulk of our analysis has been concerned with this second alternative.

The inherent danger of a policy to meet short-run shortages of manpower through a commensurate expansion of training facilities is that the policy is likely to engender the long-run problem of over-supply. In the social and natural sciences this lesson was brought home forcefully during the late 1960s, and its impact is felt to this day. That currently advocated additions to medical school capacity may well lead one to overshoot any reasonable long-run target of the physician supply was illustrated with the aid of Figure 2–2.

It is true that a surplus of professional manpower does not usually spell serious social problems other than the economic dislocation and the disappointment experienced by those who chose to invest their human capital in a potentially overcrowded field. It may be argued that disappointments of this sort are natural features of an economic system in which individuals are free to invest their time and wealth in any manner they see fit, and that it is not the government's role to protect individuals from the economic consequences of poor investment decisions. In the present context, this might be interpreted to mean that the government should always provide for a generous supply of medical school places, letting the applicants themselves bear the potential risk of under- or unemployment upon graduation. The trouble with this prescription is that the economic consequences of a physician surplus are not likely to befall the individual physician at all, or that they certainly will not be borne by physicians as much as by their patients and the general taxpayer.

It is well known that the market for physician services is one in which suppliers normally tend to have considerable influence over supply prices (fees), or, where prices are somehow constrained at given levels, over the demand for their services at given price levels. Under these circumstances the very existence of a physician surplus is likely to remain hidden from view until it becomes truly extreme. In the meantime, the surplus is apt to remain camouflaged by inefficiency in the production of better health (through the prescription and delivery of unnecessary services) and by inefficiency in the production of health services (through wasteful use of physician time). Either type of inefficiency will drive up the cost of normal health maintenance, and that cost is, of course, borne wholly by patients or by those who indirectly pay on their behalf.

As far as the delivery of unnecessary services is concerned, the preceding proposition is self-evident and requires no elaboration. With respect to the second type of inefficiency, however, it may be theorized that the physician himself must surely absorb any loss from waste in the use of his own time.[a] Unfortunately, the empirical evidence on this point is not reassuring. As was suggested by the data in Tables 2-5 and 2-6, and as has been argued by many observers of the health-care market, the cost of this type of inefficiency tends to be passed on to consumers as well. Fees in overdoctored areas are typically high enough to compensate physicians for the cost of internal inefficiency.

It is a natural tendency among professionals to view the resource-intensity of their services as an index of their quality. On this notion inefficiencies of the sort described above—and the cost increases to which they lead—are all too readily depicted as manifestations of "superior product quality." This is a tendency not only in the area of health services, but in almost all professional services, notably advanced-technology engineering and higher (including medical) education. The assumption implicit in such rationalization seems always to be that the extra quality so purchased is worth its price, an assertion the laity is ill-equipped to dispute. Where a proposition of this sort is proffered by those who stand to gain from its acceptance, however, some skepticism is clearly in order. Objectively viewed, many so-called "quality gains" achieved through higher resource intensity of the production process may in fact not be worth their sometimes substantial cost. In thinking about health manpower requirements, this possibility must constantly be kept in mind.

The apparent ability of price increases or of changes in the resource-intensity of medical treatments to compensate physicians for the cost of inefficiency (or of underemployment) not only tends to drive up the cost of health

[a]If the market for physician services were perfectly competitive, this would indeed be the case.

maintenance under conditions of excess supply, it also robs the income figure of its ability to signal conditions of oversupply to potential entrants into the profession. It must be expected that as long as physician incomes remain high, potential entrants will see no reason to shun the profession even in the face of rumors or concrete knowledge of oversupply.[b] The demand for medical educations will therefore be higher than it would be in the absence of this so-called "market failure." And if the demand for medical educations exceeds the available capacity of medical schools, concerned medical educators may argue in all sincerity—as some recently have—for increased public subsidization of the supply side to restore the market they face to a more "reasonable" balance. As was noted in Chapter Two, legislators find it difficult to reject such well-intentioned pleas.

Critics of the preceding arguments frequently raise the rhetorical questions: Precisely what is meant by an excess supply of physicians? How can one ever know that there are enough or even too many physicians? And given the lack of precision in the application of medical science to human illness, what in fact is an "unnecessary service"? These are fair questions, but they do cut both ways. The fact is that in an area as complex as the delivery of medical care, it is nearly impossible to offer an objective universally agreed upon standard of the "right" number of physicians for a given population. There are simply no easily ascertained, objective market criteria on which to develop such a standard.

In markets for most ordinary commodities, the appropriate number of suppliers is one just capable of meeting society's aggregate demand for these commodities at their prevailing, *market-determined* prices. American society is accustomed to viewing this objective criterion as a reasonable definition of "need." The propriety of applying this criterion to physician services is, however, widely questioned, for the consumption of these services has come to be viewed as a basic human right to be financed out of public funds when necessary. One need not be opposed to this philosophy to observe that its implementation can have some undesirable side effects. Where the consumption of a commodity is largely or wholly financed through the public sector and on a piece-rate (that is, fee-for-service) basis, the act of delivering the commodity inevitably becomes a key to the public treasury. In the health-care sector, suppliers can use that key all the more freely because consumers themselves are frequently unable to judge how much care is enough and how much is too much. Under these circumstances, determination of the "right" amount of consumption per capita and the "right" number of suppliers for a given population ultimately becomes a political judgment. In the case of physician care, for example, the "right" number of physicians per capita will turn out to be that number which

---

[b]The fact that general surgeons in this country continue to enjoy relatively high incomes in the face of reportedly widespread excess supply lends credibility to this hypothesis.

can be adequately supported out of the budget allocation consumers collectively see fit to set aside for physicians' sustenance. The number varies directly with the size of that allocation and inversely with the average income per physician the nonphysician sector is asked to transfer to physicians as a group.

In Chapter Two it was indicated that a ratio of between 250 to 300 physicians per 100,000 population would require an annual budget allocation of between $113 and $135 (in 1973 dollars) per capita (or between $400 and $500 per family of four) just to cover the physicians' customary *average net income*—that is, just to maintain physicians at their customary station in life. The true budget costs would, of course, be higher still, for in addition to the physicians' desired *net income*, their professional expenses (such as office space, equipment, and automobiles) must ultimately be borne by consumers as well.[c] One way to test whether 250 and 300 physicians per 100,000 population are too many or too few might be to ascertain consumers' attitudes toward this transfer of purchasing power. If that sum is lower than a generally acceptable maximum, then a case for expanding the physician supply is indicated. Given the potentially large "good Samaritan" component of physician-care, it can always be assumed that work will expand to accommodate the expanded supply of manpower. The current clamor over the high cost of physician care, however, suggests that a figure much lower than those mentioned above is deemed excessive.[d] This circumstance has clear implications for the number of physicians Americans truly wish to support—support, that is, at the incomes physicians customarily demand for their services and seem to be able to extract from society even under conditions of excess supply.

As became apparent in our review of health manpower forecasting during the past several decades (Chapter Two), those who point to a chronic shortage of medical manpower generally do not offer a robust definition of physician "requirements" either. It was observed, for example, that during the period under review there has been a gradual but steady escalation in what is considered a "minimum adequate physician-population ratio," a trend that continues unabated. The trend could be explained by parallel increases in the per capita demand for physician services, were it not for the fact that these increases have been more or less offset by concomitant gains in physician productivity (Chapter Three).

If one examines the methodology of past manpower forecasts more closely, it appears that most of the escalation in projected physician require-

[c]It is recognized that not all of a physician's professional expenses would be eliminated were he to withdraw from medical practice. Some of his aides, for example, might have to be transferred to lend greater support to the remaining pool of medical manpower.

[d]In 1970, the per capita expenditure on physician services was $65.28. This figure, however, excludes the income earned by professionally active physicians in hospitals and medical schools. On the other hand, it includes the professional expenses of office-based physicians. These expenses are typically equal to between 50 and 70 percent of net income (or 30 and 40 percent of gross income).

ments reflects a tendency to take the highest regional physician-population ratio prevailing at the time of the forecast as a national target for future years. This approach, however, virtually guarantees perennially perceived physician shortages at the aggregate level, for there is good reason to believe that geographic inequality in the physician-population ratio will persist regardless of the aggregate supply of physicians.

Use of the highest regional physician-population ratio as a national standard is presumably intended to assure all Americans the same level of health care enjoyed by residents in the most richly endowed region at the time of the forecast. Unfortunately, the approach also leads one to posit the organization of medical practice in that region as a national standard. If one compares richly and poorly endowed regions in terms of the rate of physician-visits per capita and of the number of visits per physician (Tables 2-5 and 2-6) one is led to the disturbing conclusion that consumers in the better endowed region may not benefit commensurately from their regions' higher physician endowment. Instead the data in Tables 2-5 and 2-6 support the previously offered hypothesis that much of the relatively more generous manpower endowment is absorbed by relatively greater inefficiency in the use of that manpower. Although comparisons such as that presented in Tables 2-5 and 2-6 of Chapter Two must be interpreted with caution, the fact that the rate of physician-patient contacts per capita does not seem to differ among poorly, moderately well, and richly endowed regions should give one pause. Indeed, the pattern observed in these tables raises the question of how one can speak at all meaningfully of a "physician shortage" without reference to the relative efficiency with which the existing pool of medical manpower is used.

If one incorporates the average productivity of physicians explicitly into one's forecast for future physician requirements (as is done in equation 2-5 and Figure 2-3 of Chapter Two) one discovers that future requirements are enormously sensitive to even small changes in assumed productivity growth. Precisely what is a "small change" in this context is of course a good question. Indeed, many observers of the health system suggest that it is a good question also how the term "physician productivity" can be defined in the first place. These questions were explored at some length in Chapter Three.

On the surface it might seem that the only sensible definition of physician productivity would be one based on the ultimate impact the physician has on his patients' health. In Chapter Three that proposition was rejected on two grounds. First, an outcome-based measure of physician output is rarely practical in empirical applications because so many factors other than a physician's intervention influence his patients' health status. Furthermore, it can be argued that an outcome-based measure of physician output is not really relevant from the viewpoint of health manpower policy. One's interest in that context centers solely on the role of physician productivity as a determinant of future physician requirements.

Given that focus, it is more appropriate to define physician productivity strictly in terms of the ability of physicians to meet society's demand for medical *services*, where the latter are viewed as intermediary products used by patients in the production of "better health." On this definition one would view as a productivity gain any development enabling a given pool of physicians to meet the demand for health services by an increased population or to accommodate increases in per capita demand for health care by a given population. On the other hand, any development enabling physicians to enhance the overall health status of their patients *without* thereby reducing their patients' demand for physician time does not qualify, on this definition, as a productivity gain. Such a development would of course be taken as a gain in the physician's ability to induce "better health," and it would therefore be welcomed; but since it does nothing to reduce the number of physicians deemed necessary for a given population, the development would not be particularly relevant from the more narrow perspective of health-manpower policy, a viewpoint maintained throughout this book.

As noted above, an examination of past trends in physician-productivity—with physician output measured either by expenditures on physician services or by rates of physician-patient visits—suggests that productivity gains during the past several decades have generally tended to keep pace with growth in the per capita demand for physician services (Chapter Three). Unfortunately it is difficult to pinpoint the sources of past productivity growth, so that it is equally difficult to ascertain exactly what the past in this respect portends for the future. Two opposing views have emerged on that question: one, according to which there is little hope for future gains in physician productivity; and the other, according to which physician productivity can probably be increased for decades to come. As potential sources of such gains, the optimists generally cite a shift toward prepayment for comprehensive care, the formation of group medical practices, the substitution of paramedical for medical manpower and the substitution of capital equipment for all types of health manpower. In Chapter Four, the relative merits of these proposed changes were examined in the light of available empirical evidence bearing on the issue, and on the basis simply of economic theory.

Economic theory suggests that, in comparison with the fee-for-service reimbursement of physicians, prepayment for comprehensive health care ought to induce physicians to exercise greater economy in the prescription of medical services (including those produced by themselves) and to produce those services actually being rendered as efficiently as possible. There is some evidence that where health-care delivery is financed through prepayment, the expected economies are in fact reaped and that they translate themselves into lower health-manpower requirements per capita. It must be added, however, that this evidence is almost invariably drawn from large prepaid group-practice plans operated in densely populated areas. These plans may not be representative of conditions likely to emerge under a nationwide system of prepayment.

Much of the evidence adduced in support of prepayment, incidentally, is commonly adduced also in support of group medical practice *per se*. As was argued in Chapter Four, however, a distinction must always be made between the purely economic effects of prepayment, on the one hand, and the technology of health-care production in a group practice setting, on the other. Empirical evidence that might demonstrate the economic superiority of group practice *per se* is very thin and inconclusive at best. Furthermore, there are persuasive theoretical arguments against the notion that group practice *per se* will ever be a source of economies in the use of health manpower in general, and of medical manpower in particular. In Chapter Four this proposition—perhaps startling to some—was developed at some length.

A similarly pessimistic conclusion was reached in Chapter Four concerning the potential effects of capital equipment on physician productivity. It was argued that the infusion of capital into medical practice typically enhances the physician's ability to improve his patients' health, but that it does not normally yield any economies in the number of physicians required to meet the demand for health services by a given population. That avenue, then, is one on which the formulators of the nation's health manpower policy ought not to place too much hope either.

The preceding considerations leave one with the conclusion that the substitution of paramedical for medical manpower is probably the most effective way of enhancing the average productivity of American physicians. It is this mechanism on which the formulators of the nation's health manpower policy should place primary emphasis. Even a casual glance at the evidence bearing on that proposition—such as the data in Tables 4-7 to 4-9 of Chapter Four— persuades one that the productivity gains to be had in this way are sizeable indeed. This conclusion is strengthened by the production-function estimates presented in Chapter Six.

The production-function estimates presented in Chapter Six indicate to what extent it seems *technically* feasible to increase physician productivity through health manpower substitution in medical practices. By their very nature such productivity gains come at a price—the support personnel to whom certain tasks now performed by physicians are to be delegated. In the very short run, during which the supply of physicians is absolutely fixed, a society plagued by a shortage of physician services may well be inclined to *maximize* the average productivity of physicians in this way, paying whatever price (in the form of support personnel) that maximum entails. In the longer run, however, the supply both of physicians and of their aides is variable. In that time context, a rational health manpower strategy would clearly not be simply to maximize average physician productivity, but instead to encourage use of that combination of health manpower which minimizes the total cost of delivering a given set of physician services. In Chapter Seven an attempt was made to identify such least-cost manpower combinations for alternative assumptions about the relative costs of physicians and of their support personnel.

As was noted in Chapter Seven, a variety of alternative cost concepts may be used in the search for least-cost manpower combinations. The estimates presented in the chapter are based on the so-called average direct transfer costs per M.D. office visit, a definition of costs that is identical to the average price consumers (or third party payers) have to pay per M.D. office visit. Using this definition of costs it was found that for empirically plausible physician target incomes and aide salaries, average direct transfer costs per office visit tend to reach a minimum at a staffing pattern of between 3.5 and 4.5 aides per physician (where the term aide is understood to include registered nurses, technicians, office aides, and other personnel traditionally used in physician's practices, but to exclude the newly emerging variants of "physician extenders"). Another way of putting this is that for given average prices per office visit, the physician's hourly net income is maximized at these estimated optima.

Using the production-function estimates presented in Chapter Six, it was estimated in Chapter Seven that, were American physicians to increase their support staff from the current average of about 1.75 aides per physician to the apparent optimum level of about 4, then average physician productivity (as measured by rates of patient visits or patient billings) could be expected to increase by between 30 and 50 percent over current levels, depending upon the medical specialty being considered. Given the high sensitivity of future physician requirements to even modest increases in physician productivity, this estimated productivity potential appears substantial indeed.

Toward the end of Chapter Seven we briefly explored the policy implications of our analysis. There are basically two extreme postures one could adopt in the formulation of a public health manpower policy. First, one could develop the policy as essentially a reaction to what is viewed as exogenously determined shortages (or surpluses) of particular types of health manpower. On this approach one would respond to a predicted shortage by subsidizing the construction of additional training facilties and/or the entrants into health manpower training programs. The policy response to a predicted surplus, on the other hand, might be either to do nothing or at most to eliminate whatever subsidies to health manpower training have been and are being granted. Errors in the pursuit of this policy are unlikely to be viewed symmetrically. The overriding goal will inevitably be not to err on the downward side—for example, not to permit reductions in the physician-population ratio—even if this means occasional errors on the upward side. The approach tacitly ratifies whatever particular use the health-care sector chooses to make of the available health manpower.

At the other extreme, health policymakers might develop their policies against the standard of some preconceived "ideal" health-delivery system and consciously seek to drive the health-care sector toward this ideal, if that sector cannot be expected to do so on its own volition. This might be attempted either through outright and pervasive direct regulation of individual components of the health-care sector—for example, the mandating of regional networks of health-care facilities or the prescription of optimal staffing patterns for hospitals, nursing homes, and medical practices—or more indirectly through the design of a set of financial incentives likely to elicit desired modes of conduct from the providers of health services (and, of course, from their patients as well). On this approach it might be possible to insist on efficiency in the use of whatever health manpower is available to the health-care sector.

Although public health manpower policy in this country does not fit either of these models perfectly, it seems traditionally to have tended more toward the first of these models, at least until very recently. This approach to health manpower policy is discernible also in current legislation encouraging the development of new types of allied health manpower. The assumption or hope underlying such efforts still seems to be that if only the public sector facilitates the production of such personnel, the private health-care delivery system will eagerly and properly use it. One peculiar feature of this development, however, is that the demand for it seems to have originated essentially from outside the medical profession itself; the impetus seems to have come primarily from educators and health policy planners.[2] In other words, public policy in this case seems once again to have focused primarily on the supply of health manpower without commensurate efforts to understand or to influence the demand for it.

The main thrust of our discussion in Chapter Seven—and implicitly throughout this book—has been to argue for a shift in health manpower policy away from the traditional focus on the *supply* of physicians or of allied health manpower and toward the determinants of the *demand* for physician-support personnel. A variety of policy measures in this area were discussed toward the end of Chapter Seven. They involve, on the one hand, certain legal and social constraints now deterring physicians from using physician-support personnel to the extent that is economically efficient and medically sound. Efforts to remove existing legal constraints to more extensive task delegation are, in fact, already underway in many states. Just as important, but so far neglected, is the need to educate consumers to the merits of task delegation so as to overcome consumer resistance to treatment by paramedical personnel.

One suspects, however, that future health manpower policy will also have to include the exertion of economic pressure on medical practitioners, literally forcing the latter to organize their practices efficiently. As was noted in Chapter Seven, such pressure would have to take the form of price controls, and it would have to be coupled with some form of external control over the service intensity and quality of medical treatments. The physician's current economic environment appears to be one in which incomes can be maintained by substituting price increases for resource efficiency. Such an environment is not likely to be conducive to efficiency in the production of health care, even in the absence of consumer resistance to task delegation and of legal constraints on medical practices.

In the final analysis, the problem faced by health policy planners is not only the question of whether or not the physician-support personnel to be trained in the future will actually be used by physicians. It also involves the question of *how* that personnel will be used. These questions lead one to consider the objectives pursued by policymakers in this area. At least two distinct goals suggest themselves.

First, the objective might be to upgrade the quality of physician services. This goal would imply that the medical treatments now being dispensed by the typical American physician are of unsatisfactory quality. Presumably the intended role of physician-support personnel would not be primarily to take over tasks traditionally performed by physicians, but instead to perform new tasks physicians have hitherto neglected in their treatment of patients. In other words, the objective would be to encourage delivery of an entirely new health-care product, one including a wider range of services per episode of illness and, of course, one involving higher treatment costs.

The alternative objective would be not to upgrade the quality of the treatments now being dispensed, but instead to make treatments of an unchanged quality available to greater numbers of Americans, and to reduce the cost of these treatments. This objective would be based on the implicit assumption that those patients who have traditionally had access to physician care have generally received treatments of quite satisfactory quality. Rather than adding new services to these treatments, physician-support personnel would be expected to relieve the physicians from certain delegatable tasks now routinely performed by physicians. Physicians in turn would be able to preserve their time for those patients whose conditions truly require a physician's superior skills. This was the concept of health manpower substitution discussed in Chapter Four and illustrated there with Figure 4-1. As was illustrated in Table 7-5, this type of health manpower substitution can indeed serve to reduce the cost of physician care, if physicians are willing to share the benefits from task delegation with their patients.

Both of these objectives have at one time or another been cited as reasons for training additional physician-support personnel. It can be doubted, however, that public policies in this area have been predominantly oriented toward the first of these goals. The medical profession, at any rate, would surely object to the suggestion that the overall quality of physician care in this country is wanting and that the main role of physician-support personnel will be to upgrade that quality. One suspects that most policymakers and the American public in general concur with the profession on this point. In other words, it is reasonable to assume that current legislation on paramedical manpower has been motivated primarily by a concern over the availability and cost of physician care—that it is ostensibly oriented toward the second objective stated above.

Whether or not this second objective will ultimately be served by current health manpower policies remains to be seen. Much will depend on how well policies concerning the supply of physician-support personnel are coordinated with policies on the aggregate supply of physicians in this country. We have touched on this point repeatedly in this book, albeit in passing.

Among the diverse goals pursued by the typical medical practitioner, two are likely to predominate. First, most practitioners probably have a sincere desire to render adequate health services to their immediate community. But, second, they generally do wish to earn a substantial income in the process. Given these goals, one suspects that in areas where the physician supply is taut, physician-support personnel will generally be used in the manner originally intended in health manpower legislation. The fact that, relative to the national average, physicians in underdoctored regions are observed to employ more aides per physician, to see more patients per year, and to accept lower fees for their services lends some support to this hypothesis. It is, of course, possible that the motivation underlying this behavior is a desire for more income, and that the prevailing low fees in these regions force physicians to enhance their hourly productivity through task delegation. A more generous interpretation, however, is that the employment of aides in this case is motivated largely by a desire to serve patients who would otherwise go untreated.

It is not clear that the ostensible objective of health manpower policy will be attained in areas with a relatively abundant physician supply. In such areas patients are presumably adequately served, doctors are not over-loaded, and the need for bona fide task delegation may not be obvious. Physicians may either not employ additional support personnel at all or, if they do so, use that personnel to increase the complexity of medical treatments. In so doing, physicians may believe that more complex treatments are of superior quality and worth the added cost. They may also wish simply to increase their hourly income from the sale of added services per medical case.

This brings us back to the topic with which we began this book and this chapter, namely, the crucial role of the aggregate physician supply in determining the organization of health-care production and hence the cost of that care. One feels safe in predicting that, if current attempts to increase sub-stantially the supply of physician-support personnel are coupled with equally substantial increases in the physician supply beyond currently projected levels, we shall ultimately observe not health manpower substitution in the originally intended sense, but instead greater service intensity of physician care and increases in the cost of regular health maintenance. Bluntly put, the physician-support personnel will then represent just so many more mouths to be fed through the health-care sector, rather than substitute mouths replacing others. As noted on earlier occasions, public policymakers encouraging this develop-ment must ask themselves whether this is the result they seek to achieve and, if so, whether the added service intensity of physician care yields quality gains that are worth their costs (to patients and taxpayers).

The prevailing doctrine among politicians, newspaper editors and some health experts is that a physician surplus is more easily dealt with than a deficit. On closer examination, that notion reveals a disturbing lack of apprecia-tion for the flexibility one has in organizing the health-care production process, a flexibility that blunts the consequences of tautness in the supply of particular types of health manpower, physicians included. The doctrine also reflects insensitivity to the subtle dangers inherent in any physician surplus. As has been suggested in this book. As has been suggested in this book, these dangers are not that easily dealt with once they become manifest.

II. EFFICIENCY AND THE QUALITY OF THE PHYSICIAN'S SERVICES

Throughout this book it has been tacitly assumed that the typical American physician can increase his hourly patient load without impairing the quality of his services. As noted in an earlier chapter, this assumption troubles a good many students of the health-care sector, for there is always the possibility that by raising his hourly patient load the physician *inevitably* trades off some quality for the sake of mere quantity. If so, then the physician's effective hourly output (adjusted for changes in the quality of his care) necessarily increases less than proportionately with his hourly rate of patient visits, and the production-function estimates presented in Chapter Six would in all likelihood overestimate the effect of auxiliary personnel on physician productivity.

      This is clearly a serious problem. In a sense it is fundamental to the entire debate over the potential for future gains in physician productivity. One would be remiss, therefore, in concluding this book without addressing the issue explicitly. Unfortunately, the very concept of quality care ultimately rests on a set of value judgments on which reasonable persons can disagree. There is therefore no hope of settling the matter in a few pages, or even in a book. The best an analyst can do in this area is to lay bare the premises and value judgments on which his conclusions rest, leaving it to the reader to agree, to be persuaded, or to disagree. The remainder of this chapter should be read in that spirit.

      It has to be admitted that if a physician increases his patient load without compensating changes in the organization of his medical practice—for example without employing additional support personnel or without sub-contracting additional services to outside facilities—then he is likely to trade off the quality of his services for mere quantity, at least after a point. Diagnostic tests that ought to be performed might be skipped, medical judgments might be made on inadequate information, and patients might leave the practice without sufficient counselling on the management of their health. It is not obvious, however, why there should be a decrease in the quality if the patient load is increased through delegation of medical and clerical tasks to qualified paramedi-cal and clerical personnel. In fact, the presumption ought to be that the employ-ment of the first paramedical assistant will enhance the quality of the physician's services, if for no other reason than that the presence of even a mere paramedic tends to act as a mild form of continuous peer review.[3] And it can probably be assumed that further increases in the physician's hourly patient load, *if achieved through acceptable forms of task delegation to additional aides,* will leave the quality of the individual medical treatment essentially unimpaired, so long as the physician takes, as he does, ultimate responsibility for the services rendered by his practice. In short, there is no reason to assume, as Seymour Harris appears to do in his *The Economics of American Medicine* [1964], that a reduction in physician time spent per patient visit *ipso facto* points to a deterioration of the product being delivered [p. 132]. Surely the manner in which that reduction is brought about must be considered before judging its impact on quality.

Whether or not one finds this line of argument acceptable ultimately depends on what one views as the essence of quality care in the first place. There is a school of thought according to which the physician's personal warmth and his interaction with patients on other than strictly medico-technical grounds are themselves crucial ingredients of quality care. In its final report on physician manpower, for example, the Bane Committee [1959] issued the warning:

> If the individual physician-patient relationship is to be the meaningful personal relationship which both the medical profession and the public believe it should be, it would seem that the individual physician should be able to spend more time, rather than less, with the individual patient. Such a goal can hardly be achieved if we are to have further increases in the average patient-load of the average doctor [p. 12].

This statement clearly suggests a strong positive correlation between the quality of a physician's services and the time he spends in face-to-face contact with each of his patients. *It is equally clear that, with physician output and its quality so defined, there is no hope of increasing the physician's annual output other than by increasing the number of hours he works per year.* The health manpower policies that have emerged from this concept of quality have been examined at length in Chapter Two.

In contrast to the above conception of quality care, one may adopt the premise that the physician's technical competence (that is, his ability to *diagnose* a patient's condition and to *prescribe* the appropriate treatment) are the truly essential ingredients of the care he dispenses. Hand in hand with this notion goes the view that the most relevant consideration, from society's point of view, is that those who perceive a need for medical intervention can first of all present themselves to a physician's practice for a diagnosis of their condition—that a *visit* between patient and the physician's practice takes place. On this view it matters less how many minutes the physician actually spends in face-to-face contact with each patient, and whether it is the physician or one of his aides who prepares the diagnostic material, applies the prescribed treatment, and counsels and comforts the patient, as long as the prescription itself is medically sound.

Those who espouse the latter view—the present author included—do not deny the relevancy of the human factor in medical practice. Rather, they acknowledge with candor that the formulators of the nation's health manpower policy must, in the first instance, be sensitive to a resource constraint that inevitably forces upon society a trade-off between two quite distinct dimensions of "quality health care," namely: (1) the perceived quality of the medical treatments administered to those to whom such care is actually available (hereafter referred to as "micro-quality"), and (2) the effectiveness of the health-care sector as a whole in reaching all members of society and in improving the nation's overall health status (hereafter referred to as "macro-quality"). The existence of this trade-off explains why it is so difficult to rank alternative health-care systems in terms of some overall quality index. For systems that operate under a resource constraint—for example, the *desideratum* that the nation's health-care sector ought not to absorb more than X percent of gross national product—any overall quality index is necessarily a weighted compound of the system's micro- and macro-quality, and these weights are purely subjective. The necessity of assigning such weights also explains why it is possible for different experts to travel in Great Britain or in the Soviet Union—countries that seem to emphasize macro-quality allegedly at the expense of micro-quality—and return with either glowing reports about the quality of these nations' health systems or decry the lack of quality of British or Soviet health services. Such statements merely reflect differences in the rate at which their authors are willing to trade off micro- for macro-quality. They are value judgments pure and simple.

It is probably not unfair to suggest that the medical profession in the United States has traditionally emphasized the first of the two quality indexes mentioned above—evidently at the expense of the second. This predilection with quality in the small has reflected itself quite naturally in the distribution of medical resources among different classes in society, and also in the legal statutes governing the conduct of medical practice and the activities of paramedical personnel. As was observed in the previous chapter, these legal strictures have in all likelihood functioned as important determinants of observed physician productivity.

Authors who propose that the average patient load of the typical American physician can, in fact, be increased even beyond current levels (for example, through delegation of tasks to auxiliary personnel) can make that argument on two distinct grounds. First, they may unabashedly place relatively greater emphasis on the macro-quality of the health-care system, even if that implied some reduction in micro-quality objectively defined. These authors, however, would probably not even concede that a reduction in physician-patient contact-minutes per episode of illness necessarily points to a reduction in micro-quality if the latter is evaluated by the medical soundness of the treatment dispensed. It is interesting to note, for example, that there is as yet no consensus even among medical practitioners on how best to measure the quality of individual medical treatments. The ideal would obviously be some index based on the end result from the treatment. But for reasons already mentioned, the measurement problems inherent in that approach are almost insurmountable. The practical alternative has therefore typically been to measure micro-quality either in terms of the quality of the inputs used in the production of physician services (for example, the physician's formal training), or to assess that quality by the nature of the treatment process (for example, by the comprehensiveness or soundness of the tests applied during diagnosis). Under the first of these approaches, however, quality-conscious providers, their auditors and their patients are likely to confuse mere resource intensity of treatment with quality or, more to the point, to take the input of physician time per patient visit as an index of the latter's "quality," irrespective of the organization of the physician's practice. The index of "medical soundness" advocated here is thought to be one based on the process approach.

It may, of course, be argued that in our society the socially relevant index of (micro-) quality is not one based on strictly objective medical criteria, but one that is rooted in the preferences and perceptions of the patient. "Presumably," it may be argued, "the individual cares (and is willing to pay for) not only the right to see a physician, but the manner in which he is treated, the time taken to explain the need for any given therapeutic action, etc., as well as the 'medical soundness' of the prescribed treatment." [4] This is an important objection, but it is vulnerable on several points.

First, it is never suggested by those who advocate greater efficiency in medical practice that patients be treated rudely, be denied psychological support, or be sent away without proper counselling. It *is* suggested that a brief physician-patient encounter need not be a rude one and that information concerning the management of the patient's health (including explanations accompanying therapeutic action) can often be furnished by persons other than the physician. And it is also suggested that not every patient contact with a physician's practice *must* involve face-to-face contact with a physician—a pattern that is still the norm in American medical practice.

This response may be criticized on the grounds that American patients are conditioned to heed only the advice of the physician and that they are simply not receptive to the type of manpower substitution proposed here. That objection, however, reflects the implicit assumption that consumer preferences and perceptions are an immutable state of nature and not a target for public policy as well. The fact is that the preferences of American consumers are highly malleable, so malleable in fact as to cause alarm among some social thinkers. One would therefore expect American consumers to be receptive also to careful instruction on what is and what is not a crucial element of medically sound and high-quality care, particularly if that instruction were to come from the medical profession itself. It should never be overlooked that the formulators of the nation's health manpower policy do have the option either of merely responding to consumers contemporary preferences and perceptions or of changing them through consumer education. Any serious effort in that direction on the part of either the medical profession, or of the public sector, or of the media has yet to be made.

A second major flaw in the argument cited above is the assumption that American consumers are actually "willing to pay for" highly personalized, highly time-intensive and hence highly expensive physician-patient contacts. That suggestion is startling. To be sure, some Americans are able and willing to pay for such care. But one common thread running through the entire public discussion on the American health-care crisis is that a great many Americans are either *unable* or *unwilling* to pay for even a minimally adequate amount of physician services, presumably because the personally borne cost of these services far exceeds the personal benefits expected therefrom.

The rebuttal to that response might be that, if some members of society are unable or unwilling to bear the cost of what is perceived as high-quality care, the proper policy response is not to lower quality until costs are sufficiently low, but instead to collectivize that cost through universal health insurance and to maintain high quality in the process. This author whole-heartedly endorses a policy of that sort, and he would even be willing to pay his fair share of its cost. Unfortunately, there is disturbing evidence also that Americans are unwilling collectively to finance that kind of medical care for the aged, for the indigent, or for themselves. Mounting concern on the part of legislators over the ever-rising cost of publicly funded health-care programs is a matter of public record. The easiest way to control the cost of these programs is, of course, to saddle the covered populations with co-payments of various sorts. Such a provision is in fact a prominent feature of the current Medicare program.

There is evidence that these co-payments, small as they are absolutely, have effectively barred the poorer of the aged from access to adequate physician care.[5] It is probably small comfort to those so excluded that, had they had access to physician services, these services would have been of high quality (as popularly conceived). Given the budget constraints under which the health system operates, how much more rational and, ultimately, how much more humane would it be to see public policy directed instead at ways to increase physician productivity, even if that lowers the average input of physician time per patient visit and the quality of physician care as popularly and currently perceived.

It is sometimes feared that a push for greater efficiency in health-care production will ultimately lead to a two-tier health system under which health care for the poor differs from that received by the rich. The scenario being envisaged is that patients whose health services are partly or wholly sub-sidized with public funds are more likely to be treated by paramedical personnel working in large health-care centers than those who are financially able to opt out of public programs and can afford highly physician-intensive care rendered in more traditional practice settings. Even if (as has been assumed throughout this book) the services rendered to the poor are of sound quality by any objec-tive medical criterion, it may be argued that "society as a whole may well be concerned with whether health care rendered to the poor differs markedly from the type of care rendered more fortunate members of society."[6] This also is an important objection, but it, too, is open to question.

First, while *some* social thinkers may be concerned over the emer-gence of a two-tier health system and would prefer one under which all citizens receive the same kind of care, it can be doubted that this sentiment is wide-spread in society as a whole or even among society's legislative representatives. The fact is that in this country as well as abroad society as a whole has not so far evinced a strong preference for a completely egalitarian distribution of medical services or, for that matter, of any other kind of professional services. There has been, and is likely to continue to be, a multi-tier system of health care, of legal services, of financial services, and even of pedagogic services. Admittedly, virtually every politician in this country has at one time or another endorsed the much-mouthed dictum that "every American should have access to health care of highest possible quality." But such statements deny the existence of the inescapable trade-off described earlier and can hence be dismissed as illogical at best and insincere at worst. Indeed, the degree of insincerity can be gauged by the fact that so many of these very same politicians have no compunction whatever in legislating rules that altogether eclipse some of the aged and some of the poor from adequate health-care.

Even if at some time in the future politicians believed their own rhetoric and legislated a national health scheme designed, in theory, to render health services of a *uniform*[e] perceived quality to all Americans, one would suspect that at least some members of the higher-income classes would be willing to pay extra premiums for services of a different perceived quality. These consumers might conceivably be restrained from purchasing such care by limiting the health-care provider system to one or a few types of provider facilities. But, first, it is not clear whether artificial constraints of this sort do themselves rest on an acceptable ethical foundation and, second, it may be doubted that such constraints would long remain effective. *Ultimately one's choice among alternative health systems is not one between a one-tier system and some multi-tier system, but instead among alternative multi-tier systems. The argument boils down to one's conception of an acceptable bottom tier.*

[e]This uniform level would clearly not be the highest possible level of micro-quality.

Rather than reinforcing among the poor the impression that any multi-tier system inevitably short-changes them, it would be more realistic— and of greater help to the poor—to permit the development of a pluralistic health-care delivery system under which those who can afford it can purchase health services that suit their various fancies, while those who cannot afford this luxury are nevertheless assured access to all necessary health care. Since such care would be publicly financed, it would surely not be unreasonable to insist that it be produced efficiently, subject, of course, to the satisfaction of some objective standard of acceptable quality. At the same time, every effort should be made to persuade consumers that efficiency in the production of health care need not come at the expense of quality (objectively defined), while maintenance of high quality (subjectively defined) has traditionally come at the expense of universal access to health care. This proposition may strike the reader as unduly temerarious or even wicked; it may appear less so when one considers realistic alternatives.

To sum up at this point: Proposals to enhance physician productivity through health manpower substitution rest on the idea of shortening the duration of physician-patient contact per patient visit (and per medical case) through task delegation, and devoting the physician-time so freed to the provision of additional patient visits. Critics of this idea deem it to be largely self-defeating. Reductions in physician-time per patient-visit, it is argued, *ipso facto* spell a reduction in the quality of physician care and hence in the true physician output per patient visit. On this premise, production analyses based on patient visits as an output measure are inherently suspect and not really helpful in the formulation of health-manpower policy.

In the preceding discussion we have raised essentially two objections to this line of reasoning. First, we have argued that even if a reduction in the physician-intensity of medical treatment inevitably entailed some reduction in the quality of the treatment, one may nevertheless ask the question: At what price quality? This question is always worth asking in health care, in education, in the aerospace sector, or in any other area of economic activity heavily subsidized out of the public purse.

Our second objection to the "quality" argument was that the very conception of quality underlying the argument rests on value judgments with which one can disagree. It is a notion of quality that has traditionally led to an undue emphasis on the quality of care rendered to those who actually have had access to physicians, and it has generated amazing tolerance for the persistence of wide gaps in coverage. Furthermore, it is a kind of quality for which an increasing number of Americans are either unwilling or unable to pay, individually or collectively, and social thinkers had better think twice before mandating it through public policy. Given the current clamor over the ever-rising cost of health maintenance in this country, a more realistic conception of quality would be one based on the objectively determined medical soundness of a physician's services rather than on the time he personally devotes to their production. It is a conception of quality on which this book implicitly rests.

NOTES

1. In an address to the Association of American Medical Colleges, for example, Dr. Charles C. Edwards, Assistant Secretary for Health, Department of Health, Education and Welfare, recently suggested: "I think that clearly we have moved beyond the point at which concerns about a doctor shortage were genuine, if somewhat exaggerated. Even more significant is the possibility [that] we may well be facing a doctor surplus in this country." Quoted in *The New York Times,* January 13, 1974, p. 58). The Secretary's position is not necessarily inconsistent with the National Institutes of Health's estimation that the country currently is about 30,000 physicians short of what is deemed an adequate supply. The secretary's estimate is obviously future-oriented. As was shown in Figure 1–2 of Chapter One, in the near future a surplus may develop even if there were something of a physician shortage at the moment.
2. Todd [1972], p. 61.
3. Alan Gregg [1956], p. 60, quoted in Somers and Somers [1961], p. 115.
4. Communication from an anonymous referee concerning earlier work by the author.
5. See U.S. Department of Health, Education and Welfare, Social Security Administration [1973], especially p. 5.
6. Communication from an anonymous referee concerning earlier work by the author.

Appendix A

A Model for Forecasting the Future Supply of Physicians and Derivation of Age-Specific Mortality Rates for Physicians

The supply of active physicians at some future time t can be written as the sum

$$M_t = \sum_{j=1}^{n} (a_{tj} S_{tj}) \tag{A-1}$$

where S_{tj} is the number of physicians who had graduated j years prior to t and are alive at time t; a_{tj} is the percentage of those physicians who are professionally active at time t; n denotes the maximum number of years after graduation any physician survives; and t denotes time measured in calendar years with the base-year in the forecast set equal to $t = 0$. Variable S_{tj} can be further defined as

$$S_{tj} = \begin{cases} \prod_{r=1}^{j} (b_r) \cdot G_{t-j} & \text{for } j < t, j \leqslant n \\[2em] \prod_{r=(j-t+1)}^{j} (b_r) \cdot S_{t-j}^o & \text{for } t \leqslant j \leqslant n. \end{cases} \tag{A-2}$$

In that expression, G_{t-j} (for $j < t, j \leqslant n$) denotes the number of physicians who will graduate in calendar year $(t-j)$; S_{t-j}^o (for $t \leqslant j \leqslant n$) denotes the number of physicians who had graduated in calendar year $(t-j)$ and who were reported to be alive at time $t = 0$, the base-year in which the forecast is made; and b_r denotes the proportion of physicians who were alive $(r-1)$ years after graduating and who survive the rth year. (Further on, b_r is defined as the proportion of physicians who were alive on their $(r+26)$th birthday and who survived to their $(r+27)$th birthday.)

259

In the absence of more precise information, it is best to assume that the parameters a_{tj} and b_r remain constant over the forecast horizon. Since the values of S_{t-j}^o are predetermined at the time the forecast is made, the future supply of active physicians becomes solely a function of one's assumptions about the time path of future graduations, G_t, $t > 0$.

The supply projections in Figures 1-2 and 2-2 are based on equations (A-1) and (A-2). The base year chosen for these projections is 1970. Values of S_{t-j}^o were obtained by applying the age distribution of active and inactive medical doctors (M.D.'s) in 1970 to the total of 348,000 active and inactive M.D.'s and osteopaths (D.O.'s) reported to be alive on December 31, 1970. These base-year values of S_{t-j}^o include foreign-trained physicians already practicing in the United States by the end of 1970. Table A-1 presents the 1970 age distribution of physicians in the United States and the total number of M.D.'s and D.O.'s in each age interval. Estimates for parameters a_{tj} are presented in Table A-2.

Throughout this analysis it is assumed that all physicians were exactly 26.5 years old at the time of their graduation from medical school and that they were 27 years old on December 31 of their graduating year. This assumption is consistent with the observation that the median age at graduation from American medical schools has been between 26 and 27 years for most of this century [Blumberg, 1971, pp. 60-61]. If in Table A-2 one denotes December 31, 1967 as $t = 0$, then the activity coefficients in that table can be linked to chronological age and applied to column (2) of Table A-1 to yield column (4) in that table—the number of M.D.'s and D.O.'s assumed to be professionally active in the base year. In using column (4) as estimates of S_{t-j}^o it is assumed that physicians are uniformly distributed within each age interval and that the

Table A-1. Age Distribution and Activity Status of Physicians (M.D.'s and D.O.'s) on December 31, 1970

Age of Physician (1)	Number of Physicians Active and Inactive (2)	Percent of Total (3)	Number of Active Physicians (4)
Under 30	40,200	11.5%	40,012
30–34	48,024	13.8	47,735
35–39	45,936	13.2	45,771
40–44	42,804	12.3	42,427
45–49	42,804	12.3	42,342
50–54	32,015	9.2	31,515
55–59	28,885	8.3	27,978
60–64	24,710	7.1	22,807
65–69	17,050	4.9	14,363
70–74	8,700	2.5	6,422
75 and over	17,050	4.9	9,849
Total	348,178	100.0%	321,372

Sources: Total number of active and inactive physicians—*United States Statistical Abstract 1972*, Table 70. Column (3)—American Medical Association [1971], Table 5, p. 15.

Table A-2. Distribution of Physicians by Year of Graduation and Activity Status, United States, December 31, 1967

Year of Graduation (1)	Assumed Age Interval as of Dec. 31, 1967 (2)	Number of M.D.'s Alive (3)	Number of M.D.'s Inactive (4)	Proportion Active (5)
Prior to 1915	80 or older	7,610	3,882	0.490
1915–19	79–75	5,782	1,956	0.662
1920–24	74–70	9,573	2,018	0.789
1925–29	69–65	14,916	1,820	0.878
1930–34	64–60	20,904	976	0.953
1935–39	59–55	26,869	560	0.979
1940–44	54–50	32,593	390	0.988
1945–49	49–45	31,013	301	0.990
1950–54	44–40	37,717	319	0.992
1955–59	39–35	43,642	275	0.994
1960–64	34–30	50,113	295	0.994
1965–67	29–27	26,238	106	0.996

Sources: Columns 1, 3 and 4—American Medical Association [1968b], Table 19, p. 158.

"activity coefficient" for a given age interval applies to each age-cohort within that interval.

Since the time path of future graduations, G_t, will be assumed explicitly in preparing any forecast from equations (A-1) and (A-2), the only set of parameters that remains to be estimated are the survival rates, b_r. Although subscript r for these parameters refers to years after graduation, the assumption that all physicians are 27 years old in December of their graduating year (and the further assumption that all physicians graduated in a given year stay alive at least to the end of that year) translates parameters $(1 - b_r)$ into age-specific one-year mortality rates. Thus, $(1 - b_3)$ would be the proportion of physicians who were alive on their 29th birthday but died during the following year, and $(1 - b_r)$ is the proportion who were alive on their $(r + 26)$th birthday and did not survive to their $(r + 27)$th birthday.

The majority of physicians in this country are white males. It may therefore be reasonable to approximate $(1 - b_r)$ by the age-specific mortality rates for white males in this country. These rates are published regularly in the *Statistical Abstract of the United States*. There is reason to believe, however, that the mortality rates for white males in general exceed those for physicians alone, especially if one thinks three to four decades ahead.

First, age-specific mortality rates tend to be a function of socio-economic status. A study of 1960 data by Evelyn Kitagawa [1972] has shown that males with 4 years of college education experienced a cumulative death rate between the ages from 25 to 64 about 70 percent below that for all white males in that age interval. Blumberg also has argued that physicians as a group tend to be healthier than white males in general and hence should exhibit correspondingly lower mortality rates [1971, p. 61].

Second, statistics on the entering classes in American medical schools indicate that the percentage of female students has been increasing in recent years. During most of the postwar years women graduates have amounted to between 5 and 7 percent of all medical graduates [Blumberg, 1971, p. 60]. About 17 percent of the entering class of 1972-73, however, were women ["Medical Education in the United States 1972-73" in the *Journal of the American Medical Association*, November 19, 1972]. It is one of nature's cruelties that age-specific mortality rates for males tend to be almost twice as high as those for women in the age span under consideration here. If the percentage of women graduates should increase substantially during the next several decades, age specific mortality rates for American physicians would have to be adjusted accordingly.

In the supply projections in Figures 1-2 and 2-2, no adjustment has been made for any probable change in the future sex mix of medical graduates. This is clearly conservative. However, the projections are based on one-year age-specific mortality (or survival) rates estimated specifically from data for *physicians* alive during the 1960s. The remainder of this Appendix presents the derivation of these rates, a subject matter probably of some interest in its own right.

Table A-3 presents four-year survival rates estimated from data published originally by the American Medical Association [1968b, tables 9-27), and presented also in Blumberg [1971, p. 66]. Consider now the cohort of physicians who graduated in 1959, and was reported to be alive on December 31, 1963. Assume further that 99.7 percent of this cohort survived the four-year interval to December 31, 1967. On the assumption that every physician in this cohort was 27 years old in December 1959 and hence 31 years old in December 1963, the number of these physicians still alive in 1967 ($N_{67}^{(59)}$) can be written as

$$N_{67}^{(59)} = N_{63}^{(59)} \left(b_{32} b_{33} b_{34} b_{35} \right) \tag{A-3}$$

where $N_{63}^{(59)}$ denotes the number of 1959 graduates who were alive in December 1963 and, in general, b_y denotes the proportion of physicians who lived to age $(y - 1)$ and survived the following year. Equation (A-3) can, of course, be restated as

$$0.997 = \frac{N_{67}^{(59)}}{N_{63}^{(59)}} = \left(b_{32} b_{33} b_{34} b_{35} \right) \tag{A-4}$$

If one is willing to assume that the four age-specific, one-year survival rates in equation (A-4) are identical, then the value of each is given by $[N_{67}^{(59)} / N_{63}^{(59)}]^{\frac{1}{4}}$. Alternatively, one might assume that these four rates stand in the same relationship to one another as do the age-specific mortality rates for white males in general. Denoting the latter by the general symbol m, one would then express equation (A-4) as

$$0.997 = \frac{N_{67}^{(59)}}{N_{63}^{(59)}} = b^4 \left(\frac{m_{33} m_{34} m_{35}}{m_{32}^3} \right), \tag{A-5}$$

from which one would obtain the value of the common element $b = b_{32}$ as $[N_{67}^{(59)} m_{32}^3 / N_{63}^{(59)} m_{33} m_{34} m_{35}]^{1/4}$, and the value of, say, b_{34} as bm_{34}/m_{32}. In this way, one can infer from Table A-3 estimates of the one-year, age-specific survival rates for physicians in the age span from 32 to 35 years. In empirical analyses, the refinement suggested with equation (A-5) is easy to make, but consequential only at high ages.

Consider now the cohort of physicians who graduated in 1958 and whose survivors were 32 years old in December of 1963. Lacking more precise information, one may assume that this cohort also was characterized by a four-year survival rate of 0.997 during 1963–67, so that one can posit the relationship

$$0.997 = \frac{N_{67}^{(58)}}{N_{63}^{(58)}} (b_{33} b_{34} b_{35} b_{36}), \tag{A-6}$$

from which the implicit age-specific survival rates can be obtained just as before. (They will, of course, be equal to the previous set unless the adjustment in equation (A-5) is made.) It is clear, then, that except for the first few years, one generally obtains four estimates of each age-specific, one-year survival rate, and

Table A-3. Number of U.S.-Trained Physicians Surviving the Period from December 31, 1963 to December 31, 1967

Year of Graduation (1)	Assumed Age on Dec. 31, 1963 (2)	Number Alive on Dec. 31, 1963 (3)	Number Alive on Dec. 31, 1967 (4)	Proportion Surviving the Four-Year Period (5)
Prior to 1915	76 or more	11,751	7,087	0.603
1915–19	75–71	6,805	5,262	0.773
1920–24	70–66	9,256	7,888	0.852
1925–29	65–61	14,865	13,291	0.894
1930–34	60–56	20,341	18,895	0.929
1935–39	55–51	23,697	22,668	0.957
1940–44	50–46	30,200	29,444	0.975
1945–49	45–41	27,133	26,776	0.987
1950–54	40–36	30,359	30,054	0.990
1955–59	35–31	33,605	33,509	0.997

Source: Columns 1, 3 and 4—American Medical Association [1968b], Table 27, p. 188.

these estimates need not be the same, as is more readily evident from Table A-4. Row index i in Table A-4 is equal to 64 minus the year during which the corresponding cohort of physicians graduated, and variable X_i is the corresponding four-year survival rate $(N_{67}^{(64 - i)} / N_{63}^{(64 - i)})$. Finally, for the sake of expositional convenience the one-year age-specific survival rates with double subscripts are defined so that b_{ir} denotes the proportion of physicians who were alive on their $(r + 26)$th birthday and survived the following year, *with b_{ir} being estimated from the ith cohort* (that is, physicians who graduated in calendar year $(1964 - i)$).

The age-specific survival rates, b_r, used in the forecasting model (A-1) and (A-2) have been calculated from Table A-3 in the manner set forth above and in Table A-4. Specifically, b_r is the average

$$b_r = \sum_{i=1}^{49} (b_{ir})/n_r \tag{A-7}$$

where n_r is the number of positive elements in column r of Table A-4 (usually equal to 4). In making these estimates, it has been assumed that physicians who graduated in 1960–63 were characterized by the same four-year survival rate as were those who graduated in 1959, a somewhat conservative assumption. The age-specific mortality rates $(1 - b_r)$ emerging from this exercise are shown in Table A-5, as are the cumulative survival rates for medical graduates, defined as

$$C_r = \prod_{s=1}^{r} (b_s) \tag{A-8}$$

In this expression, C_r denotes the proportion of physicians still alive r years after graduation (or on their $(r + 27)$th birthday). By way of contrast, Table A-4 also presents one-year age-specific mortality rates and cumulative survival rates for U.S. white males in general.

As is seen from Table A-5, the estimated age specific mortality rates for physicians are indeed lower than those for white males in general throughout the interval from 27 to 75 years of age. The estimated differences in the cumulative survival rate by age 64, however, is nevertheless much smaller than that estimated by Kitagawa in a comparison of mortality rates of college-educated males with those of all white males. A number of explanations for this apparent inconsistency are possible. First, it may well be the case that age-specific mortality rates for physicians are indeed higher than those for college-educated males in general. Such a phenomenon could be explained by the relatively greater stress under which many physicians work. An alternative explanation, however, may lie in the nature of the data files on which the raw statistics in Table A-3 are based.

Table A–4. Schema for the Estimation of One-Year, Age-Specific Survival Rates (b_r) for U.S. Physicians

Characteristics of ith Cohort — Yr. of Grad.	Age in Dec. '63	Four-Year Survival Rate '63 to '67	Row i	Percentage of ith cohort alive at age (27 + r − 1) and also at age (27 + r) — b_{ir} — Col. r = 1	2	3	4	5	6	7	8	9	...	48	49
1963	27	X_1	1	b_{11}	b_{12}	b_{13}	b_{14}						...		
1962	28	X_2	2		b_{22}	b_{23}	b_{24}	b_{25}					...		
1961	29	X_3	3			b_{33}	b_{34}	b_{35}	b_{36}				...		
1960	30	X_4	4				b_{44}	b_{45}	b_{46}	b_{47}			...		
1959	31	X_5	5					b_{55}	b_{56}	b_{57}	b_{58}		...		
1958	32	X_6	6						b_{66}	b_{67}	b_{68}	b_{69}	...		
.	.	.	.							.	.	.			
1918	72	X_{46}	46										...	$b_{46,48}$	$b_{46,49}$
1917	73	X_{47}	47										...	$b_{47,48}$	$b_{47,49}$
1916	74	X_{48}	48										...	$b_{48,48}$	$b_{48,49}$
1915	75	X_{49}	49										...		$b_{49,49}$
Estimated One-Year Survival Rates		b_r		b_1	b_2	b_3	b_4	b_5	b_6	b_7	b_8	b_9	...	b_{48}	b_{49}
Age to which physicians Survive			27 + r	28	29	30	31	32	33	34	35	36	...	75	76

Table A-5.   Estimated One-Year Age-Specific Mortality Rates and Cumulative Survival Rates for White Males and for U.S. Physicians

| | | Deaths per 1,000[a] | | Proportion of Those Alive at Age 27 Surviving to Age $(r + 27)$ | |
| | | Physicians $(1 - b_r)10^3$ | White Males $(1 - m_r)10^3$ | Physicians C_r^P | White Males C_r^{WM} |
r	Age				
1	28	0.82	1.76	0.99918	0.99824
2	29	0.75	1.69	0.99843	0.99655
3	30	0.72	1.66	0.99771	0.99490
4	31	0.72	1.67	0.99699	0.99324
5	32	0.73	1.70	0.99627	0.99155
6	33	0.72	1.74	0.99555	0.98982
7	34	0.71	1.81	0.99484	0.98803
8	35	0.71	1.91	0.99413	0.98614
9	36	0.72	2.05	0.99342	0.98412
10	37	1.15	2.21	0.99227	0.98195
11	38	1.59	2.40	0.99069	0.97959
12	39	2.03	2.62	0.98868	0.97702
13	40	2.47	2.87	0.98624	0.97422
14	41	2.46	3.15	0.98381	0.97115
15	42	2.66	3.47	0.98120	0.96778
16	43	2.84	3.82	0.97841	0.96409
17	44	3.03	4.21	0.97544	0.96003
18	45	3.22	4.63	0.97230	0.95558
19	46	3.20	5.08	0.96918	0.95073
20	47	3.96	5.59	0.96534	0.94541
21	48	4.71	6.14	0.96079	0.93961
22	49	5.46	6.76	0.95555	0.93326
23	50	6.22	7.45	0.94960	0.92630
24	51	6.22	8.21	0.94369	0.91870
25	52	7.37	9.04	0.93674	0.91039
26	53	8.50	9.93	0.92878	0.90135
27	54	9.64	10.93	0.91983	0.89150
28	55	10.80	12.04	0.90989	0.88077
29	56	10.81	13.26	0.90005	0.86909
30	57	12.62	14.55	0.88869	0.85644
31	58	14.42	15.94	0.87588	0.84279
32	59	16.21	17.47	0.86168	0.82807
33	60	18.04	19.18	0.84613	0.81219
34	61	18.06	21.04	0.83085	0.79510
35	62	20.47	23.06	0.81385	0.77676
36	63	22.88	25.18	0.79522	0.75720
37	64	25.27	27.33	0.77513	0.73651
38	65	27.58	29.46	0.75375	0.71481
39	66	27.51	31.61	0.73301	0.69222
40	67	30.25	33.80	0.71084	0.66882
41	68	32.94	36.19	0.68743	0.64461
42	69	35.96	39.00	0.66271	0.61947
43	70	39.71	42.41	0.63639	0.59320
44	71	41.55	46.36	0.60995	0.56570
45	72	45.98	46.36	0.58190	0.53948
46	73	51.04	46.36	0.55220	0.51447

Table A-5 continued

| | | Deaths per 1,000[a] | | Proportion of Those Alive at Age 27 Surviving to Age $(r + 27)$ | |
| | | Physicians | White Males | Physicians | White Males |
r	Age	$(1 - b_r)10^3$	$(1 - m_r)10^3$	C_r^P	C_r^{WM}
47	74	56.57	46.36	0.52096	0.49062
48	75	62.34	46.36	0.48848	0.46787

[a]Proportion of physicians who are alive on their $(r + 26)$th birthday but not on their $(r + 27)$th.

It is conceivable for example, that some physician names not in the American Medical Association files in December of 1967 were nevertheless alive.

Finally, it may be noted that the time path of the future physicians supply (variable M_t in equation (A-1)) is not as sensitive to assumptions about age-specific mortality rates as might be supposed *a priori*. This assertion is established in Table A-6, which presents projected physician-population ratios for the year 2000 using the baseline projection of graduations used in Figure 2-2 (Table A-8 below), and using age-specific mortality rates for all white males with each rate being scaled up or down by some proportionality factor. Table A-6 suggests that one ought not be unduly worried about moderate errors in the estimation of age-specific mortality rates for physicians.

Table A-6. Sensitivity of Physician-Supply Projections to Assumed Mortality Rates for Physicians

Assumed Change in Age-Specific Mortality Rates[a]	Implied Proportion of 27-Year-Olds Surviving to Age 65	Implied Physician-Population Ratio in Year 2000[b]	Percentage Deviation of Implied Physician-Population Ratio from that for Actual White Male Mortality Rates[c]
-30%	0.915	2.063	+2.6%
-20	0.893	2.045	+1.7
-10	0.881	2.027	+0.9
0	0.869	2.010	0
+10	0.857	1.993	-0.9
+20	0.845	1.977	-1.6
+30	0.833	1.961	-2.4

[a]For example, if the percentage change is -20 percent, each age-specific mortality rate $(1 - m_r)$ was multiplied by 0.8, for $r = 1, 2, 3, \ldots, 44$.
[b]Based on the baseline series of graduations assumed in Figure 2-2 (Table A-8).
[c]Defined as the implied ratio divided by the ratio corresponding to the unchanged white-male mortality rate, minus 1.

Table A-7. Projected Supply of U.S.-Trained Physicians if Annual Graduations Were Constrained to 15,000 (corresponds to Figure 1-2)

Year	Projected Population[a] (millions)	Graduations This Year	Supply of Physicians[b]		Active Physicians per 100,000 Population
			Alive	Active	
1975	212.2	12,353	350,524	341,287	161
1980	221.9	14,822	389,079	378,968	171
1985	233.3	15,000	428,470	417,348	179
1990	244.6	15,000	465,351	452,876	185
1995	254.3	15,000	495,766	482,653	190
2000	262.8	15,000	524,357	510,556	194
2005	270.1	15,000	550,306	535,732	198
2010	277.5	15,000	573,226	557,630	201

[a]Taken from U.S. Department of Commerce, Bureau of the Census (1972), Series E, Table 1, p. 12. After the year 2000, an annual net increase of 0.55 percent has been assumed.
[b]Excludes foreign-trained physicians entering the United States after 1970 and all physicians over 70 years old.

Table A–8. Projected Supply of U.S.-Trained Physicians under the Gerber Proposal (corresponds to Figure 2–2)

Year	Number of Graduations This Year		Number of Active U.S.-Trained Physicians per 100,000 Population[a]	
	Baseline[b]	Gerber	Baseline	Gerber
1975	12,353	12,353	161	161
1980	14,822	16,332	171	172
1985	15,805	21,555	180	189
1990	16,855	25,600	189	215
1995	16,855	25,600	197	239
2000	16,855	25,600	205	261
2005	16,855	25,600	212	282
2010	16,855	25,600	216	300
2015	16,855	25,600	220	315
2020	16,855	25,600	221	324

[a]For notes, see Table A–6.

[b]The baseline forecast of graduations is a preliminary estimate prepared by the Division of Manpower Intelligence, Health Resources Administration, Department of Health, Education and Welfare, and were conveyed to the author in private communication upon the author's request. These estimates seem to be the most reliable ones available at this time.

Although Table A–2 suggests that many physicians remain professionally active during their seventies, the projections in Figures 1–2 and 2–2 are based on the more conservative assumption that no physician works after his seventieth birthday. Furthermore, the series of graduations, G_t, excludes any foreign medical graduates entering the United States after 1970.

The population forecast used in calculating the physician-population ratio is the most recent projection published by the U.S. Department of Commerce, Bureau of the Census [1972b, Series E, Table 1, p. 12].

Figures 1–2 and 2–2 reflect forecasts on a year-by-year basis. Excerpts from these forecasts at five-year intervals are shown in Tables A–7 and A–8.

Appendix B

Input-Output and Pricing Decisions in Medical Practice: An Exploration of Alternative Theories

In Chapter One a distinction was made between two alternative theories concerning the determination of physician fees: one under which physicians are depicted as pure "price-takers," and a second according to which physicians enjoy discretionary power over the level of their fees—that is, under which they are viewed as "price-setters." Theories within each of these two categories come in several distinct guises. With some simplification, these variants can be placed into the following grid:

Physicians Are:	*A* *Fees Clear the Market* *for Physician Services*	*B* *Fees Do Not Clear the Market* *for Physician Services*
I Price-Takers	The physician sells his services in a competitive local market and reacts to market-determined local fee schedules.	There are price ceilings, or fee schedules, which are set by third-party payers, and the individual physician reacts to these fees.
II Price-Setters	The physician enjoys a monopoly in the market for his services and sets his fees as a single-price or price-discriminating monopolist. monopolist.	The physician takes whatever cases he likes, organizes his practice to suit his tastes and sets his fees so as to generate a given target income, related, presumably, to the income distribution in his locality.

This grid is not exhaustive but suffices for present purposes.

In so-called target-income models (type II-B) the physician is assumed to work under conditions of chronic excess demand [Feldstein, 1970], which *ipso facto* imputes to him discretionary power over his fees. If the physician uses a single fee schedule applied to all of his patients, the fees for individual services are probably determined on the basis of some full-cost pricing formula with a profit margin set to yield the desired overall income [Reinhardt 1970, Appendix A]. Alternatively, it may be assumed that the physician uses his discretionary power to tailor his fees to his individual patients' ability to pay—that he uses a so-called sliding-scale fee system. On the surface such a system may strike one as price discrimination. Under conditions of excess demand, however, it is more akin to a user-tax system under which the individual user's taxes are a function of his or her ability to pay and taxes are set at levels to yield a given target take. It is, in fact, the kind of system that might emerge under the optimal pricing rules suggested in Baumol and Bradford [1970].

Although excess demand models may well be descriptive of the real world—especially of the 1950s and 1960s when the overall physician supply was indeed rather taut—economists find such theories troublesome from an analytic viewpoint. The problem is that, whatever his pricing formula may be, the individual physician in these models is not subject to an effective market constraint on the demand side. His choice of the input-output rates for his practice are thus likely to be based on a mixture of personal, social, and medical considerations, and may not be linked at all to observable economic variables. Similarly, it is anybody's guess how the target income is chosen. Within the context of such models the economist's analytic tools tend to lose much of their cutting edge. As Feldstein [1973] has pointed out, for example, an equation relating the supply of physician hours or of physician services to medical fees is not appropriate under conditions of excess demand unless it can be assumed that physicians change their fees only infrequently and by lumpy amounts, and in the interim physicians adjust their supply to temporarily fixed fees [p. 51]. The fact that these models may in fact be descriptive of past periods furnishing the empirical record for current research on physician behavior is probably one reason why economists have so far had relatively little success in estimating a robust theory of physician behavior.

Models positing the condition of perennial excess demand are less troublesome if the individual physician is a pure price-taker, as would be the case in type I-B models. As far as the physician's input-output decision is concerned (including the supply of his own time) these models are identical to the type I-A model, and testable relationships can readily be derived from them after one has specified a concrete objective function for the physician. In principle the same can be said also of type II-A models, although here the entire demand function for the individual physician's services must be specified and estimated in an analysis of the physician's input-output and pricing decisions. Models of type I-A or B or type II-A must also be reconciled somehow with the notion that physicians can induce additional demand for their services at will. One assumption one could make is that, in equilibrium, the physician will have induced any additional demand for his services that can safely be induced. In that case one would have to posit implicitly fairly high physician-population ratios. An alternative hypothesis, recently suggested by Pauly [1973] is that the demand function to which the physician reacts has not necessarily been pushed by him as far up as it could safely be pushed on medical and legal grounds, because physicians may have some moral qualms about inducing the demand for their services for pecuniary reasons. If so, the position of the demand curve to which the physician reacts is a function of the number of colleagues with whom he shares a given patient pool. The notion underlying this theory is that if the local physician-population ratio rises and the physician's share of the local patient pool (and his income) falls, his moral qualms about inducing demand will be thereby eroded (for moral sentiments tend to be a normal good), and he will seek to shift the demand curve he faces further upward. On this theory, physicians may feel subject to a market constraint (partially fixed by their own moral standards) even at fairly low physician-population ratios.

As noted above, in developing the type I-A, I-B and II-A models, one must begin with an explicit assumption about the physician's objective function. In conventional production decision models for profit-maximizing business firms, the decisionmaker's own time allocation is thought to be independent of the input-output rates he chooses for the firm. This assumption can obviously not be grafted onto self-employed physicians whose production decisions implicitly determine also the number of hours they work and the number of hours of leisure available to them. It is therefore more reasonable to assume that the physician conducts his practice so as to maximize a utility function in income and leisure,

$$U = U(X, Y, L; Z) \tag{B-1}$$

where X denotes hours of leisure (defined as "hours not worked") per period, Y denotes after-tax income per period, L denotes the size of the physician's auxiliary staff, and vector Z contains parameters that determine the physician's trade-off between income and leisure.[a] Models of physician behavior based on this type of objective function have been developed and used by Feldstein [1970], Reinhardt [1970, Chapters 4 and 5], Rheinhardt and Yett [1972, Appendix A] and Sloan [1973a and 1973b].

The size of the physician's auxiliary staff is included as an argument in function (B-1) because, in contrast to a textbook business firm, the physician may attach certain psychic costs ($\partial U/\partial L < 0$) or benefits ($\partial U/\partial L > 0$) to the mere size of his staff. He may, for example, not wish to shoulder the responsi-

[a]Vector Z contains all those other factors that may influence professionals in the conduct of their practice, including those dictated by the profession's code of ethics. If one's interest is solely in the income-leisure trade-off, these other factors can be treated as parameters or variables capable of shifting the utility function in the income-leisure space. They need not be assumed away.

bility for maintaining and supervising a large staff, or may even view the presence of highly trained paramedics as an unwelcome form of quasi-peer supervision [Gregg 1956, p. 60].

In equation (B-1), variable X is defined by the time constraint

$$X = \bar{H} - H \tag{B-2}$$

where H denotes hours worked per period and $\bar{H}$ is a fixed total number of hours per period available for either work or leisure. The most general definition for the after-tax income (Y) entering the utility function would be the set of equations

$$Y = [1 - t(\Pi + I)] [\Pi + I] \tag{B-3}$$

$$\Pi = [P(Q) - S(Q)]Q - [W(L) + E(L)]L - FC(\bar{K}) \tag{B-4}$$

$$Q = f(H, L, \bar{K}; A) \tag{B-5}$$

where, in addition to the already familiar symbols,

Π = the pretax net-income per period derived from the physician's practice;

I = unearned income per period (that is, income not derived through hours worked);

$t(\Pi + I)$ = a progressive income tax rate;

Q = the rate of output (e.g., patient visits) produced by the physician's practice;

$P(Q)$ = the average price for physician charges per unit of his output (e.g., the average billings per patient visit), which is conceivably a function of the number of units he sells;

$S(Q)$ = the average expenditure on medical supplies and drugs per unit of output (e.g., per patient visit) which may also vary as a function of the output rate Q;

$W(L)$ = the average salary the physician pays his aides, which in principle may vary as a function of the number of aides he employs;

$E(L)$ = the average cost per period of those types of capital (equipment and floor space) that are complements of the aides and hence excluded from the production function; and which may also vary as a function of L;

$\bar{K}$ = that part of the physician's capital not strictly a complement to his aides (assumed to be fixed in this illustration); and

$FC(\bar{K})$ = the cost of K per period (assumed to be fixed).

Equation (B-5) will be recognized as the familiar production function—the technical constraint under which the physician operates. $W(L)$ in equation (B-4) may also be referred to as the supply of aides faced by the physician, and $P(Q)$ as the demand for his services. $P(Q)$ may simply be some constant P, in which case one would be dealing with a type I-A or I-B model. Alternatively, $P(Q)$ may decrease as a function of Q, in which case one would be specifying a type II-A model. Under the latter, one can envision two types of price behavior. The physician may set a single fee schedule and apply it to all of his patients; equation (B-4) above implies that assumption. Alternatively, the physician may price-discriminate in accordance with his patient's ability and willingness to pay by using a sliding-scale of fees. If one assumes that he is a perfect price discriminator, equation (B-4) no longer holds, and would have to be replaced by

$$\Pi = \int_{0}^{Q} P(u)du - S(Q)Q - [W(L) + E(L)]L - FC(\bar{K}) \qquad \text{(B-4a)}$$

If one assumes that K is given in the short run and the physician adapts his practice to this capital stock, H and L are the only decision variables to be considered.[b] Maximization of (B-1) subject to equations (B-2) to (B-4) then leads to the following first-order conditions:

$$\frac{\partial U}{\partial H} = -U_X + U_Y[1 - t^*][(P^* - S^*)f_H(\cdot)] = 0 \qquad \text{(B-6a)}$$

or

$$(P^* - S^*)f_H(\cdot) = \frac{U_X}{U_Y[1 - t^*]} \qquad \text{(B-6b)}$$

and

$$\frac{\partial U}{\partial L} = U_L + U_Y[1 - t^*][(P^* - S^*)f_L(\cdot) - W^* - E^*] = 0 \qquad \text{(B-7a)}$$

or

$$(P^* - S^*)f_L(\cdot) = (W^* + E^*) - \frac{U_L}{U_Y[1 - t^*]} \qquad \text{(B-7b)}$$

[b]This assumption is made for expositional convenience only and can easily be relaxed.

In these equations $f(\cdot)$ denotes $f(H, L, \bar{K}; A)$; $f_H = \partial f(\cdot)/\partial H$; and $f_L(\cdot) = \partial f(\cdot)/\partial L$. Variables marked with an asterisk are marginal taxes, costs, or revenues defined as follows:

S^* $= [\partial S(Q)/\partial Q]Q + S(Q)$—marginal outlays on supplies and drugs; (B-8)

W^* $= [\partial W(L)/\partial L]L + W(L)$—additional salary outlays occasioned by employment of the marginal aide; (B-9)

E^* $= [\partial E(L)/\partial L]L + E(L)$—marginal outlays on the equipment used by the marginal aide; (B-10)

t^* $= [\partial t(\Pi + I)/\partial(\Pi + I)](\Pi + I) + t(\Pi + I)$—the marginal income tax rate faced by the physician. (B-11)

Finally, depending upon what type of model one is considering, variable P^*—the marginal revenue associated with the marginal unit of output sold—will be

P^* $= P$—for the type I-A or I-B models (B-12a)

P^* $= [\partial P(Q)/\partial Q]Q + P(Q)$—for the single-price (fee schedule) monopolist (B-12b)

P^* $= P(Q)$—for the perfectly price-discriminating monopolist, where $P(Q)$ is the price of the marginal unit sold. (B-12c)

In principle the equilibrium (i.e., utility-maximizing) values of H and L may be obtained by solving (B-6b) and (B-7b) simultaneously for H and L. Figure B-1 depicts this solution graphically. The dotted lines represent the physician's utility function (B-1) for different levels of constant utility. These curves may be called "iso-happiness" curves. They indicate the rate at which the physician is willing to trade off leisure for income (at given levels of "utility" or "happiness"). The solid line in Figure B-1 represents the "opportunity locus" faced by the physician—that is, the rate at which technical and market constraints permit him to trade income and leisure. It is defined by equations (B-3) to (B-5) above. That the equilibrium point B determines not only the hours worked by the physician ($\hat{H}$, and hence also $\hat{X} = \bar{H} - \hat{H}$) and his income ($\hat{Y}$), but also the equilibrium value of the input of aides ($\hat{L}$), becomes more obvious when one derives the slope of the opportunity locus. First one uses equations (B-3) to (B-5) above to maximize Y with respect to L for given values of H. From the resulting first-order condition one obtains the income-maximizing value of L as a function of H and of the other parameters of equations (B-3) to (B-5). This solution—which may be denoted as some function $\hat{L}(H)$—can then be substituted for L in equations (B-3) to (B-5). If one finally replaces H by $\bar{H} - X$, the slope of the opportunity locus is given by

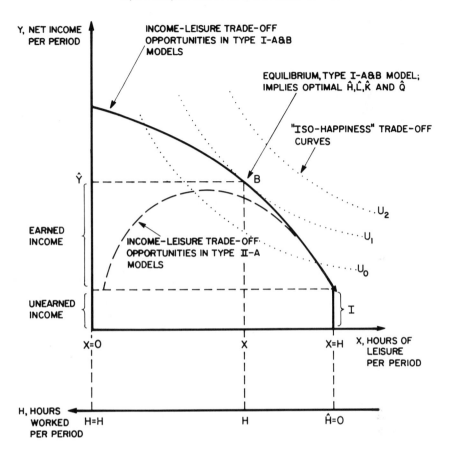

Figure B-1. Hypothetical Illustration of a Physician's Input-Output Choice

$$\frac{\partial Y}{\partial X} = -[(1 - t^*)(P^* - S^*)(f_H + f_L \frac{\partial \hat{L}(H)}{\partial H}) - (W^* + E^*)\frac{\partial \hat{L}(H)}{\partial H}] \tag{B-13}$$

In other words, for every point on the opportunity locus it is assumed that the physician optimizes the use rates of any other medical inputs.

These results are straightforward and in many ways resemble the equilibrium position of a conventional profit-maximizing business firm. The main difference lies in the fact that some of the marginal costs to which marginal revenue (P^*) is being equated include certain nonmonetary and purely subjective items—psychic costs implicit in the physician's utility function. Thus $U_X/U_Y[1 - t^*]$ in equations (B-6a and b), the physician's marginal rate of substitution between income and leisure—may be referred to as the "shadow price" of physician time. $U_L/U_Y[1 - t^*]$, on the other hand, denotes the psychic costs

($U_L < 0$) or benefits ($U_L > 0$) the physician may associate with the mere size of his auxiliary staff. These costs must be added to (or the benefits subtracted from) the monetary costs ($W^* + E^*$) associated with the employment of aides. For ordinary business firms, U_L is assumed to be zero; it may be zero for many physicians as well, as has been assumed implicitly in Figure B-1.

The ultimate objective in developing models of this sort is, of course, one's desire to predict the physician's responses to changes in observable variables and, in particular, to certain policy variables. Aside from the physician's pricing behavior, two decisions have been of particular interest to economists: the number of hours the physician decides to work (H), and the number of aides he decides to employ (L). It was noted earlier that these decisions remain something of a mystery under the target-income models. But even for the more tractable models of type I-A and B and type II-A, these decisions are characterized by highly complex (and nonlinear) equations (namely, equations (B-6b) and (B-7b) above) containing as arguments functions of the parameters in the physician's utility function (namely, U_X, U_Y and possibly even U_L). And unless the physician can be assumed to be a pure price-taker, the input decision equations for H and L contain also functions of the parameters of the demand for the individual physician's services. It is therefore not surprising that economists have found it difficult to estimate a model of physician behavior.

In a first cut at this estimation problem it is probably legitimate to sidestep some of the methodological problems cited above and to proceed with arbitrarily specified input-decision equations. This approach is followed by Sloan [1973] in his recent analysis of the input-decision equation for H. In that analysis, Sloan breaks down "hours worked per year" into "weeks worked per year" and "hours worked per week." The first of these is estimated as a linear function of after-tax income per week and certain other variables thought to characterize the physician's utility function in income and leisure. The second is related linearly to after-tax income per hour and also the other variables characterizing the physician's utility function. The income variables are, of course, thought to represent the slope of the opportunity locus facing the individual physician (the slope of the solid line in Figure B-1 and defined in equation (B-13)).

It is a well-known property of the models under discussion here that the number of hours (weeks) worked may, after a point, *decrease* with increases in hourly (weekly) remuneration—that the supply curve for physician time is backward-bending. In his analysis of physician fees, Feldstein [1970] found fairly strong evidence of a backward-bending supply curve for *physician services.* Sloan's study is not focused on physician services, but on hours worked by physicians. The study suggests a rather low overall response of physician time supplied to remuneration per unit of physician time, and only weak and somewhat inconclusive evidence of a negative response of physician time to earnings. It must be added also that the explanatory power of Sloan's estimated input-decision equations for H are rather low (with R^2 from 0.03 to 0.16). To some extent this lack of explanatory power may stem from still fairly crude data on which the analysis had to proceed; many variables thought to characterize the physician's location, for example, were statewide variables. On the other hand, it is also possible that a large number of physicians in the underlying sample worked in an economic context best described by models of the target-income variety (type II-B), and that the model underlying Sloan's empirical work (a price-taker model of the type I-A or B variety) cannot adequately represent the physician's input-output decisions, including the supply of his own time.

Although type I-A or B models may very well have little descriptive power in the context of the current health-care markets, and although estimated relationships deduced from them may be naturally inconclusive, the input decision equations one derives from them may nevertheless be put to another use, namely: the estimation of objectively optimal employment levels for aides on the basis of empirical estimates of the production function. In Chapter Seven, for example, we ask the question: *If* a physician behaved like a price-taker who sought to maximize his net income for a given number of hours he has decided to work, and for given values of P^*, S^*, W^* and E^*, how large an auxiliary staff should he employ? That estimate is obtained by solving equation (B-7b) for the income-maximizing value of L, on the assumption that $U_L = 0$. Next we turn the problem around and ask: Given values for P^*, S^*, W^* and E^*, and knowing that a physician employs, say, 1.5 aides, and assuming that $U_L = 0$, what is the implied shadow price of his leisure time? Finally, we modify the previous question to ask: *If* in addition to P^*, S^*, E^* and L it is known that the physician's shadow price of leisure is $\$Z$, then what must be the monetary equivalent of the psychic cost of employing aides ($U_L/U_Y [1 - t^*]$) for equation (B-7b) to hold? Use of the models in this way seems legitimate regardless of their power to describe physician behavior now or in the recent past.

Appendix C

Miscellaneous Tables

Table C-1.   Source Data on Regional Differences in Physician Endowments and Certain Characteristics of Private Medical Practices, United States, 1969-70

	Year	New England	East North Central	East South Central
1. Physician Endowment				
a. Total active federal and non-federal M.D.'s	1970	21,876	50,660	13,362
b. Total active federal and non-federal M.D.'s in patient care	1970	19,025	46,367	12,204
c. Total resident population, including armed forces ('000s)	1970	11,842	40,252	12,803
d. Active M.D.'s per 100,000 population	1970	185	126	104
e. M.D.'s in patient care per 100,000 population	1970	161	115	95
2. Organization of Medical Practice				
a. Average number of weeks practiced per year	1969	47.6	47.8	49.0
b. Average number of hours practiced per week	1969	52.6	52.2	52.4
c. Average number of hours per week spent in direct patient care	1969	44.7	45.0	47.0
d. Average number of patient visits per week:				
—all types of visits	1969	101.0	138.3	171.6
—office visits only	1969	71.1	100.4	123.5
e. Office visits as a percent of total visits	1969	71%	72%	72%
f. Average net income (all specialties)	1970	$38,019	$47,000	$41,963

Sources: Lines 1a and 1b: Haug, Roback and Martin [1971], Table B, p. 3, and Table D, p. 5; line 1c: *U.S. Statistical Abstract, 1972,* Table 12, p. 12; line 2a: American Medical Association [1972], Table 22, p. 57; lines 2b, 2c and 2d: American Medical Association [1971], Table 21, p. 57; line 2f: American Medical Association [1973], Table 31, p. 68.

Table C-2. Estimated Optimal Aide Employment at Alternative Input and Output Prices, Obstetricians/Gynecologists[a]

	Weekly Cost per Aide[b]			
Net Proceeds per Visit	*$70*	*$100*	*$130*	*$160*
	Based on the Office-Visit Function			
$ 5.00	4.1	3.1	_[c]	_[c]
7.00	4.5	4.0	3.4	2.6
10.00	4.8	4.5	4.2	3.8
15.00	5.1	4.9	4.7	4.4
	Based on the Total-Visit Function			
$ 5.00	4.8	4.1	3.5	2.3
7.00	5.1	4.7	4.3	3.8
10.00	5.3	5.1	4.8	4.6
15.00	5.5	5.4	5.2	5.0
	Based on the Patient-Billings Function			
–	3.9	3.7	3.5	3.3

[a]Based on the production-function estimates in Table 6–9, with G set equal to unity, $H = 60$, $OH = 35$, and all other variables, except L, set equal to their respective sample means. The 1965 sample average of gross billings per total patient visit was about $9.50; the sample average number of aides per physician was 1.51. Estimates of L for solo practitioners are only slightly below those presented here.

[b]Defined to include fringe benefits and the cost of incremental floor space.

[c]No value of L satisfies equation (6–7).

Table C-3.   Estimated Optimal Aide Employment at Alternative Input and Output Prices, Internists[a]

Net Proceeds per Visit	Weekly Cost per Aide[b]			
	$70	$100	$130	$160
	Based on the Office-Visit Function			
$ 5.00	3.8	2.7	—[c]	—[c]
7.00	4.3	3.7	3.0	1.4
10.00	4.7	4.3	3.9	3.4
15.00	4.9	4.7	4.5	4.2
	Based on the Total-Visit Function			
$ 5.00	5.0	4.4	3.6	2.1
7.00	5.4	5.0	4.6	4.1
10.00	5.7	5.4	5.2	5.9
15.00	5.9	5.8	5.6	5.4
	Based on the Patient-Billings Function			
	4.0	3.8	3.5	3.2

[a]Based on the production-function estimates in Table 6-10, with G set equal to unity, $H = 50$, $OH = 35$, and all other variables, except L, set equal to their respective sample means. The 1965 sample average of gross billings per total patient visit was about $8.70; the sample average number of aides per physician was 1.59. Estimates of L for solo practitioners are only slightly below those presented here.

[b]Defined to include fringe benefits and the cost of incremental floor space.

[c]No value of L satisfies equation (6–7).

Table C-4. Estimated Effect of Auxiliary Personnel on Physician Productivity[a]

Output Measured by:	Predicted Rate of Visits or Billings at Observed Average Rate of Aide Input	Estimated Index of Productivity at Alternative Assumed Numbers of Aides per Physician (L)					Sample Averages	
		L = 0	L = 1	L = 2	L = 3	L = 4	No. of Aides per Physician	Rate of Patient Visits or Billings
Indexes for General Practitioners								
Total Patient Visits/Week[b]	199	0.66	0.84	1.01	1.16	1.27	1.96	189
Office Visits/Week	154	0.60	0.81	1.01	1.17	1.27	—	152
Annual Patient Billings (1965–67)[c]	$60,000	0.63	0.82	1.01	1.17	1.30	—	$55,000
Pediatricians								
Total Patient Visits/Week	154	0.65	0.85	1.07	1.26	1.42	1.68	159
Office Visits/Week	130	0.61	0.84	1.07	1.25	1.35	—	133
Annual Patient Billings (1965–67)	$53,000	0.60	0.84	1.08	1.29	1.45	—	$52,200
Obstetricians/Gynecologists								
Total Patient Visits/Week	135	0.66	0.88	1.10	1.32	1.49	1.54	125
Office Visits/Week	86	0.67	0.88	1.10	1.30	1.45	—	92
Annual Patient Billings (1965–67)	$56,000	0.58	0.85	1.13	1.38	1.55	—	$57,200
Internists								
Total Patient Visits/Week	124	0.63	0.85	1.10	1.35	1.57	1.59	129
Office Visits/Week	80	0.62	0.85	1.11	1.36	1.59	—	81
Annual Patient Billings (1965–67)	$52,000	0.58	0.84	1.11	1.35	1.50	—	$51,000

[a]Calculated from the production-function estimates in Tables 6–7 to 6–10 with all inputs other than aides held constant at their sample averages, and G set equal to zero. Setting G equal to unity will not materially affect these productivity ratios.

[b]The sum of weekly office, hospital, and home visits.

[c]Annual patient billings observed for a sample of physicians surveyed in 1965 and 1967.

Table C-5.   Estimated Technically Feasible Trade-Offs between
Office-Based M.D.'s and Support Personnel, United States, 1970
and 1990[a]

	Number of M.D.'s and Support Personnel Required if the Number of Aides per M.D. (L) is equal to:				
	0	1	2	3	4
Estimated Annual Rate of Office Visits per M.D.[b]	2,681	3,699	4,821	5,938	6,911
Index Set Equal to 1.00 for $L = 1.75$	0.56	0.77	1.00	1.23	1.43
1970 Size of Resident Population: 204 million Average Annual Visits per Capita: 4.6[c]					
No. of M.D.'s required ('000s)[d]	346	251	192	156	134
No. of Aides required ('000s)	0	251	384	468	536
1990 Size of Resident Population: 245 million[e] a) Zero Growth in per Capita Demand: Av. Annual Visits per Capita: 4.6					
No. of M.D.'s required ('000s)	415	301	231	187	161
No. of Aides required ('000s)	0	301	462	562	644
b) Annual Growth in per Capita Demand: 3% Av. Annual Visits per Capita: 8.3					
No. of M.D.'s required ('000s)	756	548	421	342	294
No. of Aides required ('000s)	0	548	841	1,025	1,174

[a]Based on the assumption that physicians in 1970 employed the equivalent of the time of 2.00 aides each. For an analogous table based on the assumption that physicians in 1970 employed 1.75 aides each, see Table 7-4.

[b]Based on the productivity index for the office-visit equation estimated from the sample of internists.

[c]Office visits only.

[d]Office-based M.D.'s rendering patient care.

[e]U.S. Bureau of the Census [1972a], Series E.

Table C-6. Illustration of the Effect of Health Manpower Substitution on the Direct Costs of Furnishing an Assumed Aggregate Demand for Office Visits in 1990[a]

Assumed average annual salary per aide, and assumed contribution to nonlabor overhead and net profit per hour the physician spends in his office	*Total Cost and Cost per Office Visit if the Number of Aides per Physician Is Equal To*					
	0	*1*	*1.75*	*2*	*3*	*4*
Salary per Aide: $7,500 Contribution margin per hour:	*Total costs (billions of dollars)*[b]					
$20	$22.62	$20.60	$19.65	$19.45	$19.23	$20.20
30	33.93	29.02	26.72	26.18	24.99	25.31
40	45.24	37.44	33.79	32.90	30.75	30.60
	Average cost per office visit[c]					
$20	$11.15	$10.16	$ 9.69	$ 9.59	$ 9.48	$ 9.87
30	16.73	14.31	13.18	12.91	12.32	12.48
40	22.31	18.46	16.66	16.22	15.16	15.09
Salary per Aide: $10,000 Contribution margin per hour:	*Total costs (billions of dollars)*					
$20	$22.62	$21.85	$21.50	$21.45	$20.80	$23.17
30	33.93	30.28	28.56	28.18	27.56	28.46
40	45.24	38.70	35.63	34.90	33.32	33.75
	Average cost per office visit					
$20	$11.15	$10.78	$10.60	$10.58	$10.75	$11.43
30	16.73	14.93	14.08	13.89	13.59	14.03
40	22.31	19.08	17.57	17.21	16.43	16.64
Salary per Aide: $15,000 Contribution margin per hour:	*(Total costs (billions of dollars)*					
$20	$22.62	$24.36	$25.17	$25.46	$26.94	$29.47
30	33.93	32.78	32.24	32.18	32.70	34.76
40	45.24	41.20	39.31	38.91	38.46	40.05
	Average cost per office visit					
$20	$11.15	$12.01	$12.40	$12.55	$13.29	$14.53
30	16.73	16.16	15.90	15.87	16.12	17.14
40	22.31	20.32	19.38	19.18	18.96	19.75
Health Manpower Combinations Underlying these Cost Estimates:						
M.D.'s ('000s)	673	501	421	400	343	315
Aides ('000s)	0	501	736	800	1,029	1,260

[a]Costs cover only the office-based part of the physician's income. It is assumed that the physician works 35 hours per week and 48 weeks per year. For other footnotes, see Table 7–5.

Appendix D

The Nature of the Medical Economics Surveys

The empirical information used in Chapter Six was taken from the 1965 and 1967 nationwide surveys of physicians performed by Medical Economics, Co., publisher of the fortnightly trade journal *Medical Economics.* The information gathered by these surveys was obtained by way of mailed questionnaires. The primary purpose of the surveys is to provide the subscribers to *Medical Economics,* mostly physicians, with key economic statistics of American physicians in private practice.

In recent years, the individual physicians included in these surveys have been drawn at random, on an *N*th name basis, from the American Medical Association list of self-employed physicians, although, in some years, particular medical specialties are over-represented relative to the sampling frame.[a]

The questionnaires are mailed to the selected physicians during the early months of the survey year. They are followed by two to three additional mailings to slow respondents. The responses to the survey are then coded and keypunched by the staff of Medical Economics, Co. After coding, the individual physician is identified by number only. Moreover, Medical Economics, Co. assures the respondents that their identities will be kept in strict confidence at all times.

Since the response rates to the *Medical Economics* surveys tend to be below 50 percent,[b] the publisher's research staff normally conducts a test designed to reveal systematic differences, if any, between respondent and nonrespondents. Thus, as part of the 1967 survey, the nonrespondents were contacted, once again, by way of a briefer questionnaire covering only certain key indicators such as age, type of practice, location, income level, rate of patient visits and weekly hours in all professional activities. The test revealed

[a]The 1967 survey, for example, over-sampled pediatricians, obstetricians/ gynecologists and general surgeons.

[b]The overall response rate to the 1965 survey was 41 percent; that to the 1967 survey was 31.2 percent. In general, it has been found that the response rate to these surveys varies strongly inversely with the overall length of the questionnaire.

that, in terms of these indicators, the nonrespondents did not differ significantly from the responding physicians. In this connection, it may be mentioned also that a comparison of the *Medical Economics* data with those collected by the recently begun AMA surveys does not reveal any inconsistencies between the two series of surveys, although the response rate to the AMA survey is apparently much higher.

In short, in the absence of any compelling evidence to the contrary, it is not unreasonable to view the respondents to the *Medical Economics* surveys as broadly representative of the overall, initial sample and, indeed, of the population being sampled.

The respondents to the *Medical Economics* surveys typically cover the entire spectrum of distinct practice modes. For reasons indicated in Chapter Six, the analysis presented there was based on only those respondents who reported to be solo practitioners or members of single-specialty group practices and partnerships. Also excluded from the underlying data base were a number of responses with missing data on either inputs or output rates, and responses containing what appeared to be logically inconsistent information. An example of the latter would be a general practitioner reporting to work an average of 60 hours per week and seeing only 20 patients during that time. It was assumed that such information was the result of keypunch errors.

Table D–1 presents a brief profile of the data underlying our production function estimates.

Table D-1. Characteristics of the Data Base Underlying the Production-Function Estimates Presented in Chapter Six

Variable	General Practice	Pediatrics	Obstetrics/ Gynecology	Internal Medicine
1. Number of observations	862	270	271	296
2. Percentage of physicians in:				
−1965 survey	48%	30%	40%	53%
−solo practice	79	65	68	71
−single-specialty groups or partnerships with:				
−two members	14	19	22	17
−three members	5	12	8	8
−four or more members	2	4	2	6
3. Distribution by U.S. Census Division (percent):				
New England	4.9%	8.2%	8.8%	8.4%
Middle Atlantic	14.4	22.0	22.5	27.4
South Atlantic	12.9	14.5	17.5	10.7
East North Central	20.6	22.3	17.9	17.4
East South Central	6.4	4.3	4.6	5.0
West North Central	8.6	3.6	4.2	5.7
West South Central	8.7	8.5	6.3	4.4
Mountain	5.7	2.1	3.2	3.3
Pacific	17.9	14.5	15.1	17.7
4. Average Number of:				
Office visits/week	152	133	92	81
Hospital visits/week	31	22	32	45
House calls/week	5	4	2	3
Office hours/week	35	35	27	31
Total practice hours/week[a]	61	52	57	56
Full-time equivalent aides per physician	1.96	1.68	1.54	1.59
Gross patient billings/year[b]	$54,800	$52,200	$57,200	$51,000

[a]Total professional hours excluding time spent on research, writing, teaching and hospital-staff meetings.

[b]Reported gross income during the calendar year preceding the survey divided by the physician's reported collection ratio.

Source: *Medical Economics,* Continuing Surveys, 1965 and 1967.

Bibliography

Allen, R.G.D. *Mathematical Analysis for Economists*. London: Macmillan and Co., 1938.

American Association of Medical Colleges. *Undergraduate Medical Education, Elements—Objectives—Costs, Report of the Commission on the Financing of Medical Education*. Washington, D.C.: American Association of American Medical Colleges, October 1973.

American Medical Association. *General Report of the Commission on the Cost of Medical Care*. Vol. 1. Chicago: American Medical Association, 1964.

——*Reference Data on Profile of Medical Practice*. Chicago: American Medical Association, 1971, 1972, 1973.

Anderson, Odin W. *Health Care: Can There Be Equity? The United States, Sweden, and England*. New York: John Wiley & Sons, 1972.

——and Sheatsley, P.B. *Comprehensive Medical Insurance: A Study of Costs, Use, and Attitudes under Two Plans*. Research Series No. 9. New York: Health Information Foundation, 1959.

Arrow, Kenneth J. "Uncertainty and the Welfare Economics of Medical Care," *American Economic Review* 53 (December 1963): 941–973.

——and Capron, William M. "Dynamic Shortages and Price Rises: The Engineer-Scientist Case," *Quarterly Journal of Economics* 72 (May 1959); 292–308.

Backman, George W. *A Method for Measuring Physician Requirements, With Appraisal of Former Methods*. Washington, D.C.: The Brookings Institution, 1955.

Bailey, R.M. "Appraisal of Experience in Fee-for-Service Group Practice in the San Francisco Bay Area: A Comparison of Internists in Solo and Group Practice." Paper read before the Health Conference of the New York Academy of Medicine, April 1968.

——. "Economies of Scale in Medical Practice," in Herbert E. Klarman, ed., with the assistance of Helen H. Jaszi, *Empirical Studies in Health Economics*. Proceedings of the Second Conference on the Economics of Health. Baltimore: The Johns Hopkins Press, 1970.

293

Bane, Frank (Chairman, Surgeon General's Consultant Group on Medical Education). *Physicians for a Growing America.* Washington, D.C.: United States Government Printing Office, 1959.

Battistella, Roger M. "The Idealized Physician's Role as Perceived by People in Late Adulthood," *Inquiry* 6 (September 1969): 28–36.

"Bayne-Jones Report." See U.S. Department of Health, Education and Welfare.

Benham, L.; Maurizi, A.; and Reder, M.W. "Location and Migration of Medics: Physicians and Dentists," *Review of Economics and Statistics,* 50 (August 1968): 332–347.

Bergman, A.B.; Dassel, S.W.; and Wedgwood, R.J. "Time-Motion Study of Practicing Pediatricians" *Pediatrics* 38 (1966): 254–263.

———; Probstfield, Jeffrey L.; and Wedgwood, Ralph J. "Performance Analysis in Pediatric Practice: Preliminary Report," *Journal of Medical Education* 42 (March 1967): 249–253.

Berndt, E.R., and Christensen, L.R. "The Translog Function and the Substitution of Equipment, Structures and Labor in U.S. Manufacturing, 1929–1968," *Journal of Econometrics* (Sept. 1973), pp. 1–82.

Blank, David S., and Stigler, George J. *The Demand and Supply of Scientific Personnel.* New York: National Bureau of Economic Research, 1957.

Blumberg, Mark S. *Trends and Projections of Physicians in the United States, 1967–2002.* A Technical Report Sponsored by the Carnegie Commission on Higher Education. The Carnegie Foundation for the Advancement of Teaching, 1971.

Boan, J.A. *Group Practice.* Study prepared for the Royal Commission on Health Services, 1964. Ottawa, Ontario, Canada: Queen's Printer, 1966.

Boness, Fredrick. "Legal Constraints on the Utilization of Allied Health Personnel." Discussion Paper 73–6, Institute of Policy Analysis, La Jolla, California, October 1973.

Bradford, David F., and Baumol, William J. "Optimal Departures from Marginal Cost Pricing," *American Economic Review* 60 (June 1970): 265–283.

Brewster, A.W., and Seldowitz, E. "Medical Society Relative Value Scales and the Medical Market," *Public Health Reports* 80 (June 1965): 501–510.

Brown, Murray, ed. *The Theory and Empirical Analysis of Production.* National Bureau of Economic Research, Studies in Income and Wealth, Vol. 31. New York: Columbia University Press, 1967.

Butter, Irene. "Health Manpower Research: A Survey," *Inquiry* 4 (December 1967): pp. 5–41.

———, and Schaffner, Richard. "Foreign Medical Graduates and Equal Access to Medical Care," *Medical Care* 9 (1971): 136–143.

Canada. Royal Commission on Health Services. *Report of the Commission,* Vol. 1. Ottawa, Ontario, Canada: Queen's Printer, 1964.

The Carnegie Commission on Higher Education. *Higher Education and the Nation's Health: Policies for Medical and Dental Education.* New York: McGraw-Hill Book Co., 1970.

Charney, E., and Kitzman, H. "The Child Health Nurse (PNP) in Private Practice," *New England Journal of Medicine* 28 (December 9, 1971): 1353–1358.

Christensen, L.R.; Jorgenson, D.W.; and Lau, L.G., "Conjugate Duality and the Transcendental Logarithmic Production Function," *Econometrica* 39 (July 1971): 225–256.

Clute, K.F. *The General Practitioners.* Toronto: University of Toronto Press, 1963.

Coe, Rodney M., and Fichtenbaum, Leonard. "Utilization of Physician Assistance: Some Implications for Medical Practice," *Medical Care* 10 (November-December 1972): 497–504.

Commission on the Cost of Medical Care. *General Report.* Chicago: American Medical Association, 1964.

Davis, Karen. "A Theory of Economic Behavior in Non-Profit, Private Hospitals." Unpublished Ph.D. Dissertation, Rice University, Houston, Texas, 1969.

Densen, Paul M.; Jones, E.; Balamuth, E.; and Shapiro, S. "Prepaid Medical Care and Hospital Utilization in a Dual Choice Situation," *American Journal of Public Health* 50 (November 1960): 1710–1726.

——; Shapiro, Sam; Jones, E.W.; and Baldinger, I. "Prepaid Medical Care and Hospital Utilization: Comparison of a Group Practice and a Self-Insurance Situation," *Hospitals* 36 (November 16, 1962): 62–68, 138.

Dhrymes, P.J., and Kurz, M., "Technology and Scale in Electricity Generation," *Econometrica* 32 (July 1964): 287–315.

Dickinson, Frank G. *Supply of Physicians' Services.* Chicago: American Medical Association, Bureau of Medical Economics Research, 1951.

Diewert, W.E. "Functional Forms for Profit and Transformation Functions," *Journal of Economic Theory* 6 (June 1973): 284–316.

Diwan, R.K. "An Empirical Estimate of the Elasticity of Substitution of Production Function," *Indian Economic Journal* 12 (April-June 1965): 347–366.

Donabedian, Avedis. "Evaluating the Quality of Medical Care," *Milbank Memorial Fund Quarterly* 64 (July 1966): 166–206.

——. "An Evaluation of Prepaid Group Practice," *Inquiry* 6 (September 1969): 3–27.

——; Axelrod, S.J., and Agard, Judith. *Medical Care Chart Book.* 3rd ed. Ann Arbor: The University of Michigan School of Public Health, Bureau of Public Health Economics, 1970.

Dowling, W.L. *A Linear Programming Approach to the Analysis of Hospital Production.* Unpublished Ph.D. dissertation, University of Michigan, Ann Arbor, 1972.

Drui, Alfred B. "Methodological Issues in Measuring Ambulatory Care," *American Journal of Public Health* 63 (April 1973): 358–360.

Duncan, Burris; Smith, Ann N.; and Silver, Henry K. "Comparison of the Physical Assessment of Children by Pediatric Nurse Practitioners and Pediatricians," *American Journal of Public Health* 61 (June 1971): 1170–1176.

Egan, Douglas M. *Physician Productivity Personnel Utilization and Physician Income.* Denver, Colorado: Medical Group Management Association, 1969.

Egan, Richard L. "In Search of an Explanation," *Journal of the American Medical Association* 226 (November 1973): 991.

Ellwood, Paul M., Jr. "Restructuring the Health Delivery System–Will the Health Maintenance Strategy Work?" in *Health Maintenance Organizations: A Reconfiguration of the Health Services System.* Proceedings of the Thirteenth Annual Symposium on Hospital Affairs, Center for Health Administration Studies, University of Chicago, May 1971, pp. 2–11.

——; O'Donoghue, Patrick; Hoagberg, Earl J.; Schneider, Robert; McLure, Walter; and Carlson, Rick J. *Comparative Analysis of a Competitive HMO System with Other Health Care Delivery Systems.* (Mimeographed), 1971.

Epple, D., and Reinhardt, U.E. *Analysis of the Cost of Ambulatory Care in New York City Hospitals.* (Mimeographed), 1972.

Evans, Robert G. *Price Formation in the Market for Physician's Services in Canada, 1957–1969.* Study prepared for the Prices and Incomes Commission, Canada, 1972. Ottawa, Canada: Information Canada, 1973.

——, Parish, E.M.A. and Sully, F. "Medical Productivity, Scale Effects and Demand Creation" *The Canadian Journal of Economics* 6 (August 1973): 376–393.

Ewing, O.R. *The Nation's Health, A Ten-Year Program: A Report to the President.* Washington, D.C.: U.S. Government Printing Office, 1948.

Farrell, M.J. "The Measurement of Productive Efficiency," *Journal of the Royal Statistical Society* 120, III (1957): 253–282.

——, and Fieldhouse, M. "Estimating Efficient Production Functions under Increasing Returns to Scale," *Journal of the Royal Statistical Society* 125, II (1962): 252–267.

Fein, Rashi. *The Doctor Shortage: An Economic Diagnosis.* Washington, D.C.: The Brookings Institution, 1967.

Feldman, Marie. "Pediatric Nurse Practitioners Role in a Large Group Practice," *Hospital Topics* 50 (March 1972): 62.

Feldstein, Martin S. *Economic Analysis for Health Service Efficiency: Econometric Studies of the British National Health Service.* Amsterdam: North-Holland Publishing Co., 1967.

——. *The Rising Cost of Hospital Care.* Washington, D.C.: Information Resources Press, 1971.

——. "The Rising Price of Physicians' Services" *Review of Economics and Statistics* 52 (May 1970): 121–133.

Feldstein, Paul J. "Research on the Demand for Health Services," *Milbank Memorial Fund Quarterly* 54 (July 1966): 128–165.

——, and Severson, R.M. "The Demand for Medical Care," in American Medical

Association, *Report of the Commission on the Cost of Medical Care,*
Vol. 1. Chicago: American Medical Association, 1964, pp. 57–76.
Foundation on Employee Health, Medical Care and Welfare. *Family Medical
Care under Three Types of Health Insurance.* New York: The Foun-
dation on Employee Health, Medical Care and Welfare, 1962.
Frech, H.E., III, and Ginsburg, Paul B. "Physician Pricing: Monopolistic or
Competitive: Comment," *The Southern Economic Journal* 38
(April 1972): 573–580.
Frederick, J. Howard, M.D. "Disposables Do More than Cut Costs," *Medical
Economics* (May 27, 1968), pp. 65–69.
Freidson, Eliot. *Professional Dominance: The Social Structure of Medical Care.*
New York: Atherton Press, 1970.
Friedman, Milton. *Capitalism and Freedom.* Chicago: The University of Chicago
Press, 1962.
——, and Kuznets, Simon. *Income from Independent Professional Practice.*
New York: National Bureau of Economic Research, 1945.
Fuchs, V.R., ed. *Production and Productivity in the Service Industries.* National
Bureau of Economic Research, Studies in Income and Wealth, Vol.
34. New York: Columbia University Press, 1969.
——, and Kramer, Marcia J. *Determinants of Expenditures for Physicians'
Services in the United States, 1948–68.* Washington, D.C.: National
Center for Health Services Research and Development, 1972.
Garbarino, Joseph W. *Health Plans and Collective Bargaining.* Berkeley and Los
Angeles: The University of California Press, 1960.
——. "Price Behavior and Productivity in the Medical Market," *Industrial and
Labor Relations Review* 13 (October 1959): 3–15.
Geomet, Inc. *The Impact on Future Health Manpower Requirements and Supply
of Increasing Productivity through Use of Technological Advances.*
Geomet Report No. R–163. Rockville, Maryland: Geomet, Inc.,
1972.
Gerber, Alex. "The Medical Manpower Shortage," *Journal of Medical Education*
42 (April 1967): 306–319.
——. "Yes, There Is a Doctor Shortage," *Prism* 1 (August 1973a): 13–15, 60.
——. "Author's Reply" *Prism,* 1 (November 1973b): 6–7.
Ginzberg, Eli. "Physician Shortage Reconsidered," *New England Journal of
Medicine* 275 (July 1966).
——, with Miriam Ostow. *Men, Money, and Medicine.* New York and London:
Columbia University Press, 1969.
Glaser, William A. *Paying the Doctor: Systems of Remuneration and Their
Effects.* Baltimore: The Johns Hopkins Press, 1970.
Golladay, F.L.; Mauser, M.E.; and Smith, K.E. "Scale Economies in the
Delivery of Medical Care: A Mixed Integer Programming Analysis
of Efficient Manpower Utilization," *Journal of Human Resources*
(forthcoming in Winter issue of 1974).
Gonzalez, Arturo F., Jr. "West German Medicine: Verrrrrry Interesting,"
Prism 1 (November 1973): 39–42.
Gorham, William B. *Medical Care Prices.* Report by the Department of Health,

Education, and Welfare to the President. Washington, D.C.: U.S. Government Printing Office, February 1967.

Greenfield, H.I. *Allied Health Manpower: Trends and Progress.* New York: Columbia University Press, 1969.

Gregg, A. *Challenges to Contemporary Medicine.* New York: Columbia University Press, 1956.

Griliches, Zvi. "Estimates of the Aggregate Agricultural Production Function from Cross-Sectional Data," *Journal of Farm Economics* 45 (May 1963): 419–428.

——. "Production Functions in Manufacturing: Some Preliminary Results," in *The Theory and Empirical Analysis of Production.* National Bureau of Economic Research, Studies in Income and Wealth, Vol. 31. Edited by Murray Brown. New York: Columbia University Press, 1967.

——. "Specification Bias in Estimates of Production Functions," *Journal of Farm Economics* 39 (February 1957): 8–20.

Gross, Martin L. *The Doctors.* New York: Random House, 1966.

Grossman, Michael. *The Demand for Health: A Theoretical and Empirical Investigation.* New York: Columbia University Press, 1972.

Havighurst, Clark C. "Regulation of Health Facilities and Services by 'Certificate of Need,'" *Virginia Law Review* 59 (October 1973): 1143–1232.

Halter, A.N.; Carter, C.O.; and Hocking, J.G. "A Note on the Transcendental Production Function," *Journal of Farm Economics* 39 (November 1957): 966–974.

Hanft, Ruth S. "Reimbursement for the Services of Physician Assistants under Federal and Private Health Insurance." Paper presented to the Macy Conference on Intermediate Level Health Personnel In the Delivery of Direct Health Services, November 1972. (Processed).

Hansen, W. Lee. "An Appraisal of Physician Manpower Projections," *Inquiry* 7 (March 1970): 102–113.

——. "Shortages and Investment in Health Manpower," in *The Economics of Health and Medical Care,* Ed. S. Axelrod, Ann Arbor, Michigan: The University of Michigan School of Public Health, 1964, pp. 75–91.

Harris, Seymour E. *The Economics of American Medicine.* New York: The Macmillan Co., 1964.

Haug, J.N., and Martin, B.C. *Foreign Medical Graduates in the United States, 1970.* Chicago: American Medical Association, 1971.

——, and Roback, G.A. *Distribution of Physicians, Hospitals, and Hospital Beds in the U.S., 1967: Regional, State, County, Metropolitan Area.* Chicago: American Medical Association, 1968.

——, ——. *Distribution of Physicians, Hospitals, and Hospital Beds in the U.S., 1969,* Vols. 1 & 2. Chicago: American Medical Association, 1970.

Haug, J.N.; Roback, G.A.; and Martin, B.C. *Distribution of Physicians in the United States, 1970: Regional State, County and Metropolitan Areas.* Chicago: American Medical Association, 1971.

Heady, Earl O. *Economics of Agricultural Production and Resource Use.* Englewood Cliffs, N.J.: Prentice-Hall, 1952.

——, and Dillon, J.L. *Agricultural Production Functions.* Ames, Iowa: Iowa State University Press, 1961.

Health Maintenance Organizations: A Reconfiguration of the Health Services System. Proceedings of the Thirteenth Annual Symposium on Hospital Affairs, University of Chicago, May 1971.

Heistand, Dale L. "Research into Manpower for Health Service." *Milbank Memorial Fund Quarterly* 44, 2 (October 1966): 146–179.

Hoch, Irving. "Simultaneous Equation Bias in the Context of the Cobb-Douglas Production Function," *Econometrica* 26 (October 1958): 566–578.

Holtman, Albert G. "Another Look at the Shortage of Physicians," *Industrial and Labor Relations Review* 18 (April 1965): 423–424.

Hughes, E.F.X.; Fuchs, V.R.; and Jacoby, J.E. "Surgical Workloads in a Community Practice," *Surgery* 71 (1972): 315–372.

——; Lewit, Eugene M.; and Rand, Elizabeth H. *Operative Workloads in One Hospital's General Surgical Residency Program.* Report to the National Bureau of Economic Research, Inc., New York, 1973. (Mimeo.)

Hyde, D.R.; Wolff, P.; Gross, Anne; and Hoffman, E.L. "The American Medical Association: Power, Purpose and Politics in Organized Medicine," *Yale Law Journal* 63 (May 1954): 938–1022.

Institute of Medicine, National Academy of Sciences. *Cost of Education in the Health Professions.* Parts I and II. Washington, D.C.: National Academy of Sciences, January 1974.

Jeffers, James R.; Bognanno, Mario F.; and Bartlett, John C. "On the Demand versus Need for Medical Services and the Concept of 'Shortage,'" *American Journal of Public Health* 61 (January 1971): 46–63.

Jones, Norman H., Jr.; Struve, Charles A.; and Stefani, Paula. "Health Manpower in 1975—Demand, Supply, and Price," in U.S. National Advisory Commission on Health Manpower, *Report of the Commission,* Vol. 2, 1967, pp. 229–263.

Joorabchi, B. "Physician Migration: Brain Drain or Overflow? With Special Reference to the Situation in Iran," *British Journal of Medical Education* (March 1973), pp. 44–47.

Judek, Stanislaw. *Medical Manpower in Canada.* Ottawa, Canada: Queen's Printer, 1964.

Kehrer, B.H. and Knowles, J.C. "Economies of Scale and the Pricing of Physicians' Services." Paper delivered at the annual meeting of the Health Economics Research Organization, New York, December 1973. (Mimeo.)

Kessel, Reuben A. "Price Discrimination in Medicine" *Journal of Law and Economics* 1 (October 1958): 20–54.

Kimbell, L.J., and Lorant, J.H. "Physician Productivity and Returns to Scale." Paper presented before the American Economic Association Meetings, New York, December 29, 1973. (Mimeo.)

Klarman, Herbert E. "Approaches to Moderating the Increases in Medical Care Costs," *Medical Care* 8 (May-June 1969a): 175–190.

——. "Analysis of the HMO Proposal—Its Assumptions, Implications, and Prospects," in *Health Maintenance Organizations: A Reconfiguration of the Health Services System.* Proceedings of the Thirteenth Annual Symposium on Hospital Affairs, Center for Health Administration Studies, University of Chicago, May 1971, pp. 24–38.

——. "Economic Aspects of Projecting Requirements for Health Manpower," *Journal of Human Resources* 4 (1969b): 360–376.

——. *The Economics of Health.* New York: Columbia University Press, 1965.

Konijn, H.S. "Estimation of an Average Production Function from Surveys," *Economic Record* 35 (April 1959): 118–125.

Kovner, J.W. "A Production Function for Outpatient Medical Facilities," Unpublished Ph.D. dissertation, University of California, Los Angeles, 1968.

Lee, Roger I., and Jones, Lewis Webster. *The Fundamentals of Good Medical Care.* Chicago: University of Chicago Press, 1933.

Litman, Theodor J. "Public Perceptions of the Physicians' Assistant—A Survey of the Attitudes and Opinions of Rural Iowa and Minnesota Residents," *American Journal of Public Health* 62 (March 1972): 343–346.

MacColl, W.A. *Group Practice and Prepayment of Medical Care.* Washington, D.C.: Public Affairs Press, 1966.

Marschak, J., and Andrews, W.H. "Random Simultaneous Equations and the Theory of Production," *Econometrica* 12 (July-October, 1944): 143–205.

Mason, Henry R. "Physician Migration: Brain Drain or Overflow?," *Journal of The American Medical Association* 226 (October 22, 1973): 463.

Maurizi, A. "The Economics of the Dental Profession," Unpublished Ph.D. dissertation, Stanford University, 1967.

"Step Up Your Productivity?" *Medical Economics* (September 1968), pp. 63–154.

Monsma, George N., Jr. "Marginal Revenue and the Demand for Physicians' Services," in Herbert E. Klarman, ed., with the assistance of Helen H. Jaszi, *Empirical Studies in Health Economics.* Proceedings of the Second Conference on the Economics of Health. Baltimore: The Johns Hopkins Press, 1970.

——. "The Supply of and Demand for Physicians' Services." Unpublished Ph.D. dissertation. Princeton University. 1969.

Mountin, Joseph W.; Pennell, Elliott H.; and Berger, Anne G. "Health Service Areas: Estimates of Future Physician Requirements." Public Health Bulletin #305. Washington, D.C.: United States Government Printing Office, 1949.

Mundlak, Yair. "On Estimation of Production and Behavioral Functions," in *Studies in Mathematical Economics and Econometrics in Memory of Yehuda Grunfeld,* ed. Carl Christ et al. Stanford: Stanford University Press, 1963.

——. "Transcendental Multiproduct Production Functions," *International Economic Review* 5 (September 1964): 273–283.

——, and Hoch, Irving. "Consequence of Alternative Specification in the Estimation of Cobb-Douglas Production Functions," *Econometrica,* 33 (October 1965): 814–828.

National Advisory Commission on Health Manpower. *Report, Vols. I & II,* Washington, D.C.: U.S. Government Printing Office, 1967.

Nerlove, Marc. *Estimation and Identification of Cobb-Douglas Production Functions.* Chicago: Rand McNally and Co., 1965.

Newhouse, Joseph P. "The Economics of Group Practice," *Journal of Human Resources* 8 (Winter 1973): 37–56.

——. "A Model of Physician Pricing." *The Southern Economic Journal,* 37:2 (October 1970), pp. 174–183.

——, and Sloan, Frank A. "Physician Pricing: Monopolistic or Competitive: Reply." *The Southern Economic Journal,* 38:4 (April 1972), pp. 577–580.

Nixon, Richard. *President's Message on Health and Hospitalization.* Congressional Record, 92nd Congress, First Session, 117, Part 3, pp. 3015–3021. Washington, D.C.: U.S. Government Printing Office, 1971.

Noll, Roger G. "The Consequences of Public Regulation of Hospitals." Paper delivered to the Institute of Medicine Conference on Regulation in the Health Industry, Washington, D.C., January 1974. (Mimeo.)

Owens, Arthur. "The Economics of Partnership Practice," *Medical Economics* (June 12, 1967a), pp. 86–95.

——. "General Surgeons: Too Many in the Wrong Places," *Medical Economics* (July 20, 1973), pp. 128–133.

——. "How Do Your Practice Goals Compare?" *Medical Economics* (February 20, 1967b), pp. 65–73.

——. "How Many Doctors Are Really Working at Full Capacity?" *Medical Economics* (January 18, 1971a), pp. 85–93.

——. "Raise Fees after the Freeze? Think Twice!" *Medical Economics* (November 8, 1971b), pp. 189–197.

——. "Time Well Spent? New Norms Will Help You See," *Medical Economics* (December 6, 1971b), pp. 79–87.

——. "Why Aren't Primary-Care Doctors More Productive?" forthcoming in *Medical Economics* (June 1974).

Parker, Harry J., and Delahunt, John C. "Delegating Tasks to Physicians' Assistants: Physicians' Reactions," *Texas Medicine* 68 (October 1972): 69–79.

Pauly, Mark V. "Information and the Demand for Medical Care," December 1973. (Mimeo.)

——. "Efficiency, Incentives and Reimbursement for Health Care," *Inquiry* 7 (March 1970): 114–131.

Perrott, George S. "The Federal Employees Health Benefits Program," *Group Health and Welfare News,* Special Supplement (March 21, 1971).

——. "Utilization of Hospital Services," *American Journal of Public Health* 56 (January 1966): 62–63.

—— and Pennell, Maryland Y. "Physician Shortage Reconsidered," *New England Journal of Medicine* 275 (July 14, 1966): 85–87.

——, ——. "Physicians in the United States: Projections 1955–75," *Journal of Medical Education* 33 (September 1958).

Peterson, Paul Q., and Pennell, Maryland Y. "Physician Population Projections,

1961–75: Their Causes and Implications," *American Journal of Public Health* 53 (February 1963): 163–172.

President's Commission on the Health Needs of the Nation. *Building America's Health,* Vol. 2. Washington, D.C.: U.S. Government Printing Office, 1953.

Promoting the Group Practice of Medicine. Report of the National Conference on Group Practice, October 1967. Washington, D.C.: U.S. Government Printing Office, 1967.

Rayack, Elton. *Professional Power and American Medicine: The Economics of the American Medical Association.* Cleveland: World Publishing Co., 1967.

——. "The Shortage of Physician Services," *Industrial and Labor Relations Review* 18 (July 1965): 584–587.

——. "The Supply of Physician Services," *Industrial and Labor Relations Review* 17 (January 1964): 221–237.

Reder, M.W. "Some Problems in the Measurement of Productivity in Medical Care Industry," in *Production and Productivity in the Service Industries,* National Bureau of Economic Research, Studies in Income and Wealth, ed. V.R. Fuchs, Vol. 34. New York: Columbia University Press, 1969.

Reinhardt, Uwe E. "An Economic Analysis of Physicians' Practices." Unpublished Ph.D. dissertation, Yale University, 1970.

——. "On the Economic Characteristics of Health Maintenance Organizations," 1971. (Mimeo.)

——. "Manpower Substitution and Productivity in Medical Practice: Review of Research," *Health Services Research* (Fall 1973b).

——. "A Production Function for Physicians' Services," *Review of Economics and Statistics* 54 (February 1972a): 55–56.

——. "Occupational Licensure in the Health Care Sector," in *Canadian Higher Education in the Seventies.* Ottawa, Canada: Economic Council of Canada, May 1972b, pp. 167–175.

——. "Proposed Changes in the Organization of Health-Care Delivery: An Overview and Critique," *Milbank Memorial Fund Quarterly* 51 (Spring 1973a): 169–222.

——. "Alternative Methods of Reimbursing Non-Institutional Providers of Health Services." Paper presented to the Institute of Medicine Conference on Regulation in the Health Industry, National Academy of Sciences, Washington, D.C., January 1974. (Forthcoming in *Proceedings.*)

——, and Yett, D.E. "Physician Production Functions under Varying Practice Arrangements," Community Profile Data Center, Technical Paper No. 11 (August 1972).

Riddick, F.A.; Bryan, J.B.; Gershenson, M.I.; and Costello, A.C. "Use of Allied Health Professionals in Internists' Offices," *Archives of Internal Medicine* 127 (May 1971): 924–931.

Rimlinger, Gaston V., and Steele, Henry B. "An Economic Interpretation of the Spatial Distribution of Physicians in the U.S.," *Southern Economic Journal* 30 (July 1963): 1–12.

Roemer, Milton I. "On Paying the Doctor and the Implications of Different Methods," *Journal of Health and Human Behavior* 3 (Spring 1962): 10–19.

——; Hetherington, Robert W.; Hopkins, Carl E.; Gerst, Arthur E.; Parsons, Eleanor; and Long, Donald M. *Health Insurance Effects: Services, Expenditures, and Attitudes Under Three Types of Plan.* Bureau of Public Health Economics Research Series No. 16. Ann Arbor: School of Public Health, University of Michigan, 1972.

Rosenthal, Neal H. "The Health Manpower Gap: A High Hurdle," *Occupational Outlook Quarterly* 2 (February 1967).

Ruffin, Roy J., and Leigh, Duane E. "Charity, Competition, and the Pricing of Doctors' Services," *Journal of Human Resources* (Fall 1972).

Ruhe, C.H. William. "Present Projections of Physician Production," *Journal of the American Medical Association,* 193 (December 5, 1966): 1094–1100.

Sadler, A.M., Jr.; Sadler, B.L.; and Bliss, A.A. *The Physician's Assistant Today and Tomorrow.* New Haven: Yale University School of Medicine, 1972.

Scaer, Robert C. "There's a Doctor Surplus in our Town. Will Yours be Next?" *Medical Economics* (September 3, 1973), pp. 81–84.

Schwartz, Harry. *The Case for American Medicine: A Realistic Look at our Health Care System.* New York: David McKay Company, Inc., 1972.

Schwartz, William B. "Medicine and the Computer: The Promise and Problems of Change," *New England Journal of Medicine* 283 (December 1970): 1257–1264.

——. Testimony in Hearings before the Subcommittee on Health of the Committee on Labor and Public Welfare, U.S. Senate, 92nd Congress, First Session, on Examination of the Health Care Crisis in America, Part 3:442–463. Washington, D.C.: U.S. Government Printing Office, 1971.

Scitovsky, A.A. "Changes in the Costs of Treatment of Selected Illnesses," *American Economic Review* 57 (December 1967): 1182–1195.

Sloan, Frank A. "Lifetime Earnings and the Physicians' Choice of Specialty," *Industrial and Labor Relations Review* 24 (1970): 47–56.

——. "A Microanalysis of Physicians' Hours of Work Decisions." Paper presented at the International Economic Association Conference of Health and Medical Care, Tokyo, 1973.

——. *Supply Responses of Young Physicians: An Analysis of Physicians in Residency Programs.* Santa Monica, California: Rand Corporation, 1973. (Mimeo.)

——. "Physician Fee Inflation: Evidence from the late 1960's." Paper presented at the National Bureau of Economic Research Conference on the Role of Health Insurance in the Health Services Sector, Rochester, N.Y., May 1974. (Mimeo.)

Smith, Kenneth R.; Miller, Marianne; and Golladay, Frederick L. "An Analysis of the Optimal Use of Inputs in the Production of Medical Services," *Journal of Human Resources* 7 (Spring 1972): 208–225.

Somers, Anne R., ed. *The Kaiser-Permanente Medical Care Program: A Symposium.* New York: The Commonwealth Fund, 1971.

Somers, H.M., and Somers, A.R. *Doctors, Patients and Health Insurance.* Washington, D.C.: The Brookings Institution, 1961.

Steinwald, B., and Sloan, F.A. "Determinants of Physicians' Fees." October 1973. (Mimeo.)

Stevens, Carl M. "Physician Supply and National Health Goals," *Journal of Industrial Relations* 10 (May 1971): 119–144.

Stevens, Rosemary, and Vermulen, Joan. *Foreign-Trained Physicians and American Medicine.* U.S. Department of Health, Education, and Welfare, DHEW Publication No. (NIH) 73–325. Washington, D.C.: U.S. Government Printing Office, 1972.

Stewart, Charles T., Jr., and Siddayao, Corazon M. *Increasing the Supply of Medical Personnel: Needs and Alternatives.* Washington: American Enterprise Institute for Public Policy Research, 1973.

Stewart, William, and Pennell, Maryland Y. "Health Manpower, 1930–75," *Public Health Reports* 75 (March 1960).

Taylor, M.G. *The Administration of Health Insurance in Canada.* Toronto: Oxford University Press, 1956.

Theodore, C.N., and Haug, J.N. *Selected Characteristics of the Physician Population, 1963 and 1967.* Chicago: American Medical Association, 1968.

——; ——; Balfe, B.E.; Roback, G.A.; and Franz, E.J. *Reclassification of Physicians, 1968: New Base for Health Manpower Studies.* Chicago: American Medical Association, 1971.

Todd, C., and McNamara, M.E. *Medical Groups in the U.S., 1969.* Chicago: American Medical Association, 1971.

Todd, Malcolm C. "Medical Manpower and the Emergence of New Professions," *Texas Medicine* 68 (October 1972): 60–64.

——, and Foy, Donald F. "Current Status of the Physician's Assistant and Related Issues," *Journal of American Medical Association* 220 (June 26, 1972): 1714–1720.

United States. Congress. House. *Health Professions Educational Assistance, Hearing before the Committee on Interstate and Foreign Commerce.* 88th Congress, 1st Session, February 6, 1963.

United States. Congress. House. House Subcommittee on Public Health and Environment. Committee on Interstate and Foreign Commerce. *Hearings on the Health Professions Educational Assistance Amendments of 1971,* Parts 1 and 2. 92nd Congress, 1st Session, April 2–29, 1971.

U.S. Bureau of the Census. *Statistical Abstract of the United States.* Washington, D.C.: U.S. Government Printing Office, various years.

——. *Current Population Reports: Population Estimates and Projections. Projections of the Population of the United States by Age and Sex: 1972 to 2020.* Series P-25, No. 493. Washington, D.C.: U.S. Government Printing Office, December 1972a.

——. *Census of Housing: 1970. General Housing Characteristics.* Final Report
HC(1)-A1, United States Summary. Washington, D.C.: U.S. Government Printing Office, 1971.

——. *Census of Population: 1970. General Social and Economic Characteristics.* Final Report PC(1)-C1, United States Summary. Washington, D.C.: U.S. Government Printing Office, 1972b.

United States. Department of Health, Education, and Welfare. Office of the Secretary. *The Advancement of Medical Research and Education through the Department of Health, Education, and Welfare; Final Report of the Secretary's Consultants on Medical Research and Education.* Washington, D.C.: U.S. Government Printing Office, 1958. (Commonly referred to as the "Bayne-Jones Report.")

——. *Medical Care Prices.* A Report to the President. (Also referred to as the "Gorham Report.") Washington, D.C.: U.S. Government Printing Office, February 1967.

——, Public Health Service. *Health Manpower; Perspectice: 1967.* Washington, D.C.: U.S. Government Printing Office, 1967.

——, Bureau of Health Professions Education and Manpower Training. "Manpower Supply and Educational Statistics for Selected Health Occupations," in *Health Manpower Source Book,* Section 20. Washington, D.C.: U.S. Government Printing Office, 1969.

——, Social Security Administration, Office of Research and Statistics. *Current Medicare Survey Report; Impact of Cost-Sharing on Use of Ambulatory Services Under Medicare: Preliminary Findings, 1969. Health Insurance Statistics.* DHEW Pub. No. (SSA) 74–11702. October 10,1973.

United States. Department of Labor, Bureau of Labor Statistics. "A Study of Requirements and Supply," in *Health Manpower 1966–75.* Washington, D.C.: U.S. Government Printing Office, 1967.

——. *Manpower Report of the President: A Report on Manpower Requirements, Resources, Utilization, and Training.* Washington, D.C.: U.S. Government Printing Office, 1970.

——. *Manpower Report of the President: A Report on Manpower Requirements, Resources, Utilization, and Training.* Washington, D.C.: U.S. Government Printing Office, 1972.

United States. National Advisory Commission on Health Manpower. *Report of the Commission.* 2 vols. Washington, D.C.: U.S. Government Printing Office, 1967.

United States. National Center for Health Statistics. *Health Resources Statistics: Health Manpower and Health Facilities, 1969.* Washington, D.C.: U.S. Government Printing Office. 1970

——. *Health Resources Statistics: Health Manpower and Health Facilities, 1971.* Washington, D.C.: U.S. Government Printing Office, 1972.

——. *Vital and Health Statistics.* Series No. 10, "Data from the Health Interview Survey." Various years.

United States. President's Commission on the Health Needs of the Nation.

Building America's Health, Vol. I, "Findings and Recommendations"; Vol. II, "America's Health Status, Needs and Resources."
Washington, D.C.: U.S. Government Printing Office, 1952 and 1953.

United States. Surgeon General's Consultation Group on Medical Education.
Physicians for a Growing America. U.S. Public Health Service Pub-
lication No. 709. Washington, D.C.: U.S. Government Printing
Office, 1959.

Uyeno, Dean H. "Health Manpower Systems: An Application of the Management Sciences to the Design of Primary Health Care Teams."
Unpublished Ph.D. dissertation, Northwestern University, Evan-
ston, Illinois, 1971.

Vinod, H.D. "The Econometrics of Joint Production," *Econometrica,* 36
(April 1968): 322–336.

Walters, A.A. "Production and Cost Functions: An Econometric Survey,"
Econometrica 31 (January-April 1963): 1–66.

Weinerman, E.R. "Research into the Organization of Medical Practice," *Milbank
Memorial Fund Quarterly* 63 (October 1966): 117–118.

Weiss, J.H. "The Changing Job Structure of Health Manpower." Unpublished
Ph.D. dissertation, Harvard University, 1966.

Williamson, Oliver, E. *The Economics of Discretionary Behavior: Managerial
Objectives in a Theory of the Firm.* Englewood Cliffs, N.J.: Prentice-
Hall, 1964.

Wolfe, S., and Badgley, Robin F. *Doctors' Strike; Medical Care and Conflict in
Saskatchewan.* New York: Atherton Press, 1967.

——; ——; Kasius, R.V.; Garson, J.Z.; and Gold, R.J.M. "The Work of a Group
of Doctors in Saskatchewan," *Milbank Memorial Fund Quarterly*
65 (January 1968): 103–129.

World Health Organization. *World Health Statistics Annual,* Vol. 3. Geneva:
World Health Organization, 1972.

Yankauer, Alfred; Connelly, John P.; and Feldman, Jacob J. "Physician Productivity in the Delivery of Ambulatory Care: Some Findings from
a Survey of Pediatricians," *Medical Care* 8 (January-Feburary
1970): 35–46.

——; ——; ——. "Task Performance and Task Delegation in Pediatric Office
Practice," *American Journal of Public Health* 59 (July 1969):
1104–1117.

——; Jones, S.H.; and Hellmann, L.M. "Performance and Delegation of Patient
Services by Physicians in Obstetrics-Gynecology," *American Journal
of Public Health* 61 (August 1971).

——; ——; ——; and Schneider, J. "Performance and Delegation of Patient
Services by Physicians in Obstetrics-Gynecology," *American Journal
of Public Health* 61 (August 1971): 1545–1552.

——; Schneider, J.; Jones, S.H.; Hellman, L.M.; and Feldman, J.J., "Physician
Output, Productivity and Task Delegation in Obstetrics—Gynecolo-
gic Practices in the U.S.," *Obstetrics and Gynecology* 39 (January
1, 1972): 151.

Yost, Edward. *The U.S. Health Industry: The Costs of Acceptable Medical Care by 1975.* New York: Frederick A. Praeger, 1969.

Zeckhauser, R., and Eliastam, M. "The Productivity Potential of the Physician Assistant," *Journal of Human Resources* 9 (Winter 1974): 95–116.

Zellner, A.; Kmenta, J.; and Drèze, J. "Specification and Estimation of Cobb-Douglas Production Function Models," *Econometrica* 34 (October 1966): 784–795.

Index

About the Author

Uwe E. Reinhardt, specializing in the research area of health manpower utilization, has been a consultant to the Department of Health, Education and Welfare, the Urban Institute, and Mathematica, Inc. Currently an Assistant Professor of Economics and Public Affairs at Princeton University, Dr. Reinhardt received his undergraduate training at the University of Saskatchewan (Canada). He attended Yale University on a Woodrow Wilson Fellowship where he received his graduate degrees.